Quick Look Nursing:
Growth and Development Through the Lifespan
Second Edition

KATHLEEN M. THIES, PhD, RN
Senior Nurse Researcher
Elliot Hospital and Health System
Adjunct Associate Professor
Graduate School of Nursing
University of Massachusetts Medical Center

JOHN F. TRAVERS, EdD
Professor Emeritus
Lynch School of Education
Boston College

JONES AND BARTLETT PUBLISHERS
Sudbury, Massachusetts
BOSTON   TORONTO   LONDON   SINGAPORE

World Headquarters
Jones and Bartlett Publishers
40 Tall Pine Drive
Sudbury, MA 01776
978-443-5000
info@jbpub.com
www.jbpub.com

Jones and Bartlett Publishers
   Canada
6339 Ormindale Way
Mississauga, Ontario L5V 1J2
Canada

Jones and Bartlett Publishers
   International
Barb House, Barb Mews
London W6 7PA
United Kingdom

Jones and Bartlett's books and products are available through most bookstores and online booksellers. To contact Jones and Bartlett Publishers directly, call 800-832-0034, fax 978-443-8000, or visit our website, www.jbpub.com.

The authors, editor, and publisher have made every effort to provide accurate information. However, they are not responsible for errors, omissions, or for any outcomes related to the use of the contents of this book and take no responsibility for the use of the products and procedures described. Treatments and side effects described in this book may not be applicable to all people; likewise, some people may require a dose or experience a side effect that is not described herein. Drugs and medical devices are discussed that may have limited availability controlled by the Food and Drug Administration (FDA) for use only in a research study or clinical trial. Research, clinical practice, and government regulations often change the accepted standard in this field. When consideration is being given to use of any drug in the clinical setting, the health care provider or reader is responsible for determining FDA status of the drug, reading the package insert, and reviewing prescribing information for the most up-to-date recommendations on dose, precautions, and contraindications, and determining the appropriate usage for the product. This is especially important in the case of drugs that are new or seldom used.

Production Credits
Executive Editor: Kevin Sullivan
Acquisitions Editor: Emily Ekle
Acquisitions Editor: Amy Sibley
Editorial Assistant: Patricia Donnelly
Associate Production Editor: Wendy Swanson
Associate Marketing Manager: Ilana Goddess
Manufacturing and Inventory Control Supervisor: Amy Bacus
Composition: Auburn Associates, Inc.
Cover Design: Timothy Dziewit
Cover Illustrator: Cara Judd
Printing and Binding: Malloy, Inc.
Cover Printing: Malloy, Inc.

Library of Congress Cataloging-in-Publication Data
Thies, Kathleen M.
   Growth and development through the lifespan / Kathleen M. Thies, John F. Travers. — 2nd ed.
      p. ; cm. — (Quick look nursing)
   Rev. ed. of: Human growth and development through the lifespan / Kathleen M. Thies, John F. Travers. c2001.
   Includes bibliographical references and index.
   ISBN-13: 978-0-7637-5649-9 (pbk. : alk. paper)
   ISBN-10: 0-7637-5649-0 (pbk. : alk. paper) 1. Developmental psychology. 2. Nursing. I. Travers, John F. II. Thies, Kathleen M. Human growth and development through the lifespan. III. Title. IV. Series.
   [DNLM: 1. Human Development—Nurses' Instruction. BF 713 T439g 2009]
   BF713.T47 2009
   305.2—dc22
                                                                                                 2008008446

6048

Printed in the United States of America
12 11 10 09 08   10 9 8 7 6 5 4 3 2 1

CONTENTS

PART I: MAJOR THEORIES AND ISSUES 1

PART II: PRENATAL DEVELOPMENT 51

PART III: INFANCY 107

PREFACE

For nurses and physicians, insights into the processes of human development afford unique opportunities to further their relationships with colleagues and patients. As we move through this new century, new theories, new techniques, and new views of human nature will continue to offer hope for a more penetrating understanding of the path of human development. A major task for all nursing students is to understand human development—the characteristics, problems, and needs of people of various ages—so that they can utilize their knowledge and expertise as fully as possible to provide developmentally appropriate care to all patients and their families.

K.M.T.
J.F.T.

INTRODUCTION: THE NATURE OF HUMAN DEVELOPMENT

A person is born, grows, develops, and matures, changing from a child to an adult, and then, gracefully or otherwise, ages. What happens to the individual who undergoes such a dramatic transformation? Which influences contribute to a happy or a troubled life? Each of us, as we age, encounters problems associated with the particular time of life in which we find ourselves. Regardless of our individual circumstances, each phase of life presents difficulties that are impossible to avoid. Many of these challenges are physical and require the knowledge, expertise, and understanding of professional personnel. For those dedicated to a life of nursing, grasping the complexity of human development becomes a critical element for successful and compassionate service.

Human development is an enormously frustrating, fascinating, and almost bewildering phenomenon that produces physical and psychosocial changes throughout the life span, from conception to death. Physical changes include obvious accomplishments, such as the transformation of an apparently helpless infant into a walking, talking two-year-old. But development also encompasses less obvious psychosocial changes, such as the emergence of ever-more complex language patterns and the ability to understand obscure—even hidden—meanings. Attempting to address how these developmental changes occur leads us to search for the underlying mechanisms that explain growth and development.

DEVELOPMENTAL ORIGINS

We have attempted to unravel the Gordian Knot of development by emphasizing the role of biopsychosocial interaction in this edition. We believe this technique provides a more understandable research framework and helps to explain the complexity of development. We urge you to think of the forces that produce development as interacting in the following manner:

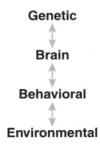

For example, seven-year-old children typically reverse their thinking; that is, they can explain how they arrived at an answer by retracing their steps. If you pour water from one bottle into a taller, thinner bottle, the level of the water will be higher. Almost all seven-year-olds, however, will tell you it is the same amount of water. When you ask them how they know, they will tell you that *they poured it back in their heads.*

These changes reflect a combination of physical forces (brain development), cognitive forces (intelligence), and psychosocial forces (environment). The interplay of these developmental influences is referred to as *biopsychosocial interactions.* (For a detailed discussion of this concept, see Dacey, Travers, & Fiore, 2009). A key to understanding human development is the search for the interactions that produce development.

DEVELOPMENTAL PERIODS

We have decided to use those developmental epochs that help readers to recall and integrate the main features of each period. Consequently, we have divided the life span as follows:

- *Prenatal period.* Topics such as fertilization techniques, genetic discoveries, the developmental milestones of the prenatal months, and many of the hazards that lead to early problems are reviewed. Our purpose is to call attention to the significant accomplishments of these months that result in an active, adaptive human being at birth.
- *Infancy (0–2 years).* Infancy is a time when physical and psychosocial changes appear with amazing rapidity. Walking and talking are two readily observable changes, but sophisticated interactions between infants and the adults around them also establish the basis of future social relationships.
- *Early childhood (2–7 years).* Growth continues at a slightly slower rate, while language and cognitive development indicate abstract ability. Peers become more important, and children acquire a good idea of who they are (sense of self) as they steadily enlarge their circle of social relationships.
- *Middle childhood (7–12 years).* The cognitive skills that enable children to engage in ever-more abstract activities (solving problems, demonstrating creativity) emerge. As their childhood world expands, they encounter increasing and varied forms of stimulation from friends, school, and the media.
- *Adolescence.* The search for identity, coupled with physical and psychosocial changes, produces an intense preoccupation with the self.
- *Adulthood.* A range of developmental tasks arise that must be mastered if successful aging is to occur. Marriage, family, health, finances, and the inevitable problems associated with aging characterize these years.

DEVELOPMENTAL ISSUES

Nature or Nurture

In the study of human development, certain themes appear with considerable regularity. One example is the issue of whether inborn tendencies (nature) or the surrounding world (nurture) exerts greater influence on development. In other words, which is more decisive for development—genes or environment? Most developmental psychologists lean toward an interplay between these two forces in shaping development: The interaction between genes and environment explains a person's development. Humans, using their genetic heritages, interact with their environments not as passive recipients, but rather as active shapers of their destinies.

The Role of Culture

The relationship of culture to human development is critical in society, as interactions with members of different cultures occur on a daily basis. Responses to others who seem different can have serious effects on achievement in school, success in work, and harmonious relationships. For example, clients from different cultures may well interact with nurses and physicians in a different manner. Their learning styles may vary, which can affect the way they think about medication. All of these differences have developmental consequences. We urge you to recognize the relationship between culture and healthy development and to search for and understand those cultural practices (e.g., parenting, attitude toward education) that promote successful nursing skills.

The Role of Gender

Gender is a powerful psychosocial factor in development. Although stereotypical thinking about males and females is slowly disappearing, if people are treated according to rigid role characteristics, then their potential is immediately limited. Children quickly construct social categories from the world around them, attach certain characteristics to these categories, and then label the categories. This process is positive, in that it helps children to organize their world. Unfortunately it may also be negative if the characteristics associated with a particular category are limiting (e.g., "Girls just can't do math").

Stability versus Change

The trade-off between stability and change is another issue that impacts the relationship between nurses and clients. Humans show amazing resiliency, which testifies to their ability to change. Yet resiliency has its limits, which testifies to the lingering effects of stability. Most developmental psychologists would argue for the presence of both stability and change.

DEVELOPMENTAL PERSPECTIVES

One way of organizing developmental data into a meaningful body of knowledge is by the use of theories. A theory is an integrated set of ideas that helps one comprehend and bring order to a mass of factual data. We urge you to select the features of each of the following theories that you believe best explains a certain aspect of development:

- *Psychoanalytic theory.* Perhaps best known because of the work of *Sigmund Freud* and *Erik Erikson,* this theory attempts to explain human development—especially personality development—as the product of unconscious forces. Erikson, while in basic agreement with Freud, placed greater emphasis on a person's environment (family, school, friends) in development.
- *Cognitive theory.* The cognitive perspective on human development has perhaps been best expressed by *Jean Piaget,* who believed that cognitive development proceeds as cognitive structures develop. The changing nature of the cognitive structures led Piaget to speculate that intellectual development comes about in a series of stages: sensorimotor, preoperational, concrete operational, and formal operational.

- *Humanistic theory. Abraham Maslow,* an adherent of the humanistic school of psychology, believed that an individual's basic needs must be satisfied if normal development is to take place. Maslow formulated a hierarchy of needs that, if satisfied, eventually would lead to self-actualization.
- *Cultural or contextual theory.* A different interpretation of cognitive development, known as the cultural or contextual perspective, was proposed by *Lev Vygotsky.* Vygotsky believed that the clues to understanding cognitive development can be found in a person's social process (i.e., the interactions that people have with those around them). *Uri Bronfenbrenner,* working within the cultural–contextual framework, stressed the importance of the environment in shaping people's lives. He proposed a system analysis of development. Identifying several systems (microsystem, mesosystem, exosystem, and macrosystem), Bronfenbrenner suggested that an individual's growth is influenced by an ever-expanding environmental network.
- *Learning theory.* Psychologists such as *B. F. Skinner* have long argued that the best explanation of development lies in learning. Skinner, using a learning perspective, argued that development proceeds when a person's behavior is reinforced. An offshoot of Skinner's work is the *social cognitive learning perspective.* Popularized by *Albert Bandura,* this perspective emphasized modeling or observational learning to explain how people behave and develop as they do. In other words, by observing the behavior of others, people learn their way through life.

As we begin our work together in this second edition of *Growth and Development Through the Lifespan,* we remain committed to the goals that guided our efforts in the first edition:

- We are intent on discussing those subjects that offer insight and understanding of life span development and that are supported by the latest and most fruitful research. We also wish to include those topics that are particularly relevant to our readers.
- We remain acutely aware of the need to provide clear application of the concepts presented throughout the book based on practical and helpful implications for providing superior health care.
- As the United States is a nation with a steadily growing immigrant population, we have increased our analysis of the role that culture plays in development.
- In attempting to reach these objectives, we have made every effort to make our work as reader-friendly and attractive as possible.

SOURCE

Dacey, J., Travers, J., & Fiore, L. (2009). *Human development across the lifespan* (7th ed.). New York: McGraw-Hill.

ABBREVIATIONS

A	adenine
ADA	Americans with Disabilities Act
ADD	attention-deficit disorder
ADHD	attention-deficit/hyperactivity disorder
AGA	appropriate for gestational age
AIDS	acquired immune deficiency syndrome
AIP	artificial insemination by partner
ART	assisted reproductive technology
BADL	bodily activities of daily living
BNBAS	Brazelton Neonatal Behavioral Assessment Scale
BPD	bronchopulmonary dysplasia
C	cytosine
CF	cystic fibrosis
cm	centimeter
CMV	cytomegalovirus
CNS	central nervous system
CVD	cardiovascular disease
dL	deciliter
DNA	deoxyribonucleic acid
DOE	Department of Energy
DSM-IV	*Diagnostic and Statistical Manual of Mental Disorders,* Fourth Edition
EDC	estimated date of confinement
EEG	electroencephalogram
ELSI	ethical, legal, and social issues
ERT	estrogen replacement therapy
ESL	English as a second language
FSH	follicle-stimulating hormone
FTT	failure to thrive
G	guanine
g	gram
GIFT	gamete intrafallopian transfer
GnRH	gonadotropin-releasing hormone
HGP	Human Genome Project
HIV	human immunodeficiency virus
IADL	independent activities of daily living
IDDM	insulin-dependent diabetes mellitus
IDEA	Individuals with Disabilities Education Act
IUD	intrauterine device
IVF	in vitro fertilization
kcal	kilocalorie
kg	kilogram
lb	pound

LBW	low birth weight
LDL	low-density lipoprotein
LEP	limited English proficiency
LH	luteinizing hormone
mg	milligram
mL	milliliter
mRNA	messenger ribonucleic acid
NAEYC	National Association for the Education of Young Children
NICHD	National Institute of Child Health and Development
NIH	National Institutes of Health
NYLS	New York Longitudinal Study
oz	ounce
PCB	polychlorinated biphenyl
PID	pelvic inflammatory disease
PIVH	periventricular–intraventricular hemorrhage
PKU	phenylketonuria
PNS	peripheral nervous system
PTSD	post-traumatic stress disorder
RDS	respiratory distress syndrome
RNA	ribonucleic acid
SAT	Scholastic Assessment Test
SES	social and economic status
SGA	small for gestational age
STD	sexually transmitted disease
T	thymidine
VLBW	very low birth weight
ZIFT	zygote intrafallopian transfer

I

Major Theories and Issues

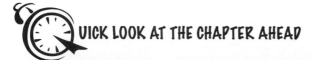

Freud's influence on theories of human development is in these areas:

- The structure of personality has three components: id, ego, and superego.
- Defense mechanisms protect the ego from unpleasant feelings, especially anxiety and guilt.
- There are three levels of awareness: conscious, preconscious, and unconscious.
- Children's control over primitive urges progresses through five psychosexual stages.
- Psychoanalysis brings into awareness unconscious conflicts, motives, and defenses so that they can be resolved.
- Early experience in childhood is the root of adult behavior and defenses.

1

Freud: Psychoanalytic Theory

TERMS

- ☐ Anal stage
- ☐ Conflict
- ☐ Conscious
- ☐ Countertransference
- ☐ Defense mechanisms
- ☐ Displacement
- ☐ Ego
- ☐ Fixation
- ☐ Genital stage
- ☐ Id
- ☐ Identification
- ☐ Latency stage
- ☐ Oedipus complex
- ☐ Oral stage
- ☐ Phallic stage
- ☐ Preconscious
- ☐ Projection
- ☐ Psychoanalysis
- ☐ Rationalization
- ☐ Reaction formation
- ☐ Regression
- ☐ Repression
- ☐ Superego
- ☐ Transference
- ☐ Unconscious

3

WHO WAS FREUD?

Born in 1856, Sigmund Freud was raised in Vienna, Austria, as the son of a Jewish merchant. After completing medical school in 1886, Freud began practicing neurology, specializing in hysteria. Concluding that its origins were sexual in nature, he developed psychoanalytic techniques to encourage patients to recall past experiences. When female patients reported prepubertal sexual encounters with their fathers, Freud struggled with deciding whether these encounters were fantasies or actual events. He underwent self-analysis, and his theory of psychosexual development ultimately evolved from this process.

Freud indulged in cocaine to relieve his depression, but his addiction to nicotine caused his death from cancer of the mouth. In 1938, he left Vienna in poor health to seek refuge from the Nazis, who had destroyed his Vienna Psychoanalytic Society. Freud died in London in 1939.

 STRUCTURE OF PERSONALITY

Freud divided personality into three components: id, ego, and superego. His concept of the **id** was influenced by Darwin. The id is the seat of instinctual drives, especially sex, food, and aggression. Operating on the pleasure principle, the id seeks immediate gratification and wants to avoid physical and psychic pain. It engages in primary process thinking, which is illogical and indulges in fantasy.

 Freud divided personality into three components: id, ego, and superego.

The id's self-serving drive for pleasure conflicts with society's norms for acceptable behavior. The **ego** emerges from this conflict, and works to keep the id out of trouble. It balances the id's drives with society's expectations by making decisions based on the reality principle—that is, delaying gratification until socially appropriate means for meeting instinctual drives can be found. The ego engages in secondary process thinking, which is realistic, and tries to solve problems.

The **superego** is the moral component of the personality. Emerging around ages 3 to 5 years, the superego represents an internalization of social standards for good and bad behavior. It is the individual's way of policing his or her own behavior. When the superego becomes too demanding, the individual feels excessive guilt for failing to meet moral perfection. In the absence of a superego, the individual feels no remorse.

 Emerging around ages 3 to 5 years, the superego represents an internalization of social standards for good and bad behavior.

 LEVELS OF AWARENESS AND DREAMS

Freud identified three levels of awareness: conscious, preconscious, and unconscious. The **conscious** consists of awareness of the present. The **preconscious** lies just below the surface, housing material that the individual knows but is not thinking about right now. The **unconscious** contains memories, thoughts, and desires of which the individual is not aware but that may have a profound influence on the person's behavior, such as hostile feelings toward a loved one. The id rests entirely in the unconscious. In his 1899 book *The Interpretation of Dreams*, Freud argued that the "royal road" to the unconscious is dreams.

CONFLICT AND DEFENSE MECHANISMS

Freud believed that the internal battles between the id, ego, and superego create **conflict** in the personality. The drives for sex and aggression are particularly conflicted because they are subject to ambiguous social norms—also known as mixed messages—and, therefore, are more likely to be unfulfilled. Unconscious internal battles produce anxiety, which can slip into consciousness and cause distress. **Defense mechanisms** (**Table 1-1**) protect the ego from unpleasant feelings, especially anxiety and guilt. They include **rationalization, repression, projection, displacement, reaction formation, regression,** and **identification**. Defense mechanisms are unconscious and are not the same thing as coping.

Defense mechanisms are unconscious and are not the same thing as coping.

STAGES OF PSYCHOSEXUAL DEVELOPMENT

Freud used the term "sexual" broadly, meaning an innate drive for physical pleasures. Freud proposed that children's control over these urges progresses through five psychosexual stages (**Table 1-2**). The failure to progress is referred to as **fixation**.

During the **oral stage** in the first year of life, the main source of pleasure is the mouth, such as sucking and biting. Adult oral fixations include smoking and eating.

The **anal stage** focuses on the toddler's pleasure in controlling bowel movements. Toilet training, which represents society's first effort to control the child's self-serving physical drives, causes conflict between child and caretakers. Adult anal fixations involve anxiety about being punished for not performing.

The **phallic stage** occurs between the third and fifth years of life. Boys find pleasure in self-stimulation and compete with their fathers for the affection of their mothers. Freud thought that girls envied boys' ability for self-pleasure and blamed their mothers for their lack of a penis. Girls compensate for this "deficiency" by forming an attachment to their fathers. The **Oedipus complex** refers to sexual desires for the parent of the opposite sex accompanied by hostility toward the parent of the same sex. This conflict coincides with the emergence of the superego. Freud believed that the resolution of this conflict is essential for healthy gender identification with the parent of the same sex. Some cross-cultural evidence supports the idea of an Oedipus complex in boys.

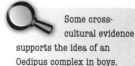

Some cross-cultural evidence supports the idea of an Oedipus complex in boys.

A stage theory focuses on discontinuity in development, because it implies that development has clearly demarcated points of change.

During the **latency stage**, from age 5 through puberty, sexual urges become suppressed as children form social relationships beyond the family, especially with peers.

Table 1-1 Defense Mechanisms

Mechanism	Explanation/Example
Rationalization	Creation of false but plausible excuses to justify behavior. Example: "Everyone else does it."
Repression	Way of keeping anxiety-producing thoughts in the unconscious. Example: "Forgetting" a troubling experience.
Projection	Attributing your thoughts, feelings, or motives to somebody else. Example: Believing a co-worker for whom you have sexual feelings has made a pass at you.
Displacement	Diverting feelings that you have toward someone away from that person and toward another person or object. Example: Yelling at your spouse when you are angry at your boss.
Reaction formation	Behaving in a way that is exactly opposite the way you feel. Example: Crusading against pornography when you secretly enjoy it.
Regression	Reverting to immature behavior. Example: Adult temper tantrums.
Identification	Aligning yourself with a person or group that you admire as a way to form a positive self-identity. Example: Joining a sorority.

The **genital stage** begins with puberty. During adolescence, sexual urges can be appropriately directed toward peers of the opposite sex. A stage theory focuses on discontinuity in development, because it implies that development has clearly demarcated points of change.

PSYCHOANALYSIS

The goal of **psychoanalysis** is to bring into awareness unconscious conflicts, motives, and defenses so that they can be resolved. Free association is the spontaneous expression of an individual's thoughts and feelings. Interpretation involves the analyst's attempt to explain the meaning of the client's experience, including the symbolism in the client's dreams. The analyst uses the client's resistance to interpretation to further understand underlying conflicts.

Table 1-2 Stages of Psychosexual Development

Stage	Age	Focus of Sexual Urges
Oral	First year of life	The mouth (e.g., sucking, biting)
Anal	Toddler	Controlling biological urges (e.g., bowel movements)
Phallic	3–5 years	Genital self-pleasure; the Oedipus complex
Latency	5 years–puberty	Suppressing urges
Genital	Puberty	Peers of opposite sex

Transference means that a patient may remind you of someone in your life and you may treat that patient in the same way that you treat that person—which may be either good or bad. Remember to treat each patient as an individual.

Transference occurs when clients relate to their analysts in ways that are similar to other significant relationships in their lives. **Countertransference** refers to the analyst's response to the client.

SOURCE

Freud, S. (1924/1952). *A general introduction to psychoanalysis* (J. Riviere, trans.). New York: Washington Square Press.

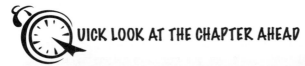

Erikson emphasized the role of the social environment in development:

- Development occurs through interacting with an ever-widening circle of people.
- There are eight stages of psychosocial development.
- Each stage is marked by a normative developmental polar crisis.
- Early negative experience is important in the development of personality, but it can be resolved at a later time.

2

Erikson: Eight Stages of the Life Cycle

Terms
- ☐ **Identity foreclosure**
- ☐ **Integration**
- ☐ **Normative developmental crisis**
- ☐ **Psychological moratorium**
- ☐ **Psychosocial development**

WHO WAS ERIKSON?

Erik Homburger Erikson was born in Germany in 1902 to Danish parents. He studied child analysis at the Vienna Psychoanalytic Institute with Anna Freud, then emigrated to the United States in 1933. There, he developed affiliations with Harvard University, Yale University, and the University of California at Berkeley, establishing Child Guidance Clinics for the treatment of childhood psychological disturbances. Erikson and his wife Joan introduced the theory of the eight stages of the human life cycle at a White House Conference in 1950, the same year *Childhood and Society* was published. Erickson wrote *Identity: Youth and Crisis* in 1968, a time of great upheaval among American youth. He died in Cambridge, Massachusetts, in 1994.

THEORY OF PSYCHOSOCIAL DEVELOPMENT

While Freud emphasized internal psychosexual conflict in personality development, Erikson recognized that the social environment plays a significant role in shaping a child's sense of self. Erikson's theory of **psychosocial development** is based on the premise that humans interact with an ever-widening circle of people, beginning with mother and ending with humankind in general.

> Erikson's theory of **psychosocial development** is based on the premise that humans interact with an ever-widening circle of people, beginning with mother and ending with humankind in general.

Each of the eight stages of the human lifecycle is marked by a **normative developmental crisis** that is resolved on a continuum between opposing positive and negative outcomes (**Table 2-1**). Personality is formed as a result of the resolution of these crises, leaving people with both strengths and weaknesses. The mature personality represents the **integration** of earlier stages of development, their crises, and resolutions, into later stages.

Unlike Freud, who was pessimistic about humans' ability to overcome an unfortunate early childhood, Erikson believed that humans rework earlier crises later in life. Their beliefs about the role of early experience are an important difference between Freud and Erikson, with Erikson being more hopeful than Freud. Reworking can be growth enhancing when the overall balance of the personality is more positive than negative. If earlier crises were poorly resolved, however, revisiting them can be disruptive, especially when doing so coincides with accidental life crises, such as illness or death.

> Their beliefs about the role of early experience are an important difference between Freud and Erikson, with Erikson being more hopeful than Freud.

THE EIGHT STAGES OF THE LIFE CYCLE

* **Trust versus mistrust.** Infants cannot meet their own needs for food, warmth, and comfort. When they can count on others—usually their mother—to meet these needs, they feel worthy of care and develop a sense of trust both in "self" and in "other." Because an attentive mother cannot meet all the child's needs at all times, even a positive resolution includes a healthy degree of mistrust. Consistently poor caregiving leaves a child with a

Table 2-1 Stages of the Life Cycle

Developmental Crisis	Period	Developmental Struggle
Trust versus mistrust	Infancy	I can trust others and thus myself versus I can't trust and my needs are unworthy.
Autonomy versus shame and doubt	Toddler	"I am," "I can," and that's good, versus "I can't" and I am bad.
Initiative versus guilt	Preschool	I can control my busyness versus what I do is bad.
Industry versus inferiority	School-aged	I can make friends and do things well versus nobody likes me and I'm stupid.
Identity formation versus identity diffusion	Adolescence	I am in tune with myself versus I am confused, a nobody.
Intimacy versus isolation	Young adult	I share who I am with special others versus I am alone and I have nothing to share.
Generativity versus self-absorption	Adulthood	I am making a contribution versus it only matters if it matters to me.
Ego integrity versus disgust and despair	Senescence	This was my life and I am okay with it versus I am filled with regret, I failed.

sense of unworthiness that can negatively influence self-identity and relationships throughout life.

- **Autonomy versus shame and doubt.** Like Freud, Erikson realized that children's ability to control their body functions poses a major developmental crisis. While toddlers attach value to exerting autonomous will, caregivers disapprove of uncivilized behaviors. In a positive resolution, toddlers gain a sense of self-pride and autonomy when adults guide them to learn approved behavior: "I am good." Even healthy toddlers experience some shame, however. The more they experience disapproval without guidance, the deeper their shame and the more they doubt their own will: "I am bad."

- **Initiative versus guilt.** Preschoolers who like to do things can do the wrong thing. Like Freud, Erikson saw this stage as the birth of a conscience. A little guilt helps children keep their initiative within bounds. However, children who are overburdened by unrealistic expectations for good behavior can only fail; they may believe they do bad things, stifling their natural inquisitiveness.

- **Industry versus inferiority.** During the latency period, children channel their energy into developing friendships and becoming good at things, such as academics and sports. They enjoy being productive and learn from their failures. Children who do not experience themselves as being competent socially, physically, or intellectually develop a sense of inadequacy and inferiority.

- **Identity formation versus identity diffusion.** Identity formation in adolescence is a cornerstone of Erikson's theory. The developmental task is to integrate childhood identifications with new biological urges, assumption of social roles, and recognition of one's abilities and limitations. During the **psychological moratorium,** adolescents try on different identities, values, and social roles. Failure to form an identity may result in identity diffusion—of feeling like a nobody, with no sense of direction or commitment to a set of

values. **Identity foreclosure** occurs when adolescents assume a preordained role without question. Erikson coined
the term "identity crisis" in reference to adolescence.

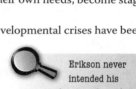

Erikson coined
the term "iden-
tity crisis" in reference to
adolescence.

- **Intimacy versus isolation.** Once young people are secure in
  their identity, they can establish intimate relationships with
  friends and loving sexual relationships. Fear of losing one's
  identity in a relationship can lead youth to avoid commitments, causing isolation and loneliness.
- **Generativity versus self-absorption.** Generative adults are productive members of society, guiding the younger generation, caring for elders, and contributing their talents for the
  betterment of all. Self-absorbed adults do not look beyond their own needs, become stag-
  nant emotionally, or lack a core set of values.
- **Integrity versus disgust.** Individuals whose resolution of developmental crises have been
  relatively positive reach old age with a sense of ego integrity.
  They accept responsibility for what life is and was—whether
  it be good, bad, or indifferent. Individuals who have been
  emotionally isolated, self-absorbed, and without a secure
  identity end life in despair and regret. Erikson believed that
  it is never too late to positively reintegrate the personality, to
  learn life's lessons, and to mature. Erikson never intended his
  stages to be viewed as what he later referred to as the
  "rosary" of development. They are a convenient heuristic,
  however.

Erikson never
intended his
stages to be viewed as what
he later referred to as the
"rosary" of development.
They are a convenient
heuristic, however.

SOURCES

Erikson, E. (1950). *Childhood and society.* New York: W. W. Norton.
Erikson, E. (1959). *Identity and the life cycle.* New York: International Universities Press.
Erikson, E. (1968). *Identity: Youth and crisis.* New York: W. W. Norton.

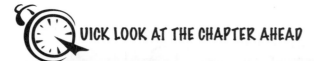

Piaget believed that cognitive development can occur only through interactions with the environment:

- Humans have a dual heredity: our physical bodies and the entire natural world, to which we must adapt.
- The constructivist perspective says that we actively construct our understanding of the world.
- The universal perspective says that all cognitive development is organized the same way within each stage.
- The components of cognition are mental structures, schemata, and operations.
- There are four stages of cognitive development: sensorimotor, preoperations, concrete operations, and formal operations.
- Development occurs through the processes of assimilation and accommodation.

3

Piaget: Universal Constructivist Perspective

TERMS
- ☐ Accommodation
- ☐ Adaptation
- ☐ Assimilation
- ☐ Concrete operational
- ☐ Formal operations
- ☐ Mental structures
- ☐ Operations
- ☐ Organization
- ☐ Preoperational
- ☐ Schemata
- ☐ Sensorimotor
- ☐ Universal constructivist

WHO WAS PIAGET?

Jean Piaget (1896–1980) spent most of his life in his native Switzerland and in France. After finishing his PhD in biology, he studied experimental psychology. In 1920, while standardizing a French version of an English intelligence test for Alfred Binet, Piaget became fascinated by children's wrong answers. Children of the same age seemed to reason incorrectly in the same way. He suspected that this phenomenon was a function of intellectual maturation, rather than quantity of knowledge. Piaget's research on children's intellectual development was guided by genetic epistemology, the study of the natural unfolding of maturational processes in organisms. For example, as an apple seed matures, it does not become more seed. Instead, it changes qualitatively—into a seedling, a sapling, and then a mature tree. Similarly, Piaget saw predictable qualitative differences in how children think about things at different ages.

Piaget wrote more than 50 books on a variety of topics, including intellectual, perceptual, and moral development in children. His basic theory is presented here in brief. While there have been many challenges to and subsequent revisions of Piaget's theory, his work continues to be a major influence in the field of child development.

UNIVERSAL CONSTRUCTIVIST THEORY

The term **universal constructivist** implies that all humans construct their understanding of the world in predictable ways. Piaget believed humans have a dual heredity: their physical bodies and the entire natural world. Humans are not passive organisms, but rather take an active role in their own development by acting on the physical environment. Piaget believed that mental life in infancy begins with motor activity. Piaget believed that development occurs only through interactions with the environment. "Constructivist" means that cognition has to be developed through experience; in other words, it is actively constructed by the child. "Universal" means not just that everyone goes through the same stages, but also that when someone is in a particular stage, that stage pertains to all areas of his or her cognitive development at the same time. The infant who swings an arm and grasps a toy is learning about controlling the body, the nature of objects, and the relationship between body and objects. The key concepts in Piaget's constructivist theory include **mental structures, organization,** and **adaptation.**

Piaget believed that development occurs only through interactions with the environment. "Constructivist" means that cognition has to be developed through experience; in other words, it is actively constructed by the child. "Universal" means not just that everyone goes through the same stages, but also that when someone is in a particular stage, that stage pertains to all areas of his or her cognitive development at the same time.

Mental Structures

Mental structures, called cognitive structures, begin with reflexes in infancy and evolve into **schemata** and then into more complex structures called **operations.** For example, infants have an innate grasping reflex that causes them to wrap their fingers around an object placed in their palms. They come to control this tendency as their nervous system matures. They begin to understand how they must grasp objects of various shapes and sizes. Their schemata for grasping a teething ring will be different from their schemata for grasping a block. Operations are made up of both schemata and cognitive structures.

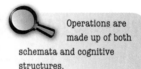

Operations are made up of both schemata and cognitive structures.

Multiple schemata are organized into structures that become increasingly efficient. For example, between infancy and age 2, mental structures are organized around children's sensory and motor interactions with the environment. Piaget referred to this part of a child's life as the **sensorimotor** period (**Figure 3-1**), the first of four stages of development. The infant matures from grasping blocks to throwing them to banging them together and then to stacking two blocks.

As children mature, higher-order structures called operations develop. Operations are the hallmarks of the last three of the four stages of development, which are collectively known as the cognitive stages: **preoperational, concrete operational,** and **formal operations** (Figure 3-1). Piaget believed there are two phases of formal operations, early (ages 11–14) and later (ages 15–19). Operations are mental actions, which allow children to interact with the environment using their minds and not just their bodies. Piaget proposed that these stages form an invariant sequence, meaning that children cannot develop formal operations until they have first developed concrete operations.

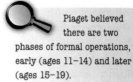

Piaget believed there are two phases of formal operations, early (ages 11–14) and later (ages 15–19).

Organization

Piaget believed that humans have a natural and innate tendency to organize their relationship with the environment. Just as the sapling becomes part of the tree, emerging schemata are integrated into existing ones, causing a reorganization of the whole structure. Each reorganization is of a higher order, reflecting greater coordination and complexity with cognitive maturity. Stacking two blocks evolves into building block cities and eventually an appreciation for the physics of architecture. Stages of development refer to predictable changes in the organization of human experience of the natural world. People organize their activities lawfully, constructing a reality that makes sense at the time.

Adaptation

Humans form cognitive structures for the purposes of adapting to the environment. To Piaget, the definition of intelligence is adaptation—that is, an ability to effectively negotiate environmental demands. Adaptation consists of the dual processes of **assimilation** and **accommodation.** When people assimilate, they incorporate an experience into existing schemata and structures. When they cannot fit an experience into existing schemata or structures, they must accommodate—that is, modify their way of thinking to fit the experience. Accommodation can be a lot of mental work; hence the famous line, "Assimilate if you can; accommodate if you must."

Accommodation can be a lot of mental work; hence the famous line, "Assimilate if you can; accommodate if you must."

Take math as an example. A first-grade student can add 3 + 2 on paper, but adding 9 + 2 requires carrying a 1 into the next column. This is a newer variation on addition. Piaget believed that there are natural limits to building structures through accommodation.

Sensorimotor Period (Newborn to 24 Months)
- Divided into six substages
- Begins with reflexive behavior; ends with symbolic thought (language)

Four major accomplishments
- Object permanence: an object or a person continues to exist even when out of sight
- Spatial relationships: in/out, up/down, gravity
- Causality: cause and effect (e.g., push the right button, Mickey Mouse pops up)
- Time: before and after (e.g., put on clean pajamas *after* a bath)

Preoperational Period (Ages 2–7)
- Animistic thinking: attributing life to inanimate objects (e.g., dolls have feelings)
- Egocentric thinking: world is created and organized around one's self
- Associationistic thinking: things that happen at the same time cause each other
- Perceptually bound: pay attention to what appears to be obvious without regard to the constraints of physics (e.g., Santa can be in two malls at once)
- Centration: attend to one piece of information at a time (e.g., only see that a glass is tall and ignore that it is also wide)

Period of Concrete Operations (Ages 7–11)
- Logical reasoning can be done mentally using rules for operation
- Ability to reverse sequences mentally (e.g., if $3+2=5$, then $5-2=3$)
- Ability to decenter when solving problems: weigh multiple pieces of information at a time (e.g., how much juice there is depends on both the height and width of the container)
- Perceive the underlying reality (physics) (e.g., Santa cannot exist in two malls at once)
- Focus on the immediate, not future oriented
- Classify objects based on at least two properties (e.g., sort baseball cards by team and position)

Period of Formal Operations (Adolescence)
- Abstract thinking: representing reality using symbols that can be manipulated mentally (e.g., symbolism in Bible stories, x in algebraic equations)
- Logical thinking more systematic: scientific method
- Metacognition: thinking about thinking
- Hypothetical/propositional reasoning: able to think "What if?", playing with different scenarios mentally, appreciate rules of logic
- Future oriented

Figure 3-1 Characteristics of the Four Stages of Development

That is, cognitive development is constrained by biological maturation. The typical first-grader cannot yet modify the cognitive structures to accommodate multiplication and division, much less algebra. But the student of algebra can still add $3 + 2$, because earlier schemata for addition have been integrated into more sophisticated mental structures.

SOURCES

Piaget, J. (1962). *Play, dreams, and imitation in childhood.* New York: W. W. Norton.

Piaget, J., & Inhelder, B. (1969). *The psychology of the child.* New York: Basic Books.

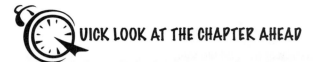

QUICK LOOK AT THE CHAPTER AHEAD

Vygotsky believed that physiological processes plus culture, and especially language, fuel development:

- Children's development occurs on two planes: within themselves and between themselves and other people.
- The mind has social origins because all mental activities result from interactions with other people.
- Learning occurs within the zone of proximal development.
- Scaffolding is how we structure the environment so that the learner can learn.

4

Vygotsky: Culture and Development

TERMS
- ☐ Internalization
- ☐ Interpsychological category
- ☐ Intrapsychological category
- ☐ Scaffolding
- ☐ Sociocultural
- ☐ Zone of proximal development

WHO WAS VYGOTSKY?

Lev Vygotsky, a Russian psychologist, has exerted a powerful influence on current developmental psychology. A theorist who thought deeply about the role of culture in development, Vygotsky was born in Russia in 1896. During his studies, he came to believe that social and cultural processes are critical for healthy growth. Although his career was abruptly terminated by his early death from tuberculosis in 1934, Vygotsky's work is more popular now than it was when he died.

Vygotsky believed that his ideas about development were truly unique (**Figure 4-1**). He argued that development proceeds from the intersection of two paths: elementary processes that are basically biological, and higher psychological processes that are essentially **sociocultural**. For example, brain development provides the physiological basis for the appearance of external or egocentric speech, which gradually becomes the inner speech children use to guide their behavior.

THE INTERACTION OF DEVELOPMENTAL MECHANISMS

Vygotsky thought that elementary biological processes are transformed into higher psychological functioning by developmental processes. Language is a good example of what he meant. Babies make a variety of sounds as they begin their language development (e.g., crying, cooing, babbling), all of which are accompanied by physical movement. Next, children point at objects (e.g., ball, cup, milk) and adults tell them the names of those objects. After children begin to speak their first words, they start to string words together, talk aloud, and, finally restrict speech much the way adults do.

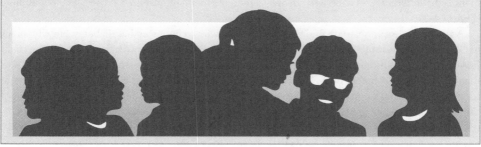

Perspective: child's cognitive development proceeds by social interactions

Basic psychological mechanism: social interactions

Role of language: moves from external to inner speech; becomes a major influence in cognitive development

Learning: biological processes plus social interactions produce learning

Problem solving: speech guides planful behavior; aided by social interactions

Figure 4-1 Vygotsky's Basic Concepts

LANGUAGE AND DEVELOPMENT

Vygotsky believed that language plays a major role in development. For example, by crying, cooing, and babbling, infants immediately begin to interact with the environment and later commence to label the objects around them. When children are approximately 3 years old, they demonstrate egocentric speech, in which they carry on conversations whether anyone is listening. Gradually, speech becomes internalized and begins to help them plan and guide their behavior.

Vygotsky gave the example of a 4-year-old child trying to get a piece of candy from a cupboard. Initially, egocentric speech guides her behavior. Standing on a stool and searching for the candy, she says aloud, "Is that the candy?" "No, I can't get it." "I need a stick." "I can move it now." She brushes the candy to the edge of the shelf. "I can get it now. The stick worked."

THE SOCIAL ORIGIN OF MIND

To understand cognitive development, Vygotsky argued that any function in a child's cultural development appears twice, on two planes: first, in an **interpsychological category** (social exchanges with others), and second, within the child as an **intrapsychological category** (using inner speech to guide behavior). He further argued that all higher functions (e.g., memory, thinking, problem solving) begin as relations between individuals.

Vygotsky used the term **internalization** to explain how external activity becomes internal activity. First, an external behavior (such as egocentric speech) is changed and begins to occur internally. Next, an interpersonal process (egocentric speech) is transformed into an intrapersonal process (inner speech). The more that children use inner speech to guide their actions, the more competent they become. Remember, however, that all mental activity results from interacting with others, which is what Vygotsky meant by the social origins of mind.

THE ZONE OF PROXIMAL DEVELOPMENT

Vygotsky defined the **zone of proximal development** as the distance between a person's actual developmental level and the higher level of potential development. The zone of proximal development is the difference between what people can do independently and what they can do with help (**Figure 4-2**).

As an example, suppose you find yourself working with a client who has diabetes, but who hates to exercise and whose diet includes too much coffee, too many sweets, and irregular meals. The client frequently complains about "feeling tired all the time." You determine what she currently does to manage her diabetes on her own. This is the lower limit of the zone. For example, she tells you that for breakfast she has a cup of coffee with real cream and sugar and nothing else. The upper limit of the zone would be her ability to eat a balanced breakfast, and to use artificial sweeteners in her coffee, as long as she has the help and support to do so. This help could be another person, or stocking her kitchen with appropriate foods that are easy to grab on her way out the door.

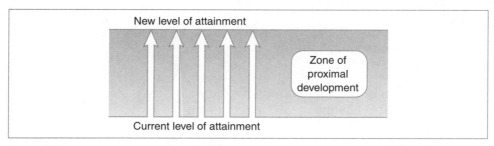

New level of attainment

Zone of
proximal
development

Current level of attainment

Figure 4-2 The Zone of Proximal Development

Progress through the zone of proximal development depends on a person's development and intellectual possibilities. In other words, one's physical abilities (in the example, the patient's disease) and mental abilities (the patient's cognitive capacity to understand the value of your suggestions) will determine the extent of her illness management.

IMPLICATIONS FOR HEALTHCARE PROVIDERS

Keep in mind several key functions that lead to successful **scaffolding.** You must capture the interest of your patients if they are to remain focused. Keep your suggestions simple; do not make the steps to reach the goal too complicated. In the example of the patient with the poor eating habits, do not overload her with nutritional information and readings, but rather remind her of the good that can come from these ideas compared to the way she has been feeling. Do not hesitate to use models, selecting individuals whom the patient admires, to illustrate how the patient can maintain good health (e.g., use magazine articles or pictures). Scaffolding your patients' zone of proximal development when you do health teaching will help them to learn more easily.

> Scaffolding your patients' zone of proximal development when you do health teaching will help them to learn more easily.

SOURCES

Vygotsky, L. S. (1978). *Mind in society*. Cambridge, MA: Harvard University Press.

Wertsch, J., & Tulviste, P. (1992). L. S. Vygotsky and contemporary developmental psychology. *Developmental Psychology*, 28, 548–557.

Bronfenbrenner introduced the idea of the ecology of human development:

- Ecology of human development is a nested arrangement of concentric social levels, beginning with the child at the center and extending outward to social and cultural beliefs and ideologies.
- The levels surrounding the child are microsystems, mesosystems, exosystems, and the macrosystem.
- Parents are not the only influence on children. Large social institutions play roles in the development of any one child.
- There are reciprocal interactions between the levels: Children influence their environments, and environments influence children's development.

5

Bronfenbrenner: Ecology of Human Development

TERMS
- ☐ **Exosystem**
- ☐ **Macrosystem**
- ☐ **Mesosystem**
- ☐ **Microsystem**
- ☐ **Reciprocal interactions**

WHO WAS BRONFENBRENNER?

Urie Bronfenbrenner, born in Russia in 1917, was a psychologist and professor at Cornell University from 1948 until his death in 2005. Through his work as president of a national task force on early childhood (1966–1967), he came to appreciate the multiple influences on children's school performance. In his 1979 book *The Ecology of Human Development*, Bronfenbrenner proposed that the culture at large plays a role in children's development through the transmission of beliefs about how children should be raised and how families should function in society. He borrowed the concepts of "ecology" and "ecosystems" from the natural sciences.

Human ecology is the study of the complex interrelationships between humans and their social environments. Using his model of human ecology, Bronfenbrenner examined the effects of a variety of social and economic factors on children's development.

THE MODEL OF HUMAN ECOLOGY

Bronfenbrenner envisioned his model of human ecology as a "nested arrangement of concentric structures, each contained within the next" (1979). Each of the concentric structures represents a level of context in which development occurs (**Figure 5-1**). There are **reciprocal interactions** between the levels. Children influence their environments, and environments influence children's development.

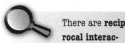

There are **reciprocal interactions** between the levels. Children influence their environments, and environments influence children's development.

The innermost structure in the concentric arrangement is the child. Bronfenbrenner recognized that children bring to their environments their own biological make-up. For example, being male or female influences how a child is perceived by others, which in turn influences the child's behavior. Temperament—especially activity level—appears to be an inborn trait. Some children rush to the top of the jungle gym, whereas others quietly dig in the sand. These children affect their parents in different ways, depending on the expectations of the parents. Parents who wanted a quiet girl may be exasperated by a highly active boy, who gets the message that he is not valued, which in turn shapes the nature of his relationship with his parents.

Working outward, the next level in the concentric structures is the **microsystem**. Microsystems are the immediate social context of a child's life—that is, the people with whom a child interacts on a regular basis. Included are parents and siblings, teachers and classmates, playmates from the neighborhood, and baby-sitters. The highly active boy may be a favorite among playmates, and the man next door may love to have him tag along when he goes to the park, but the boy may drive the teenage baby-sitter crazy.

The microsystems are embedded in the **mesosystem.** This level contains community groups such as the school, neighborhood, and other social organizations. A coach at school might recognize the athletic prowess of the highly active boy. If the boy cannot play outside because the neighborhood is unsafe or there is no coach at school, he may channel his high energy into activities that are detrimental to the community in which he lives.

Children may not be present in the **exosystem,** but these institutions—such as local governments, businesses, services, and media—nevertheless influence children's development. A school board may

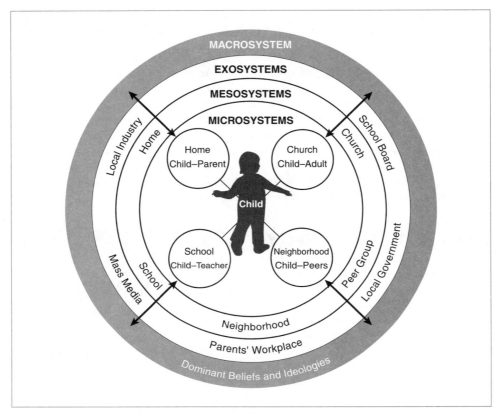

MACROSYSTEM

EXOSYSTEMS

MESOSYSTEMS

MICROSYSTEMS

Local Industry

Home

Home
Child–Parent

Church
Child–Adult

School Board

Church

Child

Mass Media

School

School
Child–Teacher

Neighborhood
Child–Peers

Peer Group

Local Government

Neighborhood

Parents' Workplace

Dominant Beliefs and Ideologies

Figure 5-1 Bronfenbrenner's Model of Human Ecology

cut funding for sports programs when the town cannot raise the revenue. The town may struggle financially when large companies move away, taking parents' jobs and the town's tax base with them. The television station may continue to cover and to glorify sports to children who can no longer participate in them. Children have an influence on these institutions as well. Teens with nothing to do can be a problem for local police.

The **macrosystem** represents the dominant beliefs and ideologies in the culture. The media cover sports because they profit financially in a capitalist society. Beliefs about children influence child-rearing practices and government policies. The cultural value placed on the primacy of the biological family has resulted in children spending years in foster homes, awaiting a reunification with unfit parents that may never come.

> The **macrosystem** represents the dominant beliefs and ideologies in the culture. The media cover sports because they profit financially in a capitalist society.

Children also influence the macrosystem. The baby-boom generation, born between 1945 and 1960, won the right to vote at age 18 by arguing that if you can be drafted, you should be able to vote for the people drafting you.

IMPLICATIONS FOR HEALTHCARE PROVIDERS

The model of the ecology of human development is responsible for our recognition of the complex effects of social and economic status (SES) of families and communities on children. SES is more than just money; it is a marker for parental education and employment and the cohesiveness of social networks. The better educated the parents, the better off the children. Educated parents work. Working parents have organizational skills and a work ethic. They introduce their children to activities that build physical, social, and academic skills. Through these activities, children develop a sense of competence and their families become part of a network of other families in the community.

Children and families of higher SES have better access to health care and to good nutrition. Children of lower SES have difficulty getting good care, have poor diets, and engage in fewer preventive efforts. As a result, the poor have a higher incidence of chronic illness (or the chronically ill have a higher incidence of being poor because it is harder for them to stay employed). It is important to understand each patient in the context of his or her ecology of human development over the period of his or her lifespan. The timing of the availability or dearth of resources and/or the effects of certain social policies can change the course of someone's life.

> It is important to understand each patient in the context of his or her ecology of human development over the period of his or her lifespan. The timing of the availability or dearth of resources and/or the effects of certain social policies can change the course of someone's life.

For example, lack of access to a dentist during childhood and adolescence may result in an adult who has very poor oral health, which in turn affects his ability to secure employment in a setting where his smile is part of his interaction with customers.

SOURCE

Bronfenbrenner, U. (1979). *The ecology of human development: Experiments by nature and design.* Cambridge, MA: Harvard University Press.

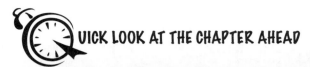

QUICK LOOK AT THE CHAPTER AHEAD

Maslow focused on how people become fully themselves:

- He developed the idea of a hierarchy of needs.
- Needs include physiological, safety, love and belongingness, esteem, and selfactualization.

6

Maslow: Humanistic Perspective on Development

TERMS
- ☐ **Deficiency needs**
- ☐ **Growth needs**
- ☐ **Hierarchy of needs**

WHO WAS MASLOW?

Abraham Maslow has long been associated with humanistic psychology, so called because of its focus on the fully human person. The great value of his work lies in its emphasis on psychologically healthy people. Maslow believed that we have much to learn from people possessing an optimistic, positive outlook.

MASLOW'S BASIC IDEAS

To understand Maslow's ideas, two principles should be remembered: (1) Maslow was interested in studying the positive, healthy personality; and (2) when individual's basic needs are satisfied, they have the energy and drive to seek higher goals. With these as his guidelines, Maslow identified a **hierarchy of needs (Figure 6-1)** that must be satisfied before people can move toward higher levels of thought, creativity, and self-fulfillment.

Of the basic needs Maslow identified—physiological, safety, love and belongingness, esteem, and self-actualization—the first four are often called **deficiency needs.** Even if these needs are satisfied, people will experience feelings of discontent or restlessness unless they are doing what they believe they should be doing. As Maslow (1987) noted, what people can be, they must be. This drive leads them to attempt to satisfy **growth needs**—that is, those self-actualization needs for truth, beauty, justice, and so on.

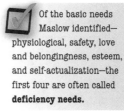

Of the basic needs Maslow identified—physiological, safety, love and belongingness, esteem, and self-actualization—the first four are often called **deficiency needs.**

THE HIERARCHY OF NEEDS

Initially, the lower, more basic needs must be satisfied before higher-level needs can be addressed. Thus satisfaction proceeds from bottom to top. Once these preeminent needs are satisfied, the search for selfactualization commences.

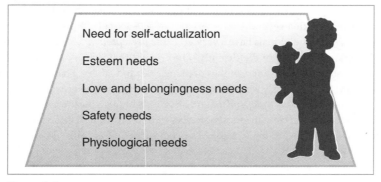

Need for self-actualization

Esteem needs

Love and belongingness needs

Safety needs

Physiological needs

Figure 6-1 The Humanistic Perspective on Development

- **Physiological needs.** Maslow's premise about the physiological was simple: A hungry or thirsty person searches for food and water more keenly than for anything else. Unsatisfied physiological needs come to dominate a person's life; everything is subordinated to efforts to satisfy them. A good example of the power of this need is a patient experiencing severe pain. Nothing matters other than the need for relief from pain.
- **Safety needs.** People need to feel physically secure from threats to their lives. When this need is unmet, any concern about higher needs is lost. For example, recently a rash of tornadoes struck southern areas of the United States. Many of the individuals interviewed were not worried about financial losses, but instead expressed their thanks that they were still alive.

  People should also be free from feelings of anxiety and fear, a need that Maslow believed was reflected in their preferences for familiar surroundings, safe jobs, and old friends. Extreme feelings of insecurity about an illness or unwarranted fear about hospitalization can often retard a patient's recovery and signal a need for constant reassurance.
- **Love and belongingness needs.** Once physiological and safety needs are met, people can turn to giving and receiving affection, building friendships, and establishing roots—in other words, to work at being accepted. These needs are not purely a drive for sexual satisfaction but rather include the notion that love involves both giving and receiving.
- **Esteem needs.** Esteem needs refer to what others think of us, as well as our opinion of ourselves. Maslow believed esteem needs reflect a desire for strength, achievement, mastery, and confidence. When these needs are met, people have positive feelings about themselves and a corresponding confidence in facing life's challenges. Maslow also believed people have a need for what he called "reputation" or "prestige." People want respect and esteem from others, but that respect or esteem must be deserved.
- **Self-actualization needs.** If all the previous needs are satisfied, humans still experience feelings of discontent and restlessness unless they are doing what they believe they are uniquely suited to do. As Maslow stated (1987, p. 22), musicians must make music, artists must paint, and poets must write if they are to find peace with themselves.

CHARACTERISTICS OF SELF-ACTUALIZED PEOPLE

From studying colleagues, friends, and historical figures such as Abraham Lincoln and Thomas Jefferson, Maslow identified several characteristics of self-actualized people (**Figure 6-2**). For example, self-actualized individuals have a very *accurate perception of reality*—an ability to judge people and situations correctly and efficiently. They *accept* themselves and others, recognizing but not being threatened by the shortcomings of themselves and others. They display considerable *spontaneity*, while simultaneously welcoming *privacy*. They are *problem centered*, not focused on themselves, and are remarkably *independent* and *creative*. Although these are the more important positive characteristics, self-actualized people also have their imperfections; they can be silly, wasteful, or thoughtless, for example. Maslow's conclusion: Self-actualized people are real, not caricatures.

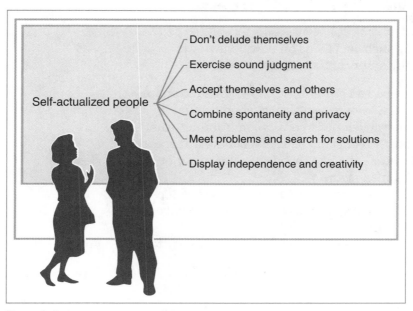

Figure 6-2 Characteristics of Self-Actualized Individuals

 ## IMPLICATIONS FOR HEALTHCARE PROVIDERS

Maslow's ideas have important implications for healthcare providers. As mentioned previously, satisfaction of a patient's needs substantially increases the chances of his or her recovery. However, healthcare providers also have the obligation to consider their own needs if they are to offer the most professional help of which they are capable. Given the potentially dangerous consequences of many diseases, they must meet their safety needs. In addition, healthcare providers should work in a situation in which their esteem needs are recognized and accepted. Maslow's hierarchy of needs is one way to prioritize nursing care. Patients who have trouble breathing may not feel safe and, therefore, may have difficulty meeting needs for belonging and mastery.

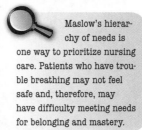
Maslow's hierarchy of needs is one way to prioritize nursing care. Patients who have trouble breathing may not feel safe and, therefore, may have difficulty meeting needs for belonging and mastery.

SOURCE

Maslow, A. (1987). *Motivation and personality* (revised by R. Frager, J. Fadiman, C. McReynolds, & R. Coc). New York: Harper and Row.

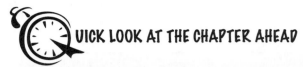

QUICK LOOK AT THE CHAPTER AHEAD

Learning theorists focus on how behavior is shaped by environmental influences:

- Pavlov paired stimulus with response to shape behavior, known as classical conditioning.
- Skinner developed operant conditioning—that is, how the consequences of a behavior increase or decrease the likelihood that the behavior will happen again.
- Bandura proposes that our behavior is shaped by what we observe in others, called social cognitive learning.
- Self-efficacy is our belief in our own ability to effect a desired outcome.

7

Pavlov, Skinner, and Bandura: Learning Perspective on Development

TERMS
- ☐ Behaviorists
- ☐ Classical conditioning
- ☐ Negative reinforcement
- ☐ Punishment
- ☐ Reinforcement
- ☐ Response
- ☐ Self-efficacy
- ☐ Social cognitive learning
- ☐ Stimulus

Learning theorists focus on behavior; consequently, they are known as **behaviorists**. They believe that unconscious forces or unseen structures do little to further our understanding of human behavior. What is needed, they claim, is a method that enables observers to measure human behavior objectively and scientifically. They argue that development proceeds through learning as humans adjust to their environments. That is, the environment either rewards, punishes, or ignores us.

To help you grasp the power and scope of the learning explanation of development, this chapter considers three learning theorists: Pavlov, Skinner, and Bandura. **Table 7-1** summarizes the key points made by each of these behaviorists.

 ## PAVLOV'S CLASSICAL CONDITIONING

One of the trials of childhood is receiving numerous injections. You may have seen pictures of children crying *before* they receive their shot. This behavior is an excellent example of **classical conditioning**, which was discovered by the Russian physiologist Ivan Pavlov (1849–1936). Children have a **response** (crying) to a **stimulus** (the injection). On later occasions, they have a response (cry) at the sight of the stimulus (the needle), or perhaps at the sight of other factors associated with the stimulus

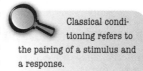
Classical conditioning refers to the pairing of a stimulus and a response.

(the person who gives the shot). Four steps in classical conditioning explain what happens here (**Table 7-2**). Classical conditioning refers to the pairing of a stimulus and a response.

 ## SKINNER'S OPERANT CONDITIONING

B. F. Skinner (1904–1990) developed an explanation of learning that stressed the consequences of behavior—what happens *after* we do something is all important.

For example, imagine a 10-year-old with a sweet tooth. His father has constantly prodded him all summer to mow the lawn: "Do it today, do it before I get home, or else." But his mother, with a shrewd understanding of human behavior, discovers that the local store carries ice cream bars that her son likes, but they are rather expensive. She promises him a package each week after he mows the lawn. By the end of the summer, the boy is cutting the grass on a regular basis with no threats, coercion, or scoldings. Skillful use of **reinforcement** greatly increased the desired behavior. Operant conditioning refers to how the consequences of a behavior increase or decrease the likelihood that the behavior will happen again.

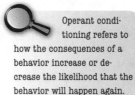
Operant conditioning refers to how the consequences of a behavior increase or decrease the likelihood that the behavior will happen again.

Table 7-1 The Major Learning Theorists

Theorist	Key Points
Pavlov	Classical conditioning; control of stimuli
Skinner	Instrumental or operant conditioning; reinforcement schedules
Bandura	Social cognitive learning; observation, modeling

Table 7-2 Pavlov's Classical Conditioning

1. US	————————————	UR
2. CS	————————————	NR
3. CS		
	————————————	UR
US		
4. CS	————————————	CR

1. injection (Unconditional Stimulus) → crying (Unconditioned Response)
2. nurse (Conditioned Stimulus) → no crying (No Response)
3. injection (US) + nurse (CS) → crying (UR) (pair US and CS)
4. nurse (CS) (remove the pairing) → crying (CR)

Operant Conditioning

Reinforcement—the consequence of behavior—is the key to under-standing Skinner's work. For example, praise is a powerful reinforcer for people. Immediately praising a patient's desirable responses (e.g., remembering to exercise at regular intervals) is reinforcement of a specific behavior.

The consequences of behavior—the reinforcers—are powerful controlling forces. We can summarize Skinner's thinking by saying, "Control the reinforcers, control the behavior." Negative reinforcers also exist. These events (also called aversive stimuli, meaning some-thing unpleasant) are *removed* after a correct response appears, and thus tend to increase the desired behavior. For example, children who neglect to do their homework are kept after school, losing their play-time. When they do what is expected—turning in homework on time—the penalty of staying after school (aversive stimulus) is re-moved, and they have their playtime returned to them (reinforce-ment). Both positive and negative reinforcement increase behavior.

Negative reinforcement should not be confused with **punish-ment,** which decreases behavior. What happens when those in au-thority withdraw a positive reinforcer (a child cannot go to the movies) or introduce something unpleasant (slapping, scolding)? Skinner believed that these conditions establish the parameters of punishment; that is, something aversive (unpleasant) appears after a response (e.g., not doing homework) or something positive (pleasant) disappears after the response. People often confuse negative rein-forcement and punishment. Negative reinforcement (sometimes called negative feedback) is not punishment. Negative reinforcement is when something unpleasant is removed, not when it is applied.

We can summarize Skinner's thinking by saying, "Control the rein-forcers, control the behavior."

Negative reinforcers also exist. These events (also called aversive stimuli, meaning something unpleasant) are *removed* after a correct response ap-pears, and thus tend to in-crease the desired behavior.

People often con-fuse negative re-inforcement and punishment. Negative reinforcement (sometimes called negative feedback) is not punishment. Negative reinforcement is when something unpleasant is removed, not when it is applied.

SOCIAL COGNITIVE LEARNING

Albert Bandura, who was born in 1925, believes that social cognitive learning occurs through observing others, even when the observer does not reproduce the model's responses during acquisition and, therefore, receives no reinforcement (Bandura & Walters, 1963). For Bandura, **social cognitive learning** means that the information people process from observing other people, things, and events influences the way they act. Observational learning has particular relevance because we know that people do not always do what they are told, but rather what they see others do.

In a classic study, Bandura and his colleagues studied the effects of live models, filmed human aggression, and filmed cartoon aggression on preschool children's aggressive behavior. The filmed human aggression involved adult models displaying aggression toward an inflated doll; the filmed cartoon aggression involved a cartoon character displaying the same behavior as the humans; the live models displayed the identical aggression as the others. Later, all the children exhibited significantly more aggression than did youngsters in a control group. Also, filmed models were as effective as live models in transmitting aggression. Bandura is the source of the concept of a "role model."

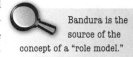

Bandura is the source of the concept of a "role model."

Bandura (1997) suggests that prestigious, powerful, competent models are more readily imitated than models who lack these qualities. Age, gender, race, educational, and socioeconomic qualities seem to be particularly effective in encouraging modeling.

IMPLICATIONS FOR HEALTHCARE PROVIDERS

Bandura's work has implications for health teaching. He suggests four ways in which our observations of other people tell us what we ourselves are capable of (i.e., our perception of our own competence): our own previous experience (I did this before, I can do it again); verbal persuasion of others (You can do it!); vicarious experience and modeling (Other people can do this, so I guess I can, too); and emotional arousal (how our own excitement, or anxiety, as we embark on a task colors our belief about the likeliness of our success). Bandura coined the phrase **self-efficacy** to describe our belief in our own ability to effect a desired outcome. You can promote patients' self-efficacy by encouraging them (verbal persuasion), introducing them to other patients like themselves (vicarious experience), and drawing on their own experiences in learning new behaviors in the past. Helping to decrease anxiety is also important.

SOURCES

Bandura, A. (1997). *Self-efficacy: The exercise of control*. New York: Freeman.

Bandura, A., & Walters, R.H. (1963). *Social learning and personality development*. New York: Holt, Rinehart & Wilson.

Dacey, J., & Travers, J. (1999). *Human development across the lifespan* (4th ed.). New York: McGraw-Hill.

- Culture is learned from birth and is shared by all members of the group who think, talk, and relate to others "like you."
- Culture, race, and ethnicity are not necessarily the same thing.
- Developmental contextualism means that culture and human development cannot be separated.
- In developmental contextualism, four forces are at work: physical setting, social influences, personal characteristics, and the influence of time.
- A cultural assessment includes communication, personal space, social organization of family and other groups, concept of time, relationship to actual or perceived control of authority, and biological variations.

8

A Cultural Perspective on Development

TERMS
- ☐ Cultural assessment
- ☐ Cultural competence
- ☐ Culture
- ☐ Developmental contextualism

Vygotsky (discussed in Chapter 4) believed in the social origins of the human mind, recognizing the importance of culture in human development. Probably the best way to think of **culture** is to view it as the sum of meanings, norms, habits, and social phenomena that give people an identity as members of a given community. It includes behavioral patterns, beliefs, attitudes, values, traditions, and other aspects of a group of people that are passed from generation to generation.

The well-known psychologist Jerome Bruner (1996) stated that culture is the framework around which humans build their minds. Human behavior emerges from unique cultural settings, which must be identified and accepted if researchers are to penetrate the secrets of development. Barbara Rogoff (1990) has studied cognitive development in children around the world; she views it as an "apprenticeship in thinking," because how children learn to think is embedded in the daily life of their unique cultural context.

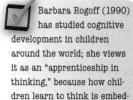 Barbara Rogoff (1990) has studied cognitive development in children around the world; she views it as an "apprenticeship in thinking," because how children learn to think is embedded in the daily life of their unique cultural context.

Table 8-1 illustrates the increasingly varied nature of the population of the United States. As a culture is dynamic and continuously changes in an effort to maintain itself, we could say that the culture of the United States itself is changing while remaining uniquely itself. It is important to remember that white, middle-class America is its own culture, and has developed over a period of time, while borrowing and integrating influences of other cultures. "Different" and "diverse" are in the eye of the beholder.

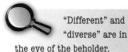 "Different" and "diverse" are in the eye of the beholder.

DEVELOPMENTAL CONTEXTUALISM

Developmental contextualism illustrates how the various cultural factors interact. This model of human development was proposed by the developmental psychologist Richard Lerner (1991) to provide a logical rationale for capitalizing on the richly diverse backgrounds of human beings. Developmental contextualism begins with the idea that all of a person's characteristics—psychological as well as biological—interact with the environment (the context in this theory). "Context" refers to four major forces of development:

- The *physical settings* of the patients, such as the home, classroom, and workplace
- The *social influences* acting on the patients, such as their families, peers, and significant others

Table 8-1 Origins of the U.S. Population; 1996–2050

	1996	2050
White Americans	73%	53%
Hispanic Americans	11%	25%
African Americans	13%	14%
Asian Americans	4%	8%
Native Americans	1%	1%

- The *personal characteristics* of the patients, such as their physical appearance, temperament, and language fluency
- The *influence of time*—that is, the changes wrought by the experiences accumulated through the years

Figure 8-1 summarizes the developmental contextual perspective.

THE IMPACT OF CULTURE

After the genocide in Rwanda in 1994, several U.S. psychologists traveled to Rwanda to help with the massive psychological problems caused by the heartrending violence. The psychologists quickly found that traditional Western therapeutic methods, such as individualized therapy, were useless. The genocide in Rwanda in 1994 was particularly painful for children who witnessed it and lost family members.

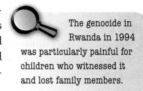

The genocide in Rwanda in 1994 was particularly painful for children who witnessed it and lost family members.

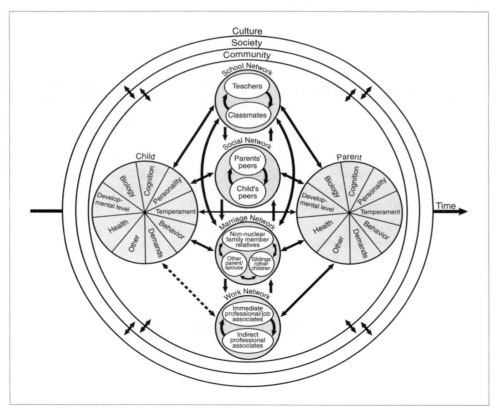

Figure 8-1 The Developmental Contextual Perspective

They also discovered that urging patients to "talk it out" simply did not work. Using native songs, dances, and storytelling, which their patients found natural and comforting, proved to be much more effective. Successful programs in Africa demand that practitioners help restore social supports and relationships. Understanding the attitudes, customs, and behaviors—in other words, the culture—of individuals is important if you are to interact positively with them.

IMPLICATIONS FOR HEALTHCARE PROVIDERS

Developing **cultural competence** is very important for healthcare providers. Culturally competent care is the adaptation of care in a manner that is congruent with the patient's culture. It is a conscious process of developing awareness, skills, and sensitivity. It begins by doing a **cultural assessment**, which includes the following areas of human behaviors and beliefs:

- **Communication:** not just what language people use, but how they talk with each other (e.g., use of eye contact; how to address men versus women, and elders versus children; and the use of formal and informal language). Example: There are more than 30 million Americans for whom English is not the primary language, of them approximately 6 million have "limited English proficiency" (LEP).
- **Physical:** preferences for personal physical space; to shake hands or not; standing and sitting postures; which parts of the body can and should not be touched; modesty and clothing. Example: The Hmong people do not want to be touched on the head for spiritual reasons.
- **Social organization:** how the "family" defines itself; how decisions are made; who cares for children, elders, and the sick; the relationship between family and the larger society such as schools and local government; beliefs about roles; rituals and rites of passage. Example: In some Asian families, decisions are made by the matriarch.
- **Time:** clock time (events occur when scheduled by the clock) versus social time (events occur when they occur); orientation to the past, present, and future. Time orientation has implications for punctuality, planning, and even delay of gratification. Example: Do not be surprised when West African patients arrive at 2 P.M. for a 1 P.M. appointment. The appointment begins in its own time.
- **Environmental control:** relationship to external agents as helpful or menacing authority figures (e.g., government, clerics, the police, doctors); relationship to the natural world (e.g., animals are part of the family); sense of destiny or fate versus self-determination. Example: Refugees from Eastern Europe may be afraid of the police and social workers.
- **Biological variations:** quantifiable "racial" differences in health that are significant and can be traced to a combination of common genes and environment (e.g., Tay-Sachs disease among Ashkenazi Jews or sickle cell disease among West Africans).

Healthcare providers must be open to learning about cultural differences and preferences. There is always concern that teaching providers about a particular culture can lead to learning stereotypes, but not teaching about culture leaves the provider ignorant of important factors to consider while caring for patients. Become familiar with cultures that are part of your own day-to-day practice by talking with patients, colleagues who are from those cultures, and others who have expertise and insight to offer. Learn another language. Learn how to best work with an interpreter; do not assume that everything is translated as you might expect. Be sensitive to the fact that people who are new to a country may be experiencing a dizzying experience of acculturation. Beware of even well-meaning stereotypes. Ask yourself, What is influencing *my* thinking?

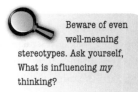

Beware of even well-meaning stereotypes. Ask yourself, What is influencing *my* thinking?

SOURCES

Bruner, J. (1996). *The culture of education.* Cambridge, MA: Harvard University Press.

Lerner, R. (1991). Changing organism–context relations as the basic process of development: A developmental contextual perspective. *Developmental Psychology, 27*(1), 27–32.

Rogoff, B. (1990). *Apprenticeship in thinking: Cognitive development in social context.* New York: Oxford University Press.

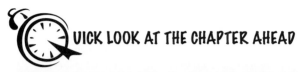
- In general, differences between males and females in areas of intellectual performance are so small as to be of little practical importance.
- Verbal and mathematical ability consists of many subcategories of performance; gender differences in the subcategories tend to cancel each other out in the larger picture.
- Gender differences in physical aggression first appear between ages 2 and 3, with boys being more aggressive than girls.

9

Gender Differences

TERMS
- ☐ Effect size
- ☐ Gender differences
- ☐ Spatial perception

Gender is the most salient human characteristic. Males and females are far more similar than they are different. Nevertheless, humans are drawn to differences and tend to exaggerate their relevance, giving rise to stereotypes.

Research on gender differences relies on meta-analysis. Researchers use the means and standard deviations for males and females reported in many studies to calculate an **effect size**. Effect size is measured in comparison to "no effect," as in "gender has no effect on aggression." Large-scale studies report gender differences in terms of variance, a statistical measure of how much of one variable (aggression) can be explained by another variable (gender).

 Effect size is measured in comparison to "no effect," as in "gender has no effect on aggression." Large-scale studies report gender differences in terms of variance, a statistical measure of how much of one variable (aggression) can be explained by another variable (gender).

When researchers look for **gender differences**, they examine the distribution of the scores for males and females. Most often, the distributions overlap. The area in which they do not overlap is the area of statistical difference. A small difference may be statistically significant, yet be of no practical importance in terms of explaining the difference or justifying interventions to eliminate it.

In 1974, Maccoby and Jacklin reported four areas of male–female differences: verbal ability, quantitative ability, spatial ability, and aggression. Since then, meta-analyses have challenged or explained those differences.

INTELLECTUAL PERFORMANCE

A popular stereotype is that girls are verbal and intuitive, whereas boys are math oriented and logical. Research shows there are no gender differences in IQ. A few differences in performance on subtests have been found, but they are smaller than stereotypes propose. Beware of stereotypes: There are actually few real differences between males and females.

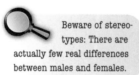 Beware of stereotypes: There are actually few real differences between males and females.

Verbal Ability

Girls develop language more rapidly than boys, placing them at an advantage in reading, spelling, and writing during the early grades. Boys are more likely to have language-related problems, such as dyslexia, which further widens the perceived gap between them and girls in elementary school. The difference in performance on verbal tasks is small, with gender accounting for only 1% of the variance in meta-analyses.

By adolescence, girls still have an advantage in terms of verbal ability, but the differences are more complex. Adolescent girls do better than boys on subtests of synonyms, speech production, and word knowledge; adolescent boys do better than girls with analogies. The Scholastic Assessment Test (SAT) in verbal ability has been heavily weighted with analogies, giving boys a slight advantage. In summary, gender differences in verbal ability are too small to be of practical importance (Lips, 1997).

Mathematical Ability

Girls have a slight advantage over boys in arithmetic computation during the elementary school years; boys do better with problem solving. Real differences emerge during high school and college, when boys' relative skill in problem solving gives them the advantage with more complex math problems. On one meta-analysis of more than 100 samples, for example, the distribution of male and female scores overlapped so closely that the difference was almost negligible (Friedman, 1989). When samples are drawn from the general population, no difference between males and females appears. In some studies, females outperform males. When samples are drawn from more gifted students, males outperform females.

The differences found between males and females in meta-analyses may be attributed to that small subgroup of males who are unusually precocious. Even so, only 1% to 5% of the variance can be explained by gender, and that gender gap has decreased in recent years as schools have paid more attention to girls' development in math (Hyde, Fennema, & Lamon, 1990). Why boys outnumber girls among the mathematically brilliant is unclear. Brain organization, social expectations, achievement motivation, and opportunity may be factors.

Spatial Ability

Spatial perception refers to the ability to locate horizontal and vertical planes in a field with conflicting information (**Figure 9-1**). Differences favoring males are small during childhood, but become larger during adulthood. Mental rotation refers to the ability to mentally visualize a three-dimensional object's rotation in space (**Figure 9-2**). Males score higher than females on this ability across the life span. Women seem to have an advantage over men on spatial tasks that depend on perceptual speed, such as matching objects (Brannon, 1996).

Experience with spatial tasks plays a role in performance on spatial tasks (Baenninger & Newcombe, 1989). Boys who grow up building things have had more experience manipulating objects with their hands and their minds than have girls. When girls participate in training exercises, their performance on spatial tasks improves.

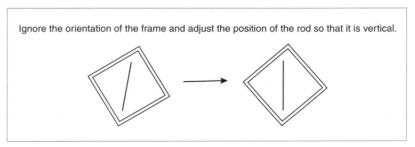

Ignore the orientation of the frame and adjust the position of the rod so that it is vertical.

Figure 9-1 Rod and Frame Test

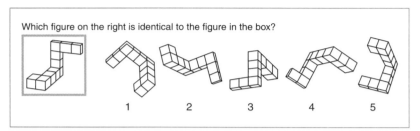

Which figure on the right is identical to the figure in the box?

1   2   3   4   5

Figure 9-2 Mental Rotation

SOCIAL BEHAVIOR: AGGRESSION

Gender differences in the display of aggressive behavior first appear between ages 2 and 3, and persist across the lifespan. Boys engage in more overt physical aggression, especially during adolescence, whereas girls are more indirect, displaying hostility and verbal aggression. Meta-analyses indicate differences are greatest in situations where social expectations for males and females either endorse or restrict physical behavior (Eagly & Steffen, 1986).

Boys' tendency toward physical aggression also may be promoted by their culture. Girls develop more verbal aggression.

Physical aggression is related to power; men justify aggression when their superior status is being challenged. For women, physical aggression is about inflicting harm, not defending their status, making them more reluctant to fight. Boys' tendency toward physical aggression also may be promoted by their culture. Girls develop more verbal aggression.

SOURCES

Baenninger, M., & Newcombe, N. (1989). Role of experience in spatial test performance: A meta-analysis. *Sex Roles, 20*, 327–343.

Brannon, L. (1996). *Gender*. Boston: Allyn & Bacon.

Eagly, A., & Steffen, V. (1986). Gender and aggressive behavior: A meta-analytic review of the social psychological literature. *Psychological Bulletin, 100*, 309–330.

Friedman, L. (1989). Mathematics and the gender gap: A meta-analysis. *Review of Educational Research, 59*, 185–213.

Hyde, J., Fennema, E., & Lamon, S. (1990). Gender differences in mathematics performance: A meta-analysis. *Psychological Bulletin, 107*, 139–155.

Lips, H. (1997). *Sex and gender* (3rd ed.). Mountain View, CA: Mayfield.

Maccoby, E., & Jacklin, C. (1974). *The psychology of sex differences*. Stanford, CA: Stanford University Press.

- In the United States, the federal government determines poverty based on family income relative to family size and composition.
- The poverty threshold for a family of two adults and two children was $19,874 in 2005.
- The table shows the U.S. statistics on poverty for 2005 (latest data before press).
- Neighborhoods with a large number of poor households tend to have poor schools.
- Schools that have functioned successfully under different economic conditions emphasize academics, are embedded in their communities, and provide a safe and encouraging environment for children.

10

A Social Class Perspective on Development

TERMS
☐ **Feminization of poverty**

Any society exerts an enormous influence on the development of its members, and this influence is conveyed in ways that are subtle but powerful. While money may or may not make you happy, it definitely gives you access not only to basic needs, such as food, clothing, and shelter, but also to the advantages children need to develop to their fullest potential in a postindustrial society, such as medical and dental care, transportation, and a good education. Poverty is about more than money.

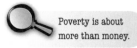

Poverty is about more than money.

To determine a person's poverty status, the U.S. Census Bureau compares the person's total family income in the last 12 months with the poverty threshold appropriate for that person's family size and composition. If the total income of that person's family is less than the threshold appropriate for that family, then the person is considered poor or "below the poverty level," together with every member of his or her family. The poverty threshold, which is reset each year, is determined by multiple factors. The interaction of poverty, children, and education is a burning issue for our society. First, however, we address the extent of poverty itself. In 2005, the poverty threshold for a family of two adults and two children in the United States was $19,874.

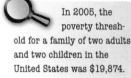

In 2005, the poverty threshold for a family of two adults and two children in the United States was $19,874.

THE CULTURE OF POVERTY

Table 10-1 presents the total number of people living in poverty in the United States, by age and race. To summarize the statistics (U.S. Census Bureau, 2007):

- The official poverty rate in 2006 was 12.3%, not statistically different from 2005.
- In 2006, 36.5 million people were in poverty, again not statistically different from 2005.
- Poverty rates remained statistically unchanged for blacks (24.3%) and non-Hispanic whites (8.2%) between 2005 and 2006; however, the rate decreased for Hispanics from 21.8% in 2005 to 20.6% in 2006.
- The poverty rate rose between 2000 and 2004 (11.3% to 12.7%) before declining to 12.3% in 2006. This compares with a poverty rate for 1959 of 22.4%, the first year for which poverty rates are available.
- The 2006 poverty rate for children younger than age 18 (17.4%) remained higher than for people ages 18 to 64 years old (10.8%) and for elders aged 65 and older (9.4%).

Table 10-1 Poverty Rates by Age and Race, 2006

Category	No. (millions)	%
Persons	36.4	12.3
Age <18 yr	12.8	17.4
Age 18–64	20.2	10.8
Age 65 and older	3.4	9.4
Race—non-Hispanic white	16	8.2
Race—black	9	24.3
Race—Hispanic	9.2	20.6

Source: U.S. Census Bureau (2007).

- The rates for children younger than age 18 and ages 18 to 64 years old were unchanged statistically, although the rate for elders (9.4%) was a decrease from 2005 (10.1%).
- Families with a female head of household and no husband have a much higher poverty rate (28.3%) than married couples (4.9%) or families with a male head of household and no wife (13.2%).

Although lack of an adequate income is what springs to mind when we think of poverty, it is important to remember that individuals and families living in poverty are extremely diverse. More young families and single women are living in poverty than ever before. The prevalence of poverty among women has reached new heights, a trend frequently referred to as the **feminization of poverty**. Healthcare providers often work with women on welfare, for example, and see the negative effects of poverty on pregnant women, both physically and psychologically.

Two factors help explain the higher rate of children living in poverty compared to adults (**Figure 10-1**). First, poor families have more children per adult than the population as a whole does. For example, 55.7% of poor families with children have only one adult, but only 13.9% of nonpoor families with children have one adult. Second, poor families with children have more children on average (2.24 per family) compared to nonpoor families with children (1.79) (Betson & Michael, 1997).

THE EFFECTS OF POVERTY ON CHILDREN

Poverty has devastating effects on all aspects of development: physical, cognitive, and psychosocial. Americans have always been firm believers that schools are the means for students to turn their lives around. But today we must objectively ask: How good are the schools that these children attend? Jonathan Kozol (1992, 2006), an outspoken critic of U.S. schools, has written two biting commentaries on classroom conditions in schools that are mostly attended by poor children. Students are crowded into small, squalid spaces, and in some cities overcrowding is so bad that schools function in abandoned factories. In one school, Kozol recounts, students eat their lunches in what was once the building's boiler room. Reading classes are taught in what used to be a bathroom; there are no microscopes for science classes; one counselor serves 3600 students in the elementary grades. In the

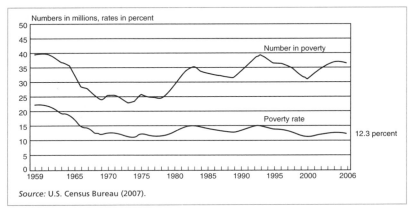

Source: U.S. Census Bureau (2007).

Figure 10-1 Child and Poverty Rates, 1959–2006

high school of the same district, there is a single physics section for 2200 students; two classes are being taught simultaneously in one classroom. Kozol refers to these shortcomings as "savage inequalities" inherent in the "apartheid of schooling in America."

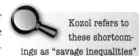
Kozol refers to these shortcomings as "savage inequalities" inherent in the "apartheid of schooling in America."

Economic differences among school systems are also reflected in access to educational technology, certainly one of the gateways to future success. Commitment to a technological education, however, requires a substantial investment for acquiring equipment and software. Some schools, owing to fiscal restraints, may find it necessary to cut supplies and expense budgets, resulting in smaller amounts and less-sophisticated equipment and software being available to their students. The resulting "technology gap" (the gulf between schools that can afford basic or more elaborate equipment and supplies and those that cannot) may well widen the already existing gap between quality of schooling for those students in poorer versus wealthier areas.

Nevertheless, some schools have functioned successfully under difficult economic conditions. They typically share the following characteristics:

- The schools place an emphasis on academic achievement.
- The schools manifest a capacity to react swiftly to the social and emotional needs of their students.
- The school atmosphere is safe and orderly, but not restrictive.
- The schools display an open and encouraging attitude toward active parental participation in the running of the school.
- A true partnership exists between school administrators and all staff personnel.
- The schools maintain a close relationship with the community, which furthers the achievements of students. Good schools promote children's development.

Good schools promote children's development.

IMPLICATIONS FOR HEALTHCARE PROVIDERS

Poverty hurts children in a range of ways difficult to identify because the poor are *not* all alike. For example, the African American youth living in an urban ghetto experiences a quite different set of problems than a malnourished, chronically diseased white child in Appalachia. Although approximately 8% of U.S. children are poor for more than 6 years, more than 30% of children experience poverty at some time in their life.

When working with poor children, you should look for undiagnosed acute and chronic health problems and their effect on development. For example, untreated ear infections may impair hearing, and anemia and nutritional deficiencies can rob children of the energy they need to grow and learn. Similarly, poor adolescents may not receive treatment for sexually transmitted diseases (STDs) or have access to prenatal care.

Impoverished and homeless children experience numerous health problems, usually resulting from a lack of medical care. As of 2004, nearly 47 million Americans (about 16%) did not have health insurance, up by 7 million from 2000. Approximately 11.7% of children younger than age 18 did not have health insurance; with white children accounting for the lowest percentage of these uninsureds (11.4%) and Hispanic children the highest (24.9%.) When working with poor children, you should look for undiagnosed acute and chronic health problems and their effect on development. For example, untreated ear infections may impair hearing, and anemia and nutritional deficiencies can rob children of the energy they need to grow and learn. Similarly, poor adolescents may not receive treatment for sexually transmitted diseases (STDs) or have access to prenatal care.

SOURCES

Betson, D., & Michael, M. (1997). Why so many children are poor. *Future of Children, 72*, 25–39.

Kozol, J. (1992). *Savage inequalities*. New York: Harper Collins.

Kozol. J. (2006). *The shame of the nation: The restoration of apartheid schooling in America*. New York: Crown Publishing Group.

U.S. Census Bureau. (2007). *Income, poverty, and health insurance coverage in the United States: 2006*. Washington, DC: U.S. Department of Commerce.

PART I • QUESTIONS

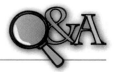

For each of the following questions, choose the **one best** answer.

1. Development is best explained by a model that
   a. concentrates on one aspect of development.
   b. uses behavior as its focus.
   c. includes biological, psychological, and social influences.
   d. restricts itself to the observable.

2. Humans have a remarkable potential for change, but resiliency has
   a. limitations.
   b. defined markers.
   c. unlimited capacity.
   d. known characteristics.

3. A 10-year-old girl peeks in her older sister's diary, but later feels guilty. She tells herself, "I shouldn't have done that. It wasn't right." According to Freud, which moral component of the personality is responsible for her feelings about her behavior?
   a. Id
   b. Ego
   c. Superego
   d. Preconscious

4. What is Freud's "pleasure principle"?
   a. The notion that unconscious forces govern our behavior is the pleasure principle.
   b. Childhood pleasures have a strong influence on adult personality.
   c. Individuals act to gratify instinctual desires and to avoid pain.
   d. Personality is shaped by how individuals indulge their sexual urges.

5. Erikson's theory of psychosocial development is based on
   a. the notion that the personality develops early in childhood.
   b. the premise that humans interact with an ever-widening circle of people.
   c. the need to avoid developmental crises.
   d. the idea that early social experiences determine later ones.

6. Which of the following crises in the life cycle is the cornerstone of Erikson's theory?
   a. Trust versus mistrust
   b. Autonomy versus shame and doubt
   c. Initiative versus guilt
   d. Identity formation versus identity diffusion

7. Which of the following statements refers to Piaget's universalist constructivist theory?
   a. Humans passively assimilate their understanding of the world.
   b. Humans construct reality through their interactions with the environment.
   c. Humans have inborn schemata that help them understand the world.
   d. Humans construct reality by being acted on by the environment.

8. What is Piaget's definition of "adaptation"?
   a. Intelligence
   b. Assimilation and accommodation
   c. Ability to effectively negotiate environmental demands
   d. All of the above

9. In his explanation of cognitive development, Vygotsky stressed
   a. assimilation.
   b. social interactions.
   c. reinforcement.
   d. schema.

10. Vygotsky believed language gradually becomes _____ and directs behavior.
    a. structured
    b. pragmatic
    c. internalized
    d. reinforced

11. In Bronfenbrenner's model of human ecology, the school, neighborhood, and peer group belong in which system?
    a. Microsystem
    b. Mesosystem
    c. Exosystem
    d. Macrosystem

12. The American cultural value placed on the primacy of the biological family is an example of a(n)
    a. microsystem.
    b. mesosystem.
    c. exosystem.
    d. macrosystem.

13. Maslow believed that our needs are best seen as a(n)
    a. ellipse.
    b. hierarchy.
    c. interlocking circle.
    d. polygon.

14. Using our abilities to the limits of our potential refers to
    a. assimilation.
    b. accommodation.
    c. conditioning.
    d. self-actualization.

15. The environment responds to human behavior and either reinforces it or eliminates it. This theory is known as
    a. operant conditioning.
    b. classical conditioning.
    c. social cognitive learning.
    d. connectionism.

16. The importance of modeling is emphasized in
    a. operant conditioning.
    b. classical conditioning.
    c. social cognitive learning.
    d. connectionism.

17. It is important to remember that different is not
    a. unique.
    b. deficient.
    c. appreciated.
    d. diffuse.

18. _____ is a belief that interactions among all aspects of development require analysis.
    a. Piagetian psychology
    b. Operant conditioning
    c. Social cognitive learning
    d. Developmental contextualism

19. Which of the following is an example of between-group differences in gender research on language development?
    a. Girls develop language more rapidly than boys.
    b. Girls do better than boys on subtests of anagrams, synonyms, speech production, and word knowledge.
    c. Although dyslexia is more common in boys, some girls develop dyslexia.
    d. Gender accounts for 1% of the variability in language development.

20. Research on aggression supports which of the following statements?
    a. Boys are more hostile than girls.
    b. For men, physical aggression is about inflicting harm.
    c. For women, physical aggression is about defending their social status.
    d. Physical aggression is related to perceptions of social power.

21. Which of the following is *not* associated with homelessness?
    a. Hunger and poor nutrition
    b. Developmental delays
    c. Health problems
    d. Lowered intelligence

22. A major characteristic of successful schools in poor economic locations is
    a. an emphasis on academic achievement.
    b. classroom television.
    c. building conditions.
    d. proximity to the center of the city.

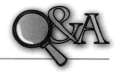

PART 1 · ANSWERS

1. **The answer is c.** The complexity of development demands an explanatory model that recognizes the interactions among the multiple levels that shape growth and development. Explanations that concentrate on only one topic are not adequate.

2. **The answer is a.** No one can tolerate intense stress indefinitely. Some of the secrets of resiliency still elude researchers.

3. **The answer is c.** Emerging around ages 3–5 years, the superego represents an internalization of social standards for good and bad behavior. It is the individual's way of policing his or her own behavior. The 10-year-old girl has internalized social standards for privacy, and feels guilty knowing that she has willfully violated those standards.

4. **The answer is c.** As the most primitive component of personality, the id is the seat of instinctual drives, especially sex, food, and aggression. Operating on the pleasure principle, the id seeks immediate gratification and wants to avoid physical and psychic pain. The drives for sex and aggression are particularly conflicted because they are subject to ambiguous social norms. Freud developed the concept of defense mechanisms, which humans use to protect the ego from unpleasant feelings, especially anxiety and guilt.

5. **The answer is b.** Erikson recognized that the social environment plays a significant role in shaping a child's sense of self. His theory of psychosocial development is based on the premise that humans interact with an ever-widening circle of people, beginning with the mother and ending with humankind. The eight stages of the life cycle are marked by normative developmental crises, the resolution of which form the personality.

6. **The answer is d.** Erikson's concept of the identity crisis in adolescence is the cornerstone of his theory. He believed that most adolescents go through a serious struggle in achieving a self-identity. The developmental struggle is to integrate childhood identifications with new biological urges, assumption of social roles, and recognition of one's abilities and limitations. Failure to form an identity may result in identity diffusion—that is, of feeling like a nobody, with no sense of direction or commitment to a set of values.

7. **The answer is b.** The term "universal constructivist" implies that all humans construct their understanding of the world in predictable ways. Humans are not passive organisms, but rather take an active role in their own development by acting on the physical environment. Piaget believed that mental life in infancy begins with motor activity. The infant who swings an arm toward and finally grasps a toy is learning about controlling the body, the nature of objects, and the relationship between the body and objects.

8. **The answer is d.** To Piaget, the definition of intelligence *is* adaptation—that is, an ability to effectively negotiate environmental demands. Adaptation consists of the dual processes of assimilation and accommodation. When people assimilate, they incorporate an experience into existing schemata and structures: "Oh, I know this. It's just like that." When they cannot fit an experience into existing schemata or structures, people must accommodate—that is, modify their way of thinking to fit the experience. Accommodation can be a lot of mental work; hence the famous line, "Assimilate if you can; accommodate if you must."

9. **The answer is b.** Vygotsky's belief in the power of social interactions to shape development distinguished his work from the work of other theorists such as Piaget.

10. **The answer is c.** For Vygotsky, egocentric speech becomes internalized and helps to direct behavior. Speech is seen as playing a central role in cognitive development.

11. **The answer is b.** The microsystem of the family is embedded in mesosystems, which include community groups in general, such as the school, neighborhood, peer group, and church or other social organizations.

12. **The answer is d.** The macrosystem represents the dominant beliefs and ideologies in the culture at large. Beliefs about children in the society at large influence child-rearing practices and government policies. For example, the cultural value placed on the primacy of the biological family has resulted in children spending years in foster homes, even when reunification with biological parents may not be in the child's best interests.

13. **The answer is b.** Maslow believed that a hierarchy best represents humans' needs, given that satisfaction of one need leads to the next. Each need can be partially satisfied before the drive to satisfy the next need begins.

14. **The answer is d.** The highest goal for humans is to be actually doing what they could be doing (self-actualization). Otherwise, a sense of restlessness and wondering will persist.

15. **The answer is a.** Skinner's interpretation of learning rests on the power of the environment to shape behavior. Careful control of the environment supposedly leads to positive (even ideal) development.

16. **The answer is c.** Bandura's work on social cognitive learning has led to increased acceptance of the use of models to shape development. When properly presented, modeling can be a powerful tool in leading to desired behavior.

17. **The answer is b.** We are all different to someone else. Consequently, individuals should not be judged by their appearance, language, or other outward characteristics.

18. **The answer is d.** Modern developmental psychologists are turning away from theories that focus on one aspect of development. Instead, they have sought explanations that recognize and analyze the complexities of human development.

19. **The answer is a.** In research, differences are addressed in several ways. One way is to distinguish between-group from within-group differences, group differences from individual differences, and differences that are statistically significant but of no practical importance. For example, girls develop language more rapidly than boys do (between-group difference), but there is a lot of variation among girls regarding their performance on tests of different types of language ability, such as anagrams and word knowledge (within-group differences). Even though dyslexia is more common in boys than girls, some girls do develop dyslexia (individual differences). Gender accounts for 1% of the variability in language development. This finding is statistically significant, but not necessarily important enough to justify developing special interventions for boys.

20. **The answer is d.** Boys engage in more overt physical aggression, especially during adolescence, whereas girls are more indirect, displaying hostility and verbal aggression. Physical aggression is related to perceptions of social power, with men perceiving that aggression is justified when their superior status is being challenged. For example, fighting among males is more about standing up for oneself than about inflicting harm. For women, physical aggression is about inflicting harm, not defending their status, making them more reluctant to fight.

21. **The answer is d.** Social class can often lead to misperceptions. A person's intelligence is not reflected by his or her social status.

22. **The answer is a.** Research has demonstrated that a focus on achievement is a feature of successful schools in deprived areas. Almost any other characteristic is secondary.

II

Prenatal Development

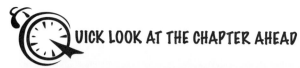

- The flow of genetic information in normal cells is from DNA to RNA to protein.
- The double helix is the name for DNA.
- DNA contains nucleotide bases A, T, G, and C.
- The complete set of DNA is the human genome, which consists of chromosomes.
- Each chromosome is comprised of many genes.
- Gene sequences instruct cells to make protein from RNA templates—a process called translation.
- Errors in translation can result in serious, life-threatening illnesses.

11

Genes, Chromosomes, and DNA

TERMS

- ☐ **Alleles**
- ☐ **Chromosomes**
- ☐ **Codominance**
- ☐ **Deoxyribonucleic acid (DNA)**
- ☐ **Dominant genes**
- ☐ **Genes**
- ☐ **Genome**
- ☐ **Genotype**
- ☐ **Nucleotide bases**
- ☐ **Phenotype**
- ☐ **Recessive genes**
- ☐ **Transcription**
- ☐ **Translation**

THE DOUBLE HELIX

All the instructions needed to direct the activities of cells are contained within **Deoxyribonucleic acid (DNA),** which is a winding double helix structure resembling a twisted ladder. DNA is made of chemical building blocks called nucleotides. Nucleotides consist of 1) a sugar molecule (a deoxyribose), 2) a phosphate group, and one of four **nucleotide bases** (A, T, G, and C). The double helix of DNA has two linked polynucleotide strands (the sides of the ladder), which are complements of one another. How the nucleotide bases are arranged side by side results in the DNA sequence along each strand (e.g., AATTCCGGA). Adenine (A) and thymine (T) always link together, as do guanine (G) and cytosine (C). This leads to four possible complementary pairings: AT, TA, GC, and CG. Each "rung" of the ladders is made up of two nitrogen bases, pared together by nitrogen bonds, holding the double helix together (**Figure 11-1**). *Each* cell in the human body contains about 6 feet of tightly coiled DNA.

CHROMOSOMES

The **genome** is an organism's complete set of DNA. The human genome consists of 46 **chromosomes**. Normal somatic cells (i.e., the cells that make up the major organs and body systems) contain 46 chromosomes arranged in 23 pairs, one of each pair is inherited from each parent. One of the 23 pairs is the sex chromosomes; the 22 other pairs are autosomes. Autosomes control most body traits, whereas sex chromosomes determine gender as well as other traits. Females contain two X chromosomes: XX. Males contain one X chromosome and one Y chromosome: XY.

GENES

Each chromosome is comprised of many **genes.** The largest chromosome has 2968 genes. The average human gene consists of 3000 nucleotide base pairs, but the largest known human gene, dystrophin, has 2.4 million bases alone. Given that there are 20,000 to 30,000 human genes, there are billions of base pairs. The key is the sequence in which the base pairs are arranged, because these are the cell's instructions on how to make the proteins necessary for life.

THE GENETIC CODE: DNA, RNA, AND PROTEINS

The flow of genetic information in normal cells is from DNA (the double strand) to RNA (ribonucleic acid, one strand) to protein. Cells contain several kinds of RNA: messenger RNA (mRNA), transfer RNA (tRNA), and ribosomal RNA (rRNA). All cellular RNA is synthesized according to instructions given by DNA templates. The synthesis of RNA from its DNA template is called **transcription,** whereas the synthesis of a protein from an RNA template is **translation.**

The human body is comprised of proteins, and proteins consist of amino acids, of which there are 20 kinds. Some proteins comprise the structural material for the human body (e.g., muscle,

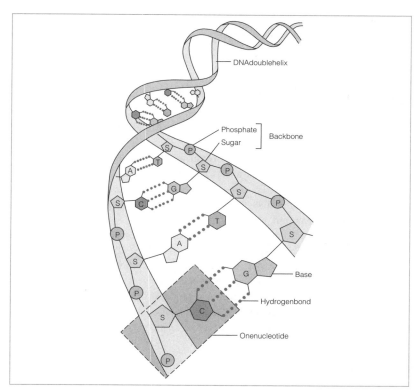

Figure 11-1 The Double Helix

skin, blood cells), and others (e.g., enzymes, hormones, insulin) regulate chemical reactions. If the body cannot synthesize proteins, it cannot live.

The constellation of all proteins in a cell is called proteome. Unlike the relatively unchanging genome, the dynamic proteome changes from minute to minute in response to tens of thousands of intra- and extracellular environmental signals. DNA contains all the information required to make the correct amount of protein at the correct time, thus controlling all metabolic activities in day-to-day life, beginning with embryogenesis.

The genetic code is the relation between the sequence of nucleotide bases in DNA (or its RNA transcript) and the sequence of amino acids in proteins. Amino acids are encoded by groups of three bases (code words, also called codons—e.g., CGG) starting from a fixed point. There are 64 possible codons; for most amino acids, there is more than one. Protein synthesis is called translation, because information present as a nucleic acid sequence is translated into a different language—the sequence of amino acids in a protein.

Given that proteins typically comprise from 100 to 1000 amino acids, the frequency at which an incorrect amino acid is incorporated in the course of protein synthesis must be *less* than 10^{-4}. In

Any mistake in forming, transferring, or reading the mRNA template can cause protein synthesis to go awry, with potentially deadly consequences for the organism.

other words, translation must by highly accurate. Any mistake in forming, transferring, or reading the mRNA template can cause protein synthesis to go awry, with potentially deadly consequences for the organism.

UNDERSTANDING GENETIC TRAITS

When genes have a variety of coded possibilities the are called **alleles.** Some genes—for example, eye color—have two alleles. In Mendelian genetics, if you inherited one brown allele and one blue allele, you have brown eyes. Brown is the **dominant gene** in this heterozygous pairing. To have blue eyes, you must have inherited two blue alleles, a homozygous pairing. Blue is the **recessive gene**. Two brown-eyed parents can have a blue-eyed child if both parents are heterozygous; that is, both have one brown allele and one blue allele. The child inherits the blue gene from each even though it was not expressed in either parent.

There are other patterns to genetic inheritance. **Codominance** occurs when a gene has multiple alleles that are expressed. For example, blood type has three alleles. Type AB blood has two codominant alleles—for A antigen and B antigen—and one, O, in which no antigen is expressed. Other patterns include incomplete dominance (crossing red flowers with white ones yields pink flowers); segregation (when two parents are heterozygous for albinism, each child has a 25% chance of being a homozygous albino); and independent assortment (when two parents are heterozygous for albinism and also for deafness, each child has a one in 16 chance of being both albino and deaf).

GENOTYPE, PHENOTYPE, AND DISEASE

Each person's genetic code is called a **genotype**; it is like a blueprint. How genotype is expressed is called **phenotype**; it is the final product. For example, two brown-eyed people have the same phenotype, but they may have different genotypes. In other words, one may be heterozygous (brown/blue) while the other is homozygous (brown/ brown).

Phenotype is influenced by factors other than genes. For example, if you are genetically coded to be 6 feet tall but are malnourished in childhood, you may not reach your genetic potential. Similarly, certain diseases (e.g., hypertension) are polygenic in origin. When or if this genotype is expressed may depend on lifestyle habits, such as smoking, lack of exercise, and consumption of a diet rich in fats. Researchers suspect that a genotypic tendency for some cancers (e.g., Hodgkin's disease) may be triggered by viral infections.

SOURCES

Cummings, M. R. (2006). *Human heredity* (7th ed.). Belmont, CA: Thomson Brooks/Cole.

Human Genome Project. (2007). *Human Genome Project information.* Retrieved March 13, 2008, from www.ornl.gov/sci/techresources/Human_Genome/home.shtml

National Institutes of Health Books. (2007). *Biochemistry.* Retrieved January 10, 2008, from www.ncbi.nlm.nih.gov/books/bv.fcgi?rid=stryer.section.704

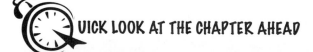

- Germ cells (gametes) divide through meiosis, forming haploid cells.
- Somatic cells divide through mitosis, forming diploid cells.
- Diploid cells have 46 chromosomes arranged in 23 pairs.
- Haploid cells have 23 single chromosomes; sperm and ova are haploid cells.
- Fertilization is an active biochemical process involving both sperm and ovum.

12

Fertilization in Utero

TERMS

- ☐ **Acrosome**
- ☐ **Acrosome reaction**
- ☐ **Capacitation**
- ☐ **Chromatids**
- ☐ **Conception**
- ☐ **Corona**
- ☐ **Diploid cells**
- ☐ **Fallopian tubes**
- ☐ **Fertilization**
- ☐ **Gametes**
- ☐ **Genetic variability**
- ☐ **Germ cells**
- ☐ **Haploid cells**
- ☐ **Meiosis**
- ☐ **Mitosis**
- ☐ **Oocyte**
- ☐ **Ovulation**
- ☐ **Ovum**
- ☐ **Polar body**
- ☐ **Secondary oocyte**
- ☐ **Somatic (body) cells**
- ☐ **Sperm**
- ☐ **Spermatids**
- ☐ **Zona pellucida**
- ☐ **Zygote**

CELL DEVELOPMENT

Conception, which is the union of a **sperm** and an **ovum**, marks the beginning of pregnancy. **Fertilization** occurs when two **germ cells** fuse to become one new cell, called a **zygote**. Germ cells are also called **gametes**. In females, they are known as egg cells, or, ova; in males, they are known as sperm cells. Gametes develop through the process of cell division called **meiosis**.

Meiosis and Mitosis

Cells are produced by either **mitosis** or **meiosis**. Human **somatic (body) cells** are **diploid cells**; that is, they have 46 chromosomes that are arranged in 23 pairs. One pair carries the sex chromosomes, and is either XX or XY. Diploid somatic cells have 46 chromosomes in 23 pairs.

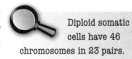
Diploid somatic cells have 46 chromosomes in 23 pairs.

Mitosis is the process by which one diploid somatic cell divides to produce two diploid somatic cells identical to the original. The DNA in the chromosomes of the original cell replicates itself. After division, each new cell has 46 chromosomes.

Meiosis is the process of cell division by which one diploid somatic cell produces four haploid gamete cells (**Figure 12-1**). Haploid cells have half the number of chromosomes of the original diploid somatic cell—that is, 23 single chromosomes instead of 46.

Two successive cell divisions occur in meiosis. First, the 46 chromosomes in the diploid somatic cell replicate. Then, rather than separate into two identical cells as in mitosis, the chromosomes intertwine and exchange genetic material. This exchange is responsible for **genetic variability**, such as eye color or height. When the cell divides, it forms two cells, each containing 23 chromosomes that are doubled in structure, but in combinations that are different from the original cell.

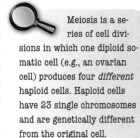
Mitosis is how one diploid somatic cell (e.g., a skin cell) divides into two diploid somatic cells genetically identical to the original (i.e., with 46 chromosomes each).

Meiosis is a series of cell divisions in which one diploid somatic cell (e.g., an ovarian cell) produces four *different* haploid cells. Haploid cells have 23 single chromosomes and are genetically different from the original cell.

At the second division, the 23 double chromosomes split in half. The two halves, called **chromatids**, move apart, forming two more cells with 23 single chromosomes each. In other words, four different **haploid cells** arise from the original diploid cell. Ova and sperm are haploid cells.

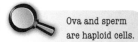
Ova and sperm are haploid cells.

Ovum

While the female fetus is still in utero, her ovarian somatic cells undergo meiosis to produce the gamete egg cells, or ova. Meiosis stops before the first division is complete. The resulting cell, called the **oocyte**, contains 46 chromosomes, which have a doubled structure. The oocyte then rests until puberty. All of a female's ova are in place by her 6th month of fetal life. A female infant is born with approximately 1 million egg cells, although half will no longer be viable by the time she reaches puberty.

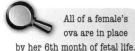
All of a female's ova are in place by her 6th month of fetal life.

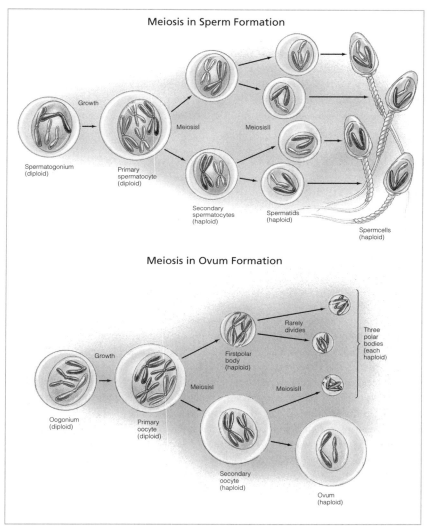

Meiosis in Sperm Formation

Growth

Spermatogonium
(diploid)

Primary
spermatocyte
(diploid)

MeiosisI

MeiosisII

Secondary
spermatocytes
(haploid)

Spermatids
(haploid)

Spermcells
(haploid)

Meiosis in Ovum Formation

Growth

Rarely
divides

Firstpolar
body
(haploid)

Three
polar
bodies
(each
haploid)

Oogonium
(diploid)

Primary
oocyte
(diploid)

MeiosisI

MeiosisII

Secondary
oocyte
(haploid)

Ovum
(haploid)

Figure 12-1 Meiosis

At puberty, the oocyte divides into two cells, with 23 chromosomes each arranged in a doubled structure. One of the cells, the **secondary oocyte**, is larger and contains more cytoplasm than the smaller cell, the first **polar body**. The second meiotic division begins at **ovulation**. The first polar body divides into two smaller ones, which disintegrate. The secondary oocyte divides into a second polar body and immature ovum, each with 23 single chromosomes. This second division is not completed until fertilization, when the immature ovum forms a nucleus in response to penetration by sperm. Ovulation represents a meiotic division.

Ovulation represents a meiotic division.

Sperm

Male gametes do not develop until puberty, when cells in the testes undergo meiosis. After the second division, there are four haploid cells, called **spermatids**. Each cell has 23 chromosomes, one of which is either an X or a Y chromosome. A spermatid loses cytoplasm; its nucleus becomes compacted, forming the head of the sperm; and a centriole develops into the tail. Sperm can remain viable in the testes for as long as 42 hours.

Sperm can remain viable in the testes for as long as 42 hours.

THE FERTILIZATION PROCESS

Before-Fertilization Status

Fertilization usually takes place in the outer third of the **fallopian tubes**. After the ovum is released, it is carried into the fallopian tubes by virtue of peristaltic movement caused by high estrogen levels. The ovum is surrounded by two membranes. The inner membrane is the **zona pellucida**, which later nourishes the newly fertilized egg. The outer membrane is the **corona**. In Latin, *zona pellucida* means "clear or bright zone," and *corona* means "crown."

In Latin, *zona pellucida* means "clear or bright zone," and *corona* means "crown."

The mature ovum is fertile for 24 hours. Sperm can survive in the female reproductive tract for 72 hours. Of the 200 to 400 million sperm released during ejaculation, only approximately 200 will reach the fallopian tubes in about 4 hours. Only one sperm may fertilize an ovum; fertilization by more than one sperm leads to embryonic death.

A sperm's success depends on several things. First, it must undergo **capacitation** while in the female reproductive track—that is, a reorganization of the chemical make-up of the sperm cell, preparing it for the acrosome reaction. The head of the sperm is covered by a cap called the **acrosome**. One result of capacitation is that the acrosomal membrane becomes destabilized.

The ovum may be selective about which sperm it allows in, based on the outcome of its capacitation, and may actually engulf the sperm, drawing in the one most compatible for a successful acrosome reaction.

Second, enzymes covering the acrosome are deposited on the outer membrane of the ovum, binding it there. The **acrosome reaction** is the process by which the sperm, using the acrosome like a drill, penetrates and passes through the zona pellucida to the oocyte. Sperm motility is also an important factor affecting this process. The zona pellucida is not a passive bystander; it has sperm receptors—enzymes that break down the corona and the acrosomal cap, facilitating the sperm's entry and passage. At the same time, acrosomal enzymes break down the zona pellucida. The ovum may be selective about which sperm it allows in, based on the outcome of its capacitation, and may actually engulf the sperm, drawing in the one most compatible for a successful acrosome reaction.

The Moment of Fertilization

As the sperm enters the ovum, the zona pellucida hardens and its sperm receptors are destroyed, so that other sperm cannot bind to or enter the ovum. Following fusion of the sperm and the oocyte, the sperm head is incorporated into the egg cytoplasm and forms a pronuclus. Meiotic division in the ovum is then completed, as the mature ovum develops a pronucleus and the second polar body is ejected.

The newly developed pronuclei of the ovum and sperm are now enclosed in a single membrane and immediately move toward each other. Their individual pronuclei each contain 23 single chromosomes, the haploid number. The pronuclei membranes disappear, allowing the chromosomes to pair up, resulting in 46 chromosomes, arranged in 23 pairs. This transformation produces the zygote, a single diploid somatic cell that contains all of the genetic material for an individual who will be different from either parent . . . and from everyone else.

 The newly developed pronuclei of the ovum and sperm are now enclosed in a single membrane.

Gender is determined at the moment of fertilization. A mature ovum can carry only the X chromosome. A sperm cell, however, may carry either the X or the Y chromosome on its 23rd chromosome. Thus the sex chromosome carried by the sperm determines the gender of the human organism. A pairing of XX results in a female child; XY results in a boy. Because the sperm cell may carry either the X or the Y chromosome, the father determines the gender of his children.

Because the sperm cell may carry either the X or the Y chromosome, the father determines the gender of his children.

IMPLICATIONS FOR HEALTHCARE PROVIDERS

For every 100 ova exposed to sperm, 84 are fertilized, 69 are implanted, 42 survive for 1 week, 37 survive to 7 weeks prenatally, and 31 survive to birth. Thus there is a 70% rate of spontaneous abortion (i.e., miscarriage) prenatally.

More males are conceived than females, in a ratio of 160:105. More male embryos die in utero, however, so that at birth the male–female ratio is 105:100. Boys are more vulnerable than girls, such that by age 18, the genders are equally represented in the population.

SOURCE

Perry, S. E., Wilson, D., Hockenberry, M. J., & Lowdermilk, D. L. (2005). *Maternal child nursing care.* New York: Elsevier Health Sciences.

- The first 2 weeks are the germinal period.
- For the first 8 weeks, the new organism is called an embryo.
- Organogenesis is 95% complete by week 8.
- Fetus is the name given to the prenatal human organism from 2 months to birth.

13

Conception to Birth

TERMS

- ☐ **Blastocyst**
- ☐ **Ectoderm**
- ☐ **Embryo**
- ☐ **Endoderm**
- ☐ **Fetus**
- ☐ **Germinal period**
- ☐ **Lanugo**
- ☐ **Mesoderm**
- ☐ **Morula**
- ☐ **Myelination**
- ☐ **Nidation**
- ☐ **Organogenesis**
- ☐ **Trophoblast**
- ☐ **Vernix caseosa**

Understanding prenatal development (**Figure 13-1**) is important for two reasons. First, the developing organism is open to environmental influences over a period of 40 weeks. The timing and nature of these influences can permanently alter the development of the fetus. Second, how development occurs prior to birth gives us information about development after birth.

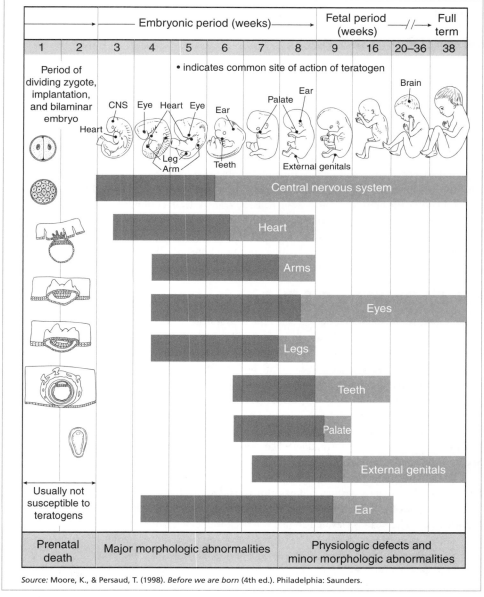

Source: Moore, K., & Persaud, T. (1998). *Before we are born* (4th ed.). Philadelphia: Saunders.

Figure 13-1 Prenatal Development

EMBRYONIC DEVELOPMENT: 0-8 WEEKS

Embryo is the name given to the fertilized ovum during the first 8 weeks of prenatal development. The first 2 weeks are also called the **germinal period**. From 3 to 8 weeks is the critical period of **organogenesis**, during which all of the major organs develop.

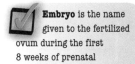
Embryo is the name given to the fertilized ovum during the first 8 weeks of prenatal development.

Germinal Period: 0-2 Weeks

0–40 hours: The fertilized ovum is called the zygote and consists of two to four cells. It rests in the fallopian tube.

40–72 hours: Having grown to 12 to 16 cells, the **morula** floats into the uterus and grows to 64 cells.

4–8 days: The **blastocyst** continues to grow to more than 100 cells. The inner cell mass becomes the human organism itself. The **trophoblast** forms between the inner mass and the environment; it will later develop into the placenta. By day 6 or 7, the blastocyst implants on the uterine wall, i.e., endometrium, in a process called **nidation**.

8–13 days: Cells separate and arrange themselves into three embryonic germ layers, which give rise to all of the major organs. The **ectoderm**—the outer layer—gives rise to the nervous system (including the brain and spine), skin, nails, hair, and salivary, pituitary, and mammary glands. The **endoderm**—the innermost layer—gives rise to the thyroid, bladder, lungs, and digestive system. The **mesoderm**—which emerges between the ectoderm and the endoderm—gives rise to the heart, circulatory and lymph systems, connective tissue, muscle, and bones. By the end of the 2nd week, the placenta, umbilical cord, and amniotic sac have taken shape.

Period of the Embryo: 3-8 Weeks

Third week: An indentation of cells, called the neural plate, forms in the ectoderm, giving rise to the brain (hindbrain, midbrain, forebrain) and neural tube (spinal cord). The chambers of the heart and blood vessels arise from a similar process in the mesoderm.

Fourth week: The heart begins to beat. Limb buds are visible. Eyes, ears, nerves, and the skeletomuscular and digestive systems begin to form. Vertebrae are present; major veins and arteries are completed. The neural tube closes. The embryo is approximately 0.5 cm long and weighs 0.4 g.

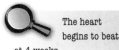
The heart begins to beat at 4 weeks.

Fifth week: Bronchial buds form; they will eventually become the lungs. Hand plates form.

Sixth week: Sex differentiation occurs. The head becomes prominent, the lower jaw fuses, and the parts of the upper jaw are present. The external ear is visible.

Seventh week: The face, eyelids, and neck form. The stomach is in position. Muscles are forming throughout the body, and neurons are developing at the rate of thousands per minute.

Eighth week: The head is elevated so that the neck is distinct. The inner and middle ear develop. The embryo moves and responds to some stimulation. Ninety-five percent of organogenesis is complete. The human organism is approximately 2 to 3 cm long and weighs 2 g. The mother is probably now aware that she is pregnant.

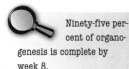
Ninety-five percent of organogenesis is complete by week 8.

FETAL DEVELOPMENT: 10–40 WEEKS

Fetus is the name given to the prenatal human organism from 2 months to birth.

> **Fetus** is the name given to the prenatal human organism from 2 months to birth.

10–12 weeks: The intestines are in position, the spinal cord is apparent, the eyes take final form, and blood forms in the bone marrow. Sex organs appear. Urine forms. The fetus is 6 to 8 cm long and weighs 19 g.

16 weeks: The fetus looks human. Bones and joints are distinct; the two halves of the brain are visible. The hard and soft palate of the mouth are differentiated. **Lanugo** (fine hair) and **vernix caseosa** (oil) begin to appear on the skin. The fetus is 12 cm long and weighs 100 g.

20 weeks: Dental enamel forms. All of the nerve cells a person will have for life are present. Sheathing of nerve fibers begins, but will not be complete until many years later. The fetus is active, kicking, sucking, and sleeping. The heartbeat is readily audible. The intestines work. The fetus is 16 to 18 cm long and weighs 300 g.

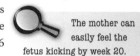

> The mother can easily feel the fetus kicking by week 20.

24 weeks: Fat begins to accumulate under the skin. Fetal activity slows as higher regions of the brain form, quieting fetal reflexes in response to random stimuli. The eyes are complete. The fetus is 23 cm long and weighs 600 g.

28 weeks: Fetal activity increases again as the brain develops. Growth slows, and fat forms beneath the skin. Fingernails appear. The eyes open, close, and respond to light. Surfactant begins to form in the lungs, allowing them to expand without collapsing. The fetus is viable, capable of breathing. The fetus is 27 cm long and weighs 1100 g.

32 weeks: The fetus responds to external sounds. Testes descend into the scrotum. The fetus looks smooth and chubby, and should be in a head-down position for delivery. The brain is 25% of its adult weight. The fetus is 31 cm long and weighs 1800 to 2100 g.

36 weeks: The fetus adds 50% of its birth weight in the last month. Growth slows and the brain becomes more convoluted, although the cerebral cortex does not yet influence volitional behavior. Lanugo hair disappears.

By 40 weeks: The fetus has smooth skin, moderate to profuse hair on its head, and lanugo hair on the shoulders only. **Myelination** of the brain begins. The fetus is 45 to 50 cm long and weighs about 3200 g. An average newborn weighs 3.2 kg (7 lb) and is 50 cm long (19.5 in).

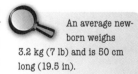

> An average newborn weighs 3.2 kg (7 lb) and is 50 cm long (19.5 in).

SOURCE

Perry, S. E., Wilson, D., Hockenberry, M. J., & Lowdermilk, D. L. (2005). *Maternal child nursing care.* New York: Elsevier Health Sciences.

- Infertility is the inability to conceive after 1 year of trying when the female is under 35 and 6 months when the female is over 35.
- Cause of infertility in males include environmental agents, problems with sperm production or transport, low sperm count and motility.
- Causes of infertility in females include problems with the production and transport of ova, endometriosis, and infections.
- Infertility can cause stress and a sense of loss and inadequacy in a relationship.

14

Infertility

TERMS
- ☐ Epididymis
- ☐ Erectile dysfunction
- ☐ Follicle-stimulating hormone (FSH)
- ☐ Infertility
- ☐ Luteinizing hormone (LH)
- ☐ Pelvic inflammatory disease (PID)

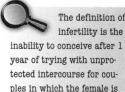

For nonprofessionals, **infertility** probably means an inability to have children. Unfortunately, it is not that simple. A couple may easily conceive their first child, yet have difficulty conceiving again. Members of a couple who had conceived with previous partners may not be able to conceive together. Estimates are that about one in six U.S. couples meet the criteria for infertility. The definition of infertility is the inability to conceive after 1 year of trying with unprotected intercourse for couples in which the female is younger than age 35 and after 6 months of trying for couples in which the female is older than age 35. **Table 14-1** presents the myths and facts about infertility.

> The definition of infertility is the inability to conceive after 1 year of trying with unprotected intercourse for couples in which the female is younger than age 35 and after 6 months of trying for couples in which the female is older than age 35.

CAUSES OF INFERTILITY

The causes of infertility can be traced to either the man or the woman (**Table 14-2**). In approximately 30% of cases, the cause is attributed to the female; in 30% of cases, the cause is attributed to the male; in 30% of cases, the cause is attributed to both; and in 10% of cases, the cause is never determined.

Possible Causes of Male Infertility

Fertility specialists have concluded that male infertility has increased in the last 50 years (especially in Western countries) and have turned their suspicions to a wide range of causes.

- **Environment:** Environmental pollutants such as polychlorinated biphenyls (PCBs) and the pesticide DDT may be partly responsible for reduced male fertility. Other environmental agents such as nicotine, alcohol, marijuana, and stress are also associated with a lowered sperm count and defective sperm.
- **Sperm production:** Endocrine disorders can upset the production and balance of key hormones, such as testosterone, estrogen, **luteinizing hormone (LH)**, and **follicle-stimulating hormone (FSH)**, thereby compromising the production of sperm. Varicoceles is a condition in which valves in the veins that carry blood away from the testicles do not function

Table 14-1 Myths and Facts About Infertility

Myth	Fact
Infertility is a woman's problem.	Infertility is a female problem in 30% of the cases, a male problem in 30% of the cases, a shared problem in 30% of the cases, and unexplained in 10% of the cases.
Fertilization is not really a problem.	More than 5 million people of childbearing age in the United States experience infertility.
Fertilization is more of a mental than a physical problem.	Infertility is a disease or disorder of the reproductive system. Psychological factors may be responsible, but only in a small number of cases.
The couple is doing something wrong.	Infertility is a medical condition, not a sexual disorder.

Table 14-2 Male- and Female-Related Infertility Problems

Male	Female
Environmental	Ovulation problems
Sperm count	Tubal blockage
Sperm interactions	Endometriosis
Infections	IUDs
Varicocele	Voluntary
Structural	Other
Voluntary	

properly. As a result, blood pools around the testicles and generates extra heat near the sperm production centers, reducing the number of sperm.

- **Sperm transport:** Approximately 10% of male infertility is due to difficulties in the sperm transport system—that is, from the testes through the **epididymis**. The passage of sperm can be blocked by scarring from previous infections, such as sexually transmitted diseases (STDs) and mumps. Surgery is typically required to remove the blockage.

> ☑ Endocrine disorders can upset the production and balance of key hormones, such as testosterone, estrogen, **luteinizing hormone (LH)**, and **follicle-stimulating hormone (FSH)**, thereby compromising the production of sperm.

- **Sperm count:** Low sperm count alone (less than 20 million sperm/mL) is *not* a cause of infertility. Many men with a low sperm count father children, although it may take a longer time. On rare occasions, a man's semen may lack sperm because of a congenital problem with the testes, or even because of an injury to the testes. Infections can also cause this condition.
- **Sperm morphology and motility:** Once a man's sperm has been judged to be healthy, attention focuses on what happens to the sperm once they enter the vagina. Indeed, any aberration in sperm capacitation, motility, and the acrosome reaction will compromise male fertility (see Chapter 12). For example, are there any antibodies present in the cervical mucus that attack the sperm before or while it undergoes capacitation? Do the sperm penetrate the cervical mucus? Does the head of the sperm (the acrosome) possess the necessary enzymes that would permit the sperm to penetrate the outer membrane of the egg? What is the nature of the sperm motility?
- **Voluntary infertility:** Estimates are that 500,000 vasectomies are performed each year in the United States. The resulting sterility is generally permanent owing to the difficulty of reversing the procedure.
- **Other causes:** Other male problems include premature ejaculation, retrograde ejaculation, impotence, and an inability to sustain an erection, known as **erectile dysfunction**.

Possible Causes of Female Infertility

When a woman is unable to conceive, the initial search for causes usually turns to the timing and functioning of her menstrual cycle.

- **Production of ova:** Polycystic ovary syndrome is an endocrine disorder in which the ovaries overproduce androgens (e.g., testosterone) as a result of overproduction of luteinizing hormone by the pituitary gland. When LH and FSH are not secreted in the proper proportions, mature eggs may not form. Insulin also plays a role. Higher-than-average insulin levels promote the production of androgens by the ovaries, and even more so in ovaries that are particularly sensitive to insulin, such as in women who are obese. Also, scarring from previous surgery for ovarian cysts and/or the effects of radiation treatment may damage the ovary, resulting in diminished egg production.

> Polycystic ovary syndrome is an endocrine disorder in which the ovaries overproduce androgens (e.g., testosterone) as a result of overproduction of luteinizing hormone by the pituitary gland.

- **Transport of ova:** The fallopian tubes, which ensnare eggs when they are released from the ovary, and through which ova travel to the uterus, may be blocked. If blockage occurs, sperm cannot travel through the tube to meet and fertilize the egg. Such a blockage can be caused by scar tissue resulting from previous surgery, such as to the bowel or bladder, and/or from STDs. For example, chlamydia is usually a silent infection that may lurk in a woman's pelvic organs. STDs can lead to **pelvic inflammatory disease (PID)**, which can cause infertility. Approximately 30% of infertility problems in women are attributed to tubal blockage.
- **Endometriosis:** Approximately 15% of all women have endometriosis, a condition in which endometrial tissue grows outside of the uterus (most often in the pelvis), leading to pain and scarring. When the tissue grows along the ovaries and fallopian tubes, the scarring interferes with their functioning. This problem is a major cause of infertility in women.
- **Intrauterine devices (IUDs):** Although discredited because of the hazards they introduce, especially the risk of infection, these conraceptive devices still are responsible for some problems seen today.
- **Voluntary infertility:** For women, sterilization takes the form of blocking or cutting the fallopian tubes to prevent passage of the egg to the uterus.
- **Other causes:** Normally, the thick cervical mucus thins in response to an increase in estradiol levels during the follicular phase of the menstrual cycle, making it easier for sperm to penetrate. If the cervical mucus is too thick or contains antibodies that attack the sperm, then fertilization is impossible. The uterus, including its shape, condition, and susceptibility to fibroids (benign tumors), can occasionally cause fertility problems.

IMPLICATIONS FOR HEALTHCARE PROVIDERS

Determining the causes of infertility requires time, effort, and careful examination by a fertility specialist. The first step is always a thorough health history and assessment for both the man and the woman, including but certainly not limited to reproductive and sexual health. Relevant questions would address how long the couple has been trying to conceive; if either has conceived children previously; use of tobacco, alcohol, recreational drugs, and medications; past injuries and illnesses; and so on. Many other health issues and lifestyle behaviors may contribute to infertility, both individually and in combination.

For many couples, dealing with infertility can cause significant emotional stress. Some may not want to discuss it outside of their relationship, as the response of family and friends may cause further distress rather than being helpful. The following suggestions may help your patients:

- Become well informed about infertility and normal responses to it.
- Allow patients to be angry and sad.
- Recognize that both members of the couple will respond differently.
- Encourage patients to reach out to friends, family, and support groups. Let them know what the patients need—and don't need.
- Improve communication within the couple relationship. The couple should not let infertility take over their lives.

SOURCES

MedlinePlus. (2008). *Infertility.* Retrieved March 13, 2008, from www.nlm.nih.gov/medlineplus/infertility.html

Perry, S. E., Wilson, D., Hockenberry, M. J., & Lowdermilk, D. L. (2005). *Maternal child nursing care.* New York: Elsevier Health Sciences.

- Assisted reproductive technology (ART) is an option for couples who are unable to conceive naturally.
- Sperm donation occurs when male sperm is artificially introduced into a woman's cervical canal. The sperm may be that of her partner or of a donor.
- Egg donation occurs when female ova are harvested from either a woman or a donor, and introduced to sperm in a specialized solution in a laboratory; the fertilized egg is then implanted into the woman's uterine lining.
- In vitro fertilization occurs by introducing sperm to ova in a specialized solution in a laboratory; the fertilized egg is then implanted into the woman's uterine lining.

15

Assisted Reproductive Techniques

TERMS
- ☐ Assisted reproductive technology (ART)
- ☐ Egg donation
- ☐ In vitro fertilization (IVF)
- ☐ Sperm donation

71

Although there is about a 90% chance of diagnosing the causes of infertility, the problem cannot always be corrected. Before seeking any **assisted reproductive technology (ART)**, couples need thoughtful analysis, extensive research, and considerable caution. **Figure 15-1** illustrates several assisted reproductive techniques.

COMMON ART PROCEDURES

Sperm Donation

When a couple determines that the problem is related to sperm, they have several choices, including **sperm donation**.

- **Artificial insemination by partner (AIP):** AIP is when a woman is inseminated with her partner's sperm. Sperm is introduced into the cervical canal or uterus, thereby avoiding any potential problems with vaginal fluids.

> ✓ AIP is when a woman is inseminated with her partner's sperm. Sperm is introduced into the cervical canal or uterus, thereby avoiding any potential problems with vaginal fluids.

- **Donor insemination:** Artificial insemination by donor sperm, or donor insemination, is used more frequently than AIP when the partner's sperm count is low, when the male partner is sterile, or when there is a background of genetic disorders, or Rh incompatibility.
- **Sperm banks:** The appeal of this technique lies in the screening processes used, which are intended to reduce the risk of sexually transmitted diseases (STDs). In 1985, mandatory screening of donors for the human immunodeficiency virus (HIV) and freezing and quarantining of semen became required (CDC, 1985), resulting in virtually no women being infected with donated semen. A 2007 study looked at 160 couples who chose sperm washing prior to artificial insemination because the male was HIV positive and the female was not: none of the women became infected with HIV (Savasi et al., 2007).

The donor's traits are carefully recorded, because most couples want to match the male partner's characteristics as closely as possible. Donors typically receive a fee of about $100

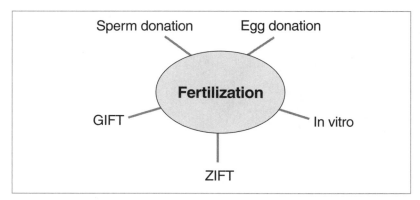

Figure 15-1 Fertilization

and are not told about the use of their sperm. They must also waive all parental rights to any children conceived with their sperm.

In Vitro Fertilization

In vitro fertilization (IVF) is a more commonly known fertilization technique. The steps in IVF are as follows:

1. The woman is usually treated with hormones to stimulate maturation of eggs in the ovary, and she is observed closely to determine the timing of ovulation (i.e., the time at which the egg leaves the surface of the ovary).
2. The physician makes an incision in the abdomen and inserts a laparoscope (a thin tubular lens through which the physician can see the ovary) to remove mature eggs.
3. The egg is placed in a solution containing blood serum and nutrients.
4. Capacitation—a process in which a layer surrounding the sperm is removed so that the sperm may penetrate the egg—takes place.
5. Sperm are added to the solution and fertilization occurs.
6. The fertilized egg is transferred to a fresh supporting solution.
7. Fertilized eggs (usually three) are inserted into the uterus.
8. The fertilized egg is implanted in the uterine lining.

During the IVF process, the woman is treated with hormones to prepare her body to receive the fertilized egg. Approximately 27,000 IVF procedures are done every year in the United States, with an estimated success rate of 20% (Marrs, Bloch, & Silverman, 1998).

Egg Donation

If a woman is unable to produce an egg, **egg donation** may be used for IVF. Donor eggs are not widely available, however, and usually come from relatives or IVF patients who donate their extra eggs. This practice in itself may be a problem because many women using IVF techniques are older, raising the possibility of chromosomal disorders in their egg cells. Also, a woman who is having difficulty with egg production may not have a particularly receptive uterine lining.

Timing is critical with egg donation techniques because uterine development must precisely match the ovarian cycle and ovulation for implantation to occur. The difficulty is increased when two women are involved. To solve the timing problem, the donor woman receives drug treatment to slow her ovulation time in an attempt to match the development of the uterine lining of the woman who is receiving the donor egg. When the match seems ideal, ovulation is triggered in the donor and her eggs are harvested, fertilized with the male partner's sperm, and inserted into the receiving woman's uterus.

Other ARTs

Many new forms of ART are now available (**Table 15-1**). Consequently, today a child may have as many as five parents: a sperm donor (father or other male), an egg donor (mother or other female), a surrogate mother, and the couple who raise the child. These new techniques raise critical legal and ethical issues.

Table 15-1 New Forms of ART

Name	Meaning
Gamete intrafallopian transfer (GIFT)	Sperm and egg are placed in the fallopian tube, a more natural environment for fertilization.
Zygote intrafallopian transfer (ZIFT)	The fertilized egg is transferred to the fallopian tube.
Cryopreservation	Embryos are frozen for future use.
Surrogacy	One woman carries another woman's embryo to term.

IMPLICATIONS FOR HEALTHCARE PROVIDERS

Couples who turn to ART usually have been diagnosed with one or more of the fertility problems discussed in Chapter 14 and typically are experiencing emotional turmoil. When working with these individuals, encourage them to learn as much as possible about their infertility problem to help them feel they have input into the process. Be alert for any signs of blame or guilt, and urge both partners to discuss problematic matters with you, thus helping them to maintain a positive relationship. Above all, impress on both partners the importance of not letting the infertility crisis take over their lives. Keep in mind that the time may come when you feel the necessity of recommending professional counseling (Marrs et al., 1997).

SOURCES

Centers for Disease Control and Prevention. (1985). Testing donors of organs, tissues, and semen for antibody to human T-lymphotropic virus type III/lymphadenopathy-associated virus. *Morbidity and Mortality Weekly Review, 34,* 294.

Marrs, R., Bloch, L. S., & Silverman, K. K. (1998). *Dr. Richard Marrs' fertility book: America's leading infertility expert tells you everything you need to know about getting pregnant.* New York: Dell.

Perry, S. E., Wilson, D., Hockenberry, M. J., & Lowdermilk, D. L. (2005). *Maternal child nursing care.* New York: Elsevier Health Sciences.

Savasi, V., Ferrazzi, E., Lanzani, C., Oneta, M., Parrilla, B., & Persico, T. (2007). Safety of sperm washing and ART oucome in 741 HIV-1-serodiscordant couples. *Human Reproduction, 22*(3), 772–777.

- The Human Genome Project occurred from 1990 to 2003. A "rough draft" of the human genome was announced in 2000.
- The goals included identifying all human genes in DNA and addressing ethical, legal, and social issues that would arise.
- Humans may have 20,000 to 30,000 genes.
- In the foreseeable future, diseases such as diabetes may be treated and even cured using gene therapy.

16

The Human Genome Project

TERMS
☐ Genome
☐ Human Genome Project (HGP)

HOW THE HUMAN GENOME PROJECT BEGAN

The **Human Genome Project (HGP)** was a 13-year-old project (1990–2003) coordinated by the US Department of Energy, the National Institutes of Health, and eventually the Wellcome Trust (UK) as well. Two gatherings of America's top biologists in the 1980s are credited as the forerunners of the HGP. In 1985, a group of scientists met at the University of California, Santa Cruz to discuss the possibility of mapping the human genome. A **genome** is all the genetic material in a human chromosome. Most of the participants at this meeting were sure it *could* be done, but were skeptical that it *should* be done because of the enormous expense. Given the widespread benefits that would come from the project, however, almost all of the scientists present agreed that it deserved continued consideration.

> A **genome** is all the genetic material in a human chromosome.

In March 1986, a meeting of international scientists took place in Santa Fe, New Mexico. This meeting is considered to be the actual beginning of the HGP. The National Institutes of Health (NIH), with the assistance of the Department of Energy (DOE), assumed leadership of the project.

GOALS OF THE HUMAN GENOME PROJECT

The goals of the HGP were:

- Identify all of the genes in human DNA
- Determine the sequences of the 3 billion chemical base pairs (A, T, C, G) that make up human DNA
- Store this information in databases
- Improve tools for data analysis
- Transfer related technologies to the private sector
- Address the ethical, legal, and social issues (ELSI) that may arise from the project

Initially, it had been estimated that there could be 50,000 to 100,000 human protein coding genes, and it would take many more than 13 years to map them. In 2003, a final draft of the completed map was announced, and in 2004, after further analysis, the estimated number of genes was lowered to 20,000 to 30,000. Different methods of counting genes, and different measures for when a gene stops and starts, account for some of the uncertainty of the exact number. In 2006, further refinements to the data were made, and will likely continue as research on the genes and chromosomes continues. Nevertheless, the surprisingly low number of genes for such a complex species has shocked scientists (the simple roundworm has 20,000 genes in its DNA). More recent research suggests that the differences between species may rest not with the numbers of genes in DNA, but how the sequences in those genes are arranged; differences in RNA may vary more among species than DNA.

ACCOMPLISHMENTS TO DATE

The following are some of the findings from the HGP:

- The average gene consists of 3000 bases, but sizes vary greatly—the largest known human gene is dystrophin at 2.4 million bases.
- The order of almost all (99.9%) nucleotides is exactly the same in all humans.

- There are about 1.4 million locations where single-base DNA differences (SNPs) occur in humans. This will help in finding chromosomal locations for disease-associated sequences and tracing human history.
- The functions are unknown for over 50% of discovered genes.
- Less than 2% of the genome encodes for the production of proteins.
- Repetitive sequences that do not code for proteins ("junk DNA") make up at least 50% of the human genome.
- Chromosome 1 has the most genes (2968), and the Y chromosome has the fewest (231).

There is much more that we do not know: exact gene number, locations, and functions; how genes are regulated; the organization of DNA sequences; the structure and organization of chromosomes; and so on. Of great interest from a healthcare perspective is the correlation of single-base DNA variations (SNPs) among individuals with disease; disease-susceptibility based on gene sequence variation; and the genes involved in complex traits and multigene diseases. Genetic research has major implications for treating such common diseases as cardiovascular disease, diabetes, and arthritis.

The 2006 Nobel Prize in medicine was awarded to two US researches, Drs. Craig Mello and Andrew Fire, who found that short snippets of RNA in the nematode worm can silence the expression of targeted genes—a phenomenon referred to as RNA interference. In the future, it may become possible to silence genes that are responsible for diabetes and other diseases in humans. Rapid progress in genome science and a glimpse into its potential applications have prompted some experts to predict that sales of DNA-based product and technologies will exceed $45 billion by 2009.

Despite these successes, the difficulty of the task that remains cannot be discounted. Although hundreds of diseases are caused by a single gene, the genetic contributions are much more obscure for thousands of others. For example, some diseases (e.g., diabetes) need an environmental trigger, whereas for other diseases more than one gene may have to be faulty.

Studies of genetic susceptibility will undoubtedly follow the same pattern. The genes that render people susceptible to certain diseases do not, by themselves, cause disease. Rather, the combination of a particular environmental factor with a particular gene is needed. Once the mechanisms that cause a susceptibility gene to spring into action are more fully understood, such preventive measures as screening techniques and drug therapy will save many lives.

IMPLICATIONS FOR HEALTHCARE PROVIDERS

Several ethical, legal, and social issues (ELSI) demand your attention. Unfortunately, this explosion of knowledge is also leading to uncertain, even dangerous, consequences. For example, if a family member is susceptible to a particular disease, do insurance companies have the legal right to deny this person, and perhaps the entire family, health insurance? How private or public is a person's medical history? Grappling with this and similar issues has led to the creation of a program for studying the ethical, legal, and social implications of the HGP—the ELSI program.

SOURCES

Human Genome Project. (2007). *Human Genome Project information*. Retrieved March 13, 2008, from www.ornl.gov/sci/techresources/Human_Genome/home.shtml

Venter, J. C., et al. (2001). The sequence of the human genome. *Science, 291*(5507), 1304–1351.

QUICK LOOK AT THE CHAPTER AHEAD

- A genetic disease is caused by abnormalities in an individual's genetic material (genome).
- There are four different types of genetic disorders: (1) single-gene, (2) multifactorial, (3) chromosomal, and (4) mitochondrial.
- Sickle cell anemia is an example of a single-gene disorder.
- Spina bifida is an example of a multifactorial genetic disorder.
- Down syndrome is an example of a chromosomal genetic disorder.
- Mitochondrial genetic disorders are rare, and can cause multiple life threatening deficits.

17

Genetic Disorders

TERMS
- ☐ Barth's syndrome
- ☐ Cystic fibrosis (CF)
- ☐ Down syndrome
- ☐ Fragile X syndrome
- ☐ Genetic disorder
- ☐ Hemophilia
- ☐ Phenylketonuria (PKU)
- ☐ Sex-linked disorders
- ☐ Sickle-cell anemia
- ☐ Spina bifida
- ☐ Tay-Sachs disease
- ☐ Turner syndrome

Genes reproduce themselves, but as cells divide, the genes do not remain identical. Specialization occurs, so that different kinds of cells are formed at different locations. In the process, mistakes sometimes happen, leading to defects and disorders that affect normal function (**Figure 17-1**). A **genetic disorder** is a disease caused by abnormalities in an individual's genetic material (genome). Four types of genetic disorders are distinguished: (1) single gene, (2) multifactorial, (3) chromosomal, and (4) mitochondrial.

A **genetic disorder** is a disease caused by abnormalities in an individual's genetic material (genome). Four types of genetic disorders are distinguished: (1) single gene, (2) multifactorial, (3) chromosomal, and (4) mitochondrial.

According to the Centers for Disease Control and Prevention (CDC; Kung, Hoyert, Xu, & Murphy, 2007), the three leading causes of infant mortality—congenital malformations, disorders related to short gestation and low birthweight, and sudden infant death syndrome—accounted for approximately 43% of all infant deaths in the United States.

SINGLE-GENE GENETIC DISORDERS

Single-gene disorders are caused by changes or mutations that occur in the DNA sequence of one recessive gene. Two carriers of a recessive gene have a one in four chance of passing on the disorder to their child.

This section discusses the incidence and characteristics of some single-gene disorders that are inherited. Certain disorders, such as Tay-Sachs disease and sickle-cell anemia, are found among specific populations because of intermarriage.

According to the Centers for Disease Control and Prevention (CDC), in 2002 the primary cause of infant deaths was congenital malformations, deformations, and chromosomal abnormalities. These errors accounted for 5630 infant deaths.

Tay-Sachs Disease

Jews of Eastern European origin are struck hardest by **Tay-Sachs disease**, which causes death by the age of 4 or 5 years. At birth, the afflicted children appear normal, but development slows by the age of 6 months, and mental and motor deterioration begin. Approximately 1 in every 25 to 30 Jews of Eastern European origin carries the defective gene, which is recessive—increasing the likelihood of passing on the disorder. Tay-Sachs disease occurs when a gene fails to produce an enzyme that breaks down fatty materials in the brain and nervous system. As a result, fat accumulates and destroys nerve cells, causing loss of coordination, blindness, and finally death.

Two carriers of a recessive gene have a one in four chance of passing on the disorder to their child.

Sickle-Cell Anemia

Sickle-cell anemia mainly affects people of African descent. It appeared thousands of years ago in equatorial Africa, and increased resistance to malaria among carriers of the defective gene. Estimates are that 10% of the African American population in the United States carry the sickle-cell trait. In patients with sickle-cell anemia, the red blood cells are distorted and angular, not round. Because of the cells' shape, they encounter difficulty in passing through the blood vessels.

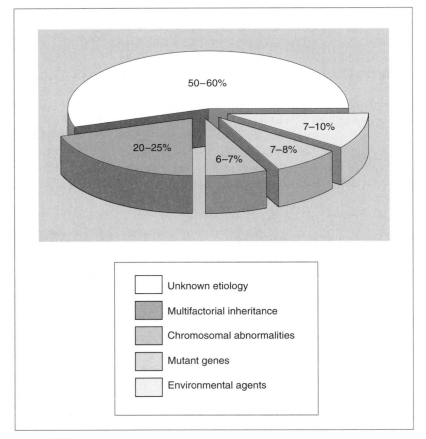

Figure 17-1 Sources of Genetic Defects

The cells tend to pile up and clump, producing oxygen starvation accompanied by considerable pain. The body then acts to eliminate these cells, and anemia results.

Cystic Fibrosis

In the population of the United States, **cystic fibrosis (CF)** is the most severe genetic disease of childhood, affecting about one in 1200 children; one in 30 individuals is a carrier. The disease causes a malfunction of the exocrine glands—the glands that secrete tears, sweat, mucus, and saliva. Breathing and digestion are difficult because of the thickness of the mucus. The secreted sweat is extremely salty, often producing heat exhaustion. Although CF has killed more children than any other genetic disease, the CF gene now has been identified, and new research offers hope concerning the detection of carriers.

Phenylketonuria

Phenylketonuria (PKU) results from the body's failure to break down the amino acid phenylalanine, which then accumulates, affects the nervous system, and causes mental retardation. Most states now require infants to be tested for PKU at birth. If phenylalanine is present in the blood, the infants are placed on a special diet that has been remarkably successful in preventing the disease.

However, this success has produced other problems. Women who were treated successfully as infants may give birth to children with mental retardation because of a toxic uterine environment. Thus, at the first sign of pregnancy, these women must return to a special diet. The person cured of phenylketonuria still carries the faulty genes.

Sex-Linked Disorders

Sex-linked disorders occur because of what is known as sex-linked inheritance. The X chromosome is substantially larger than the Y chromosome, and the female carries more genes on the 23rd chromosome than does the male. This difference helps to explain sex linkage. Think back to the difference between dominant gene and recessive traits. If a dominant gene and a recessive gene appear together, the dominant trait is expressed. An individual must have two recessive genes for the recessive trait (e.g., blue eyes) to appear. On the 23rd set of chromosomes, however, nothing on the Y chromosome offsets any negative effects of a gene on the X chromosome.

Perhaps the most widely known of the sex-linked disorders is **hemophilia**, a condition in which the blood does not clot properly. Several of the royal families of Europe were particularly prone to this condition.

Another sex-linked trait attributed to the X chromosome is color blindness. The X chromosome contains the gene for color vision. If it is faulty, nothing on the Y chromosome counterbalances the defect.

 ## MULTIFACTORIAL GENETIC DISORDERS

Multifactorial genetic disorders are caused by a combination of environmental factors and mutations in multiple genes. Some of the most common chronic disorders are multifactorial disorders: heart disease, high blood pressure, Alzheimer's disease, arthritis, diabetes, cancer, and obesity.

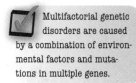
Multifactorial genetic disorders are caused by a combination of environmental factors and mutations in multiple genes.

Spina Bifida

Spina bifida means "cleft spine." This condition is an example of a birth defect likely caused by the interaction of several genes with possible environmental factors, such as insufficient folic acid in the diet of the pregnant mother. The embryo's neural tube does not close, so some of the membrane surrounding the spinal cord protrudes through this opening (meningocele) or some of the spinal cord itself protrudes

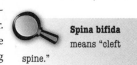
Spina bifida means "cleft spine."

(myelomeningocele), causing varying degrees of mental retardation and paralysis of the lower limbs. Spina bifida affects one in 1000 births, depending on geographic location, and affects whites of European heritage and Hispanics more often than Asians and Africans. Usually, there is no family history.

CHROMOSOMAL DISORDERS

Because chromosomes are carriers of genetic material, chromosomal abnormalities can result in disease. These diseases can be classified into one of two categories: those caused by abnormalities of number (too many or too few chromosomes) and those caused by abnormalities of structure.

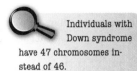
Individuals with Down syndrome have 47 chromosomes instead of 46.

Down Syndrome

An example of abnormality of too many chromosomes is trisomy 21, better known as **Down syndrome**, in which an individual has an extra chromosome, producing a total of 47 chromosomes instead of 46 (**Figure 17-2**). Down syndrome is usually due to a random event that occurs during

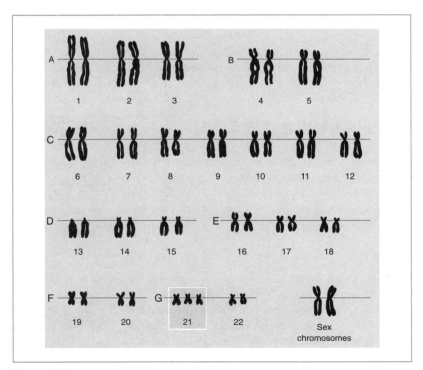

Figure 17-2 Down Syndrome (3 chromosomes in group 21)

formation of the reproductive cells (i.e., the ovum or the sperm); however, the vast majority of cases are attributed to abnormalities in the ovum, as the incidence of the syndrome is associated with increased maternal age. Chances of giving birth to a child with Down syndrome are about 1 in 750 births if the mother is between ages 30 and 35; 1 in 300 if the mother is between ages 35 and 39; and 1 in 80 if the mother is between ages 40 and 45. After age 45, the incidence jumps to 1 in 40 births.

Down syndrome, which was identified in 1866 by British physician Langdon Down, produces distinctive facial features, small hands and oral cavity, and varying degrees of mental retardation. People with Down syndrome are at higher risk for leukemia, heart and thyroid disorders, and early dementia.

Turner Syndrome

Turner syndrome is an abnormality of too few chromosomes. Females have an XO pattern, instead of XX, as a result of 45 chromosomes instead of 46. Turner syndrome occurs in 1 of every 2500 births, and is characterized by short stature, poorly developed secondary sex characteristics, and usually sterility.

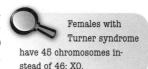
Females with Turner syndrome have 45 chromosomes instead of 46: XO.

Fragile X Syndrome

An example of abnormality of structure is **fragile X syndrome**. In 1991, scientists discovered the gene (called *FMR1* for "Fragile X Mental Retardation–1") that causes this condition. *FMR1* is located on the long arm of the X chromosome in a region of DNA that varies in length from one person to another. In some people, it is longer than usual, called a premutation. With each generation, the DNA lengthens, finally expanding to a critical length, switching off the gene so that it does not produce the protein that it normally makes.

Fragile X syndrome is the most common inherited cause of mental impairment. About 1 in 259 women carry the fragile X gene and could pass it to their children, both male and female. About 1 in 800 men carry this gene; their daughters will also be carriers, but their sons will not be. Fragile X syndrome affects 1 in 4000 males and 1 in 6000 females of all races and ethnic groups.

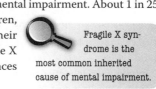
Fragile X syndrome is the most common inherited cause of mental impairment.

MITOCHONDRIAL GENETIC DISORDERS

Mitochondria are responsible for processing oxygen and converting substances from the foods we eat into energy—adenosine triphosphate (ATP)—for essential cell functions. As mitochondria have their own DNA (mtDNA), which is different from nuclear DNA, mitochondrial disorders are like an energy crisis, meaning that the cells cannot function normally. Not only is ATP not produced, but the by-products of inefficient energy conversion also become free radicals. These free radicals act like a poison inside the body, further damaging the mitochondria and, therefore, the organ systems.

More than 200 mitochondrial disorders have been identified to date. For example, **Barth's syndrome** in infants is characterized by skeletal myopathy, cardiomyopathy, short stature, and neutropenia. About one in 4000 children in the United States will develop mitochondrial disease by the age of 10 years.

IMPLICATIONS FOR HEALTHCARE PROVIDERS

There are several risk factors to keep in mind in your clinical work:

- **Advanced parental age:** Maternal age older than 35 and paternal age older than 50 are associated with an increased risk for chromosomal abnormalities.
- **History of miscarriages or stillbirths:** Couples who have experienced three or more miscarriages may carry a chromosomal problem that predisposes them to miscarriage and chromosomal abnormalities.
- **Previous children with birth defects, mental retardation, growth retardation, or neurological problems:** Any of these conditions may be an isolated event or an indicator of chromosomal or genetic disorders.
- **Family history of birth defects:** A carefully researched family history is important. Some couples worry needlessly about the possibility of a disorder arising; others ignore potential problems because of inadequate information.
- **Exposure to medications, radiation, or toxic chemicals:** Exposure to any teratogenic agent should raise concern about the chances of random abnormalities occurring.
- **Ethnic background:** Certain groups are more susceptible to specific genetic disorders.

SOURCES

Human Genome Project. (2007). *Human Genome Project information.* Retrieved March 13, 2008, from www.ornl.gov/sci/techresources/Human_Genome/home.shtml

March of Dimes. (2008). *Professionals and researchers.* Retrieved March 13, 2008, from www.marchofdimes.com/professionals/14332_1209.asp

MedlinePlus. (2008). *Genetic disorders.* Retrieved March 13, 2008, from www.nlm.nih.gov/medlineplus/geneticdisorders.html

National Institutes of Health Books. (2007). *Biochemistry.* Retrieved March 13, 2008, from www.ncbi.nlm.nih.gov/books/bv.fcgi?rid=stryer.section.704

- Teratogens are extrauterine agents that cause structural abnormalities in the embryo or fetus.
- Types of teratogens include chemicals (alcohol), maternal diseases and illnesses (rubella and diabetes), and environmental hazards (radiation).
- Fetal alcohol syndrome is a type of retardation that can result from use of alcohol during pregnancy.
- The virus for HIV/AIDS may be transmitted when maternal blood enters the fetal circulation or by mucosal exposure to the virus during labor and delivery.

18

Influences on Prenatal Development

TERMS
- ☐ **Fetal alcohol syndrome**
- ☐ **Teratogens**

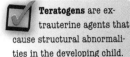

Whatever affects the mother can affect the fetus. **Teratogens** (from *teras*, meaning "monster," and *genesis*, meaning "origin") are extrauterine agents that cause structural abnormalities in the developing child. They include chemical substances, infectious diseases, and environmental hazards to which the mother is exposed during pregnancy. Some chronic health conditions, such as diabetes, are not extrauterine agents, but can nevertheless affect the fetus.

> **Teratogens** are extrauterine agents that cause structural abnormalities in the developing child.

The relationship between the timing of prenatal exposure to a teratogen and fetal development is critical. Exposure from the 3rd to 8th week—when 95% of the major organ systems form—can result in major abnormalities of vital structures, such as arms, legs, heart, and eyes. Later exposure may cause organs to malfunction. Long-term exposure (e.g., to alcohol) is most devastating of all. The effects are usually both irreversible and preventable.

CHEMICAL SUBSTANCES

Alcohol interferes with fetal cell division and growth throughout pregnancy. During the third trimester in particular, alcohol adversely alters development of the central nervous system (CNS) and brain. **Fetal alcohol syndrome** is characterized by retarded growth before and after birth; unusual facial features, such as a small head, flat philtrum (no depression between the nose and upper lip), and small widely spaced eyes; and structural abnormalities of the palate, heart, kidneys, and bladder. The most striking deficit is impaired intellectual capacity, especially mental retardation, which is often accompanied by seizures. Withdrawal from alcohol causes tremors, increased muscle tone, and irritability. Fetal alcohol syndrome is found in approximately 40% of infants born to alcoholics. There is no known minimum amount of alcohol that can be safely consumed during pregnancy. Women are best advised to abstain from alcohol if they are trying to become pregnant, and during pregnancy.

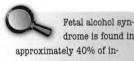

> Fetal alcohol syndrome is found in approximately 40% of infants born to alcoholics.

Cocaine increases maternal and fetal heart rates and blood pressures, decreases blood flow to the fetus, and causes uterine contractions. Complications of cocaine use during pregnancy may include fetal death, spontaneous abortion, premature birth, infants small for gestational age (SGA), and ventricular hemorrhage (bleeding into the brain). Infants also experience abnormalities of the genitourinary system and neurological irritability, such as disturbed wake–sleep cycles, increased muscle tone, difficulty being soothed, and learning disabilities.

Smoking decreases blood flow to the placenta, constricts blood vessels in the uterus, and interferes with maternal absorption of vitamins and calcium. Mothers who smoke—especially older mothers—have a higher incidence of premature birth and placenta previa (separation of the placenta from the uterine wall). Their full-term infants are also more likely to have lower birth weights.

There is no known minimum amount of alcohol that can be safely consumed during pregnancy. Women are best advised to abstain from alcohol if they are trying to become pregnant, and during pregnancy.

Medications that pregnant women use, both prescribed and over-the-counter, are also chemical substances (**Figure 18-1**). Women should consult with their health care provider regarding any medications they may take during pregnancy.

Women should consult with their health care provider regarding any medications they may take during pregnancy.

Medication (Use)	Effects on Fetus and Neonate
Benefit outweighs risk	
Aspirin (pain)	Malformations of the CNS, bones, and internal organs
Insulin (diabetes mellitus)	Malformation of the sacrum (lower spine)
Isoniazid (tuberculosis)	Increase of anomalies
Glucocorticoids, e.g., prednisone (anti-inflammatory)	Cleft palate, cardiac defects
Penicillin (infections)	No known adverse effect
Benefit versus risk uncertain	
Lithium (bipolar disorder)	Cleft palate, anomalies of the eye, goiter
Cytotoxic drugs (cancer) trimethoprim-sulfamethoxazole	Increase of anomalies
Sulfonamides, e.g., Septra (anti-infective)	Cleft palate
Aminoglycosides, e.g., gentamicin (anti-infective)	8th cranial nerve damage (hearing)
Risk outweighs benefit	
Tetracycline (antibiotic)	Inhibited bone growth, discolored teeth in childhood
Methotrexate (cancer, arthritis)	Multiple anomalies; has been used as an abortive
warfarin (i.e., Coumadin) (blood thinner)	Skeletal and facial anomalies, mental retardation
Iodide (hypothyroidism)	Congenital goiter, mental retardation

Figure 18-1 Prescription Medications During Pregnancy

The use of prescription medications during pregnancy is referred to as a managed risk. The decision to use a medication is made by weighing the benefits to the mother against the risks to the fetus, especially during the first trimester of gestation (see table). The Food and Drug Administration has developed a classification system for all medications (categories A, B, C, D, and X) that can be found in any pharmacology reference book.

INFECTIOUS DISEASES

The most common diseases that are potentially harmful to the fetus are collectively referred to by the acronym STORCH: syphilis, toxomoplasmosis, rubella, cytomegalovirus, and herpes.

Syphilis is a sexually transmitted disease (STD) that, if left untreated, will result in death for approximately 50% of fetuses during or after the second trimester. Infants who survive may be mentally retarded, blind, or deaf, or all three.

Toxoplasmosis is an infection with a microorganism (*Toxoplasma gondii*) that is transmitted to humans from animals, especially cats. It occurs in 1 or 2 of every 1000 live births. The highest risk to the fetus occurs when the mother contracts the disease in the third trimester, although she may be unaware that she is infected. Consequences may include spontaneous abortion, premature birth, SGA infants, and mental retardation.

Rubella (German measles) affects fewer than one child per 1000 live births. If a mother is infected during the first trimester, rubella can cause deafness, heart defects, and cataracts in her child.

Cytomegalovirus (CMV) belongs to the herpes simplex group. CMV infection affects 12 to 20 of every 1000 newborns. Of those children 5% to 10% have significant neurological complications, including mental retardation and hearing problems. An infected fetus may die in utero or survive with brain damage.

ENVIRONMENTAL HAZARDS

Lead contamination can cause increased rates of spontaneous abortion, fetal death, and premature birth. Infants who survive are more likely to have poor growth and neurological difficulties. Pregnant women should be excluded from working with lead. Exposure in men is associated with a decreased sperm count.

Radiation exposure is a well-known significant risk because it alters fetal cell division and growth. It has been associated with spontaneous abortions, congenital abnormalities, and mental retardation. Fetuses who are exposed are at higher risk for childhood leukemia.

MATERNAL ILLNESS

Diabetes mellitus, especially Type 1, insulin-dependent diabetes mellitus (IDDM), is characterized by increased levels of blood glucose (hyperglycemia), which crosses the placenta from mother to fetus. Maternal hyperglycemia during the 3rd to 6th weeks of gestation results in three to four times the incidence of congenital anomalies, such as heart defects and hydrocephalus. Later during pregnancy, maternal hyperglycemia stimulates insulin production in the fetus to lower the fetus's blood

In areas of the world where breastfeeding is a safer option than formulas made with impure water, women with HIV may need to weigh the risk of transmitting the virus to their infants against the benefits of breastfeeding.

glucose levels. This leads to excessive fetal growth, and infants born large for gestational age who are at risk for acute hypoglycemia after birth.

Acquired immune deficiency syndrome (AIDS) develops in infants whose mothers are infected with the human immunodeficiency virus (HIV). Although the precise mechanisms are unknown, scientists at the National Institutes for Health (NIH) think the virus may be transmitted when maternal blood enters the fetal circulation or by mucosal exposure to the virus during labor and delivery; there is a 10% to 14% chance that HIV will be transmitted through breastfeeding. In areas of the world where breastfeeding is a safer option than formulas made with impure water, women with HIV may need to weigh the risk of transmitting the virus to their infants against the benefits of breastfeeding.

In the first few months of life, infants with prenatal exposure to HIV often are without symptoms; however, they may have positive antibody titers for as long as 18 months, which indicates transfer of maternal antibodies across the placenta. By 15 months, half of these infants will have shed the maternal antibodies and remain without disease. In recent years, 90% of babies who will develop true HIV have been successfully identified by a laboratory technique called polymerase chain reaction (PCR) assay, which detects minute quantities of the virus in an infant's blood.

Many children with HIV infection are slow to reach physical and cognitive milestones, and some develop neurological problems. They are more likely to be SGA, experience failure to thrive, and are vulnerable to bacterial and viral infections.

> Although the precise mechanisms are unknown, scientists at the National Institutes for Health (NIH) think the virus may be transmitted when maternal blood enters the fetal circulation or by mucosal exposure to the virus during labor and delivery; there is a 10% to 14% chance that HIV will be transmitted through breastfeeding.

> In recent years, 90% of babies who will develop true HIV have been successfully identified by a laboratory technique called polymerase chain reaction (PCR) assay, which detects minute quantities of the virus in an infant's blood.

IMPLICATIONS FOR HEALTHCARE PROVIDERS

Education, early screening, and public health initiatives are key to preventing the sequelae of exposure to damaging substances during the prenatal period. The effects can last for a lifetime, and often prove costly economically, psychologically, and socially.

SOURCES

MedlinePlus. (2008). *MedlinePlus.* Retrieved March 13, 2008, from www.nlm.nih.gov/medlineplus

Organization of Teratology Information Specialists. (2008). *Home.* Retrieved March 13, 2008, from http://otispregnancy.org

Perry, S. E., Wilson, D., Hockenberry, M. J., & Lowdermilk, D. L. (2005). *Maternal child nursing care.* New York: Elsevier Health Sciences.

- Prematurity is determined by the relationship between gestation and weight at birth.
- Infants are *premature* if born before 37 weeks, regardless of weight.
- *Low birth weight* refers to infants weighing less than 2500 g at birth even if they are born at term.
- *Very low birth weight* refers to infants weighing less than 1500 g.
- Risk factors for prematurity include maternal age (under age 16 and older than 35); poor health habits; diabetes; problems with the placenta, uterus, or cervix; and disease.
- Complications of prematurity are often derived from the consequences of poor lung function.
- The premature infant looks like an extrauterine fetus, with thin skin, little body fat, and lanugo.
- Long-term outcomes for premature infants depend on multiple factors, but they do have an increased incidence of health and learning problems.

19

Hazards of Prematurity

TERMS
- ☐ **Appropriate for gestational age (AGA)**
- ☐ **Bronchopulmonary dysplasia (BPD)**
- ☐ **Corrected age**
- ☐ **Gestational age**
- ☐ **Lanugo**
- ☐ **Low birth weight (LBW)**
- ☐ **Periventricular–intraventricular hemorrhage (P/IVH)**
- ☐ **Premature**
- ☐ **Respiratory distress syndrome (RDS)**
- ☐ **Small for gestational age (SGA)**
- ☐ **Very low birth weight (VLBW)**

Preterm birth is responsible for almost two-thirds of infant mortality. Those preterm infants who survive are at increased risk for cerebral palsy, mental retardation, and sensory and learning impairments. They also experience more chronic health problems during infancy and childhood. These difficulties have implications for the affected individuals' social, educational, and psychological adaptation.

TERMS USED TO REFER TO PREMATURITY

The average gestational period for the human infant is 40 weeks. The date when the baby's birth is expected is called the estimated date of confinement (EDC). It is calculated by counting backward 3 months from a woman's last menstrual cycle and then adding 7 days. An infant is full term when its birth occurs between 1 week before and 2 weeks after the EDC. The infant weighs 3100 to 3400 g and is about 50 cm long at this point.

According to the World Health Organization, infants are **premature** (or preterm) if they are born before 37 weeks, regardless of their weight. **Low birth weight (LBW)** refers to infants weighing less than 2500 g at birth (5.5 lb), even if they are born at term. **Very low birth weight (VLBW)** refers to infants weighing less than 1500 g (3.3 lb); they are unlikely to be born at term.

Although the terms "premature" and "low birth weight" are often used interchangeably, the actual determination of prematurity is based on the relationship between the child's weight and gestational age (**Table 19-1**). **Gestational age** is determined through neurological and physical assessment between 2 and 8 hours after birth. Identifying the point in fetal development at which the infant was born is critical for anticipating problems in the postnatal period. The **corrected age** of a preterm infant is calculated by adding the postnatal age to the gestational age. Thus an infant who was born at 30 weeks' gestation 2 weeks ago is considered to be at 32 weeks now. However, some neonatologists have come to question this practice.

According to the World Health Organization, infants are **premature** (or preterm) if they are born before 37 weeks, regardless of their weight. **Low birth weight (LBW)** refers to infants weighing less than 2500 g at birth (5.5 lb), even if they are born at term. **Very low birth weight (VLBW)** refers to infants weighing less than 1500 g (3.3 lb); they are unlikely to be born at term.

Premature infants are considered **appropriate for gestational age (AGA)** when their weight at birth is typical for a fetus of the same gestational age. Infants are considered **small for gestational age (SGA)** when their weight is less than would be expected. Premature infants who weigh more at birth typically do better. For example, those weighing more than 2500 g who are born after 37 weeks are more likely to survive with good outcomes than those weighing less than 2000 g who are born at the same gestational age.

The younger and smaller the infant is, the less mature are the major organ systems essential for sustaining life. The key systems are those that allow for exchange of oxygen (lungs, red blood cells), absorption of nutrients (gastrointestinal tract), generation of energy for cell growth (glucose regulation), and autonomic regulation (skin integrity, body temperature, fluid volume, blood pressure, heart rate).

Table 19-1 Classification of Prematurity

Classification	Gestational Age (weeks)	Weight (g)	Characteristics
Borderline premature	36–37	2500–3200	Lanugo on skin; fewer creases on feet; genitalia not fully developed; difficulties with breathing, regulating temperature, and feeding; jaundice; 90% chance for healthy survival
Moderately premature	31–35	1500–2500	Same as borderline premature, only more so; thinner skin; more vascular problems regulating glucose, fluid volume, and red blood cell production; 50% risk for disabilities
Extremely premature	23–30	400–1400	No subcutaneous fat beneath paper-thin skin; eyes possibly fused shut; significant respiratory problems; infants < 1000 g have 70% incidence of brain hemorrhage and serious disabilities; those < 600 g likely die

COMPLICATIONS OF PREMATURITY

While many complications of prematurity are possible, the most critical organ system is the lungs. Surfactant, which begins to form at about 28 weeks' gestation, allows the alveoli to expand so that oxygen and carbon dioxide can be exchanged. Muscles in the chest wall facilitate expansion of the lungs.

Poor gas exchange at the cellular level has cascading consequences for all major organ systems. The combination of decreased oxygen perfusion, acid–base imbalances in metabolism and respiration, and related difficulties with regulation of blood flow can adversely affect the developing brain, the retinas of the eyes, and the intestines; it can also complicate the closure of the patent ductus in the heart. The long-term effects on the child's growth and development vary.

The emergence of **respiratory distress syndrome (RDS)** is related to a child's having immature lungs at birth. Because of poor oxygen exchange, the infant is easily fatigued and at risk for pneumonia. Difficulties regulating breathing and heart rate render the infant more vulnerable to stress, such as that associated with a cold room or handling. While RDS is usually self-limiting and without long-term effects, it can lead to other problems, especially if an infant requires mechanical ventilation.

Bronchopulmonary dysplasia (BPD) is a chronic lung condition that affects infants who are born prior to 28 weeks' gestation and who require mechanical ventilation for RDS, which can overexpand and traumatize underdeveloped lungs. BPD develops when infants depend on oxygen for more than 28 days and beyond 36 weeks' gestational age. A family history of asthma is also a factor. The morbidity and mortality related to BPD depends on several factors: age and weight of the infant at birth, duration of mechanical ventilation, and timing of surfactant administration. Early surfactant administration markedly decreased BPD related to oxygen toxicity in an earlier generation of premature infants. However, as smaller premature infants survive, they remain on mechanical ventilation longer, increasing exposure to pathogens and thus their mortality and morbidity risks. In general, the smaller the infant for gestational age (<32 weeks), the greater the risk.

Survivors of BPD may experience delays in physical growth and cognitive and language development, although by ages 10 to 12 years most children with BPD are developmentally normal. Many require nasal oxygen throughout childhood, which limits their physical activities and requires special arrangements at school. Children with BPD are also at risk for frequent respiratory ailments and asthma.

Periventricular–intraventricular hemorrhage (P/IVH)—bleeding into the ventricles of the brain—is the most common cause of brain damage in premature infants. Its incidence is 40% in infants weighing less than 1500 g at birth, but almost 70% in those weighing less than 1000 g. Almost all cases of P/IVH occur within 4 days of birth, but early-onset P/IVH may occur within 24 hours of birth. The cause of P/IVH lies in the relationship between an immature myocardium and immature autonomic self-regulatory mechanisms, which results in fluctuations in blood flow to and blood pressure in the brain. Respiratory distress, infection, traumatic birth, and maternal hypertension during pregnancy can also be factors.

Outcome for the infant with P/IVH depends on the extent and area of hemorrhage, as well as the presence or lack of posthemorrhage hydrocephalus. Half of infants with extensive P/IVH die; those who survive are often severely disabled. Moderate damage can cause mental retardation and neuromuscular abnormalities, such as cerebral palsy. Those infants with mild P/IVH may manifest more subtle difficulties later in childhood, such as learning or emotional disabilities.

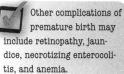
Other complications of premature birth may include retinopathy, jaundice, necrotizing enterocolitis, and anemia.

Other complications of premature birth may include retinopathy, jaundice, necrotizing enterocolitis, and anemia.

CHARACTERISTICS OF PREMATURE INFANTS

A premature infant may look like an extrauterine fetus. The skin is typically thin and almost translucent; it is possible to see veins under the skin. Some features may appear wrinkled owing to the lack of fat deposits beneath the skin. Ear cartilage is soft and flexible. There may be excessive body hair, the **lanugo** that is typically shed late in fetal development. The infant's cry is weak, and he or she may have difficulty feeding because of a poor sucking reflex. The clitoris in the female infant may be enlarged in comparison to other genitalia; the male infant may have a small scrotum that is smooth instead of with ridges. Premature infants have poor thermoregulation, compounded by a lack of physical activity.

GROWTH AND DEVELOPMENT OF PREMATURE INFANTS

The growth pattern of premature infants is adjusted for corrected age (gestational age plus postnatal age) for 2 to 3 years after birth. For example, at 6 months after birth, the corrected age of a preterm infant is 4 months; that is, the infant is expected to exhibit characteristics more typical of a 4-month-old baby. LBW babies are still smaller than average at 3 years, even when corrected age is used. By adolescence, however, most have reached their genetic potential with regard to size.

Head circumference is a good indicator of neurodevelopmental outcome. Growth of the head when accompanied by milestones in neuromotor functioning signifies that the brain is developing after birth. The critical postnatal period for catch-up growth is 6 weeks to 6 months. The smaller the head at birth, the less catch-up growth that is experienced after birth, regardless of weight and gestational age.

In recent years, improvements in medical and nursing care have increased the survival of premature infants. Of babies born at 28 weeks, approximately 80% now survive. Nevertheless, the complications associated with prematurity may have sequelae that continue into childhood or throughout life. As a rule, the more premature an infant and the smaller the birth weight, the greater the risk of complications. It must be stressed, however, that it is impossible to predict the long-term outcome for an individual baby just on the basis of gestational age or birth weight.

IMPLICATIONS FOR PARENTS AND HEALTHCARE PROVIDERS

Figure 19-1 lists risk factors that may contribute to premature birth. Many of these risk factors are preventable. Parenting a premature infant is difficult. Parents must mourn the loss of the healthy child who was not born, while anticipating the loss of the premature infant they have. Some parents may avoid becoming emotionally engaged with their infant in the neonatal intensive care unit. At first, they may focus only on hard data, such as blood gas or bilirubin levels. Later, parents may comment on the infant's behavior, such as yawning.

Figure 19-1 lists risk factors that may contribute to premature birth.

When parents note that the baby is responding to them personally, they begin to claim the child as theirs emotionally. Parents need guidance from nurses and physicians to do so. The behavioral cues of premature infants are more difficult to read than are the cues of the typical newborn. Parents may misinterpret cues or overstimulate the premature baby in an effort to interact with him or her.

It is important to understand how cues between infants and parents work so that you can facilitate the attachment process. Premature infants are at greater risk for neglect and abuse from

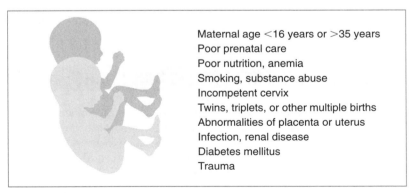

Maternal age <16 years or >35 years
Poor prenatal care
Poor nutrition, anemia
Smoking, substance abuse
Incompetent cervix
Twins, triplets, or other multiple births
Abnormalities of placenta or uterus
Infection, renal disease
Diabetes mellitus
Trauma

Figure 19-1 Risk Factors for Premature Birth

overwhelmed parents when they finally go home. Nurses are in a position to intervene early so as to promote optimal outcomes for these tiny babies.

SOURCES

Bancalari, E. & del Moral, T. (2001) Bronchopulmonary dysplasia and surfactant. *Biology of the Neonate, 80*(Suppl 1), 7–13.

Blanc, A., & Wardlaw, T. (2005). Monitoring low birth weight: An evaluation of international estimates and an updated estimation procedure. *Bulletin of the World Health Organization, 83*, 178–185.

Explaining the 2001–02 infant mortality increase: Data from the linked birth/infant death data set. (2005, January 24). *National Vital Statistics Report, 53*(12).

MedlinePlus. (2008). *MedlinePlus*. Retrieved March 13, 2008, from www.nlm.nih.gov/medlineplus

Osborn, D. A., Evans, N., & Kluckow, M. (2003). Hemodynamic and antecedent risk factors of early and late periventricular/intraventricular hemorrhage in premature infants. *Pediatrics, 112*, 33–39.

World Health Organization. (2008). *Low-birthweight infants*. Retrieved March 13, 2008, from www.who.int/whosis/indicators/2007LBW/en/

QUICK LOOK AT THE CHAPTER AHEAD

- About 2%–4% of children in the United States are adopted; about 127,000 new adoptions each year.
- In closed adoptions, biological parents have no contact with their offspring and adopted children have no knowledge of their backgrounds.
- In open adoptions, there is the option for contact with the biological parents and/or for information about them.
- Discussions with children about being adopted must be developmentally appropriate.

20

Adoption

TERMS
- ☐ Adoption
- ☐ Closed adoption
- ☐ Open adoption

Couples who remain childless despite using assisted reproduction techniques should not feel that they have exhausted all avenues. **Adoption** (to take a child of other parents voluntarily as one's own) remains an attractive option (**Figure 20-1**).

FACTS ABOUT ADOPTION

Approximately 2% to 4% of children in the United States are adopted. Since 1987, the number of adoptions per year in the United States has remained relatively constant, ranging from 118,000 to 127,000; recent data cite 127,000 adoptions in 2001. Government data indicate that in 2001, 39% of adoptions were handled by publicly funded child welfare agencies, and another 46% through private agencies. The latter include adoptions among family members, such as by a stepparent. About 15% of adoptees come from outside the United States. By comparison, in 1992, these figures were 18%, 77%, and 5%, respectively.

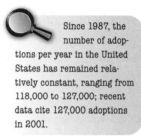

Since 1987, the number of adoptions per year in the United States has remained relatively constant, ranging from 118,000 to 127,000; recent data cite 127,000 adoptions in 2001.

In spite of competition among traditional couples, single adults, older adults, and homosexual adults, more children are available for adoption than is commonly thought. Many of these children fall into special categories: older children, minority children, and children with disabilities. While these children are available for immediate adoption, the waiting period for healthy white infants may be years.

ISSUES FACING ADOPTING PARENTS

Couples thinking about adoption should carefully consider several issues they must address when children reach various ages. Given their personalities, interests, and experiences, they will probably

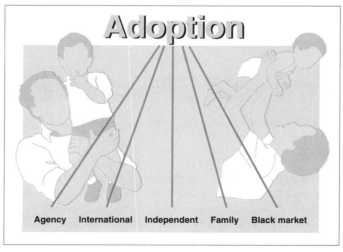

Figure 20-1 Sources of Adopted Children

be more comfortable with the thought of adopting children in one age group than with adopting children in other age groups.

Infants

Infants are the easiest to adopt because they do not have the experiences that older children bring with them. Mother–infant attachment typically proceeds normally.

Preschool Children

Children should learn that they are adopted from their adoptive parents, and not from other sources. Most parents tell children they are adopted when they are around 3 or 4 years old, depending on the child. Parents experience appreciable anxiety during this time, worrying about how and when to tell children. Once children realize they are adopted and understand what that means, the relationship with the adoptive parents inevitably changes, affecting both parents and children. Children, for example, must cope with the idea of being relinquished—not an easy task. Parents must accept the idea that their children will want to know more about their biological parents.

School-Age Children

During the 7- to 12-year period, children with improving cognitive abilities ask certain adoption-related questions: Who are my parents? Where did I come from? What did my parents look like? Where do they live? Why did they relinquish me? They may well go through a period of grieving for the loss of their family of origin.

Adolescence

With adolescence comes a host of developmental changes. Physical changes, sexual maturation, cognitive advances, and the struggle for identity become important issues for teenagers. Adopted children may be bothered by a lack of any physical similarity to their family. "Genealogical bewilderment" may haunt them, causing them to create a "hereditary ghost"—that is, some imaginary figure children create who represents what is good and desirable in their fantasy genetic past. Note that these are possibilities, nothing more.

 TYPES OF ADOPTION

Adoption may take one of two forms: closed or open.

Closed Adoption

In traditional **closed adoptions,** biological parents were completely removed from the life of their child; no contact between the parties was allowed before or during the postplacement period. The bonds between birth parents and child were legally and permanently severed; the child's history was sealed by the court. Not only did the law intervene, but in some extreme cases women were blindfolded and forced to use earplugs during birth. No chance was taken that any emotional attachments could endure.

Open Adoption

In the 1970s, the concept of closed adoption was challenged on the grounds that both children and biological parents were being needlessly harmed and subjected to unnecessary emotional problems. When a pregnant woman approaches an adoption agency today, she gets what she wants. She can insist that her child be raised by a couple with specific characteristics: nationality, religion, income, number of family members. She can ask to see her child several times each year, perhaps take the youngster on a vacation, and telephone the child frequently. The adoption agency will try to meet these demands.

This process, which is called **open adoption,** focuses on the sharing of information or contacts between the adoptive and biological parents of an adopted child, before, during, and after placement. Thus we see a new definition of adoption: the process of accepting the responsibility of raising an individual who has two sets of parents.

IMPLICATIONS FOR HEALTHCARE PROVIDERS

Healthcare providers need to attend to both the physical health and the behavioral health of adopted children and their families. For example, children who are adopted from outside the country may arrive with physical and possibly behavioral health problems, depending on their age and their care in their country of origin. It may be difficult to obtain a complete health history. Adoptive parents may underestimate the demands of caring for children with special needs.

Do not let the fact of a child's adoption lead you to conclude that an adopted child may be more susceptible to problems than any other child. The developmental outcomes of adopted children are generally positive, and research to date does not support any other conclusion. Nevertheless, do not overlook the possibility that there may be problems related to the adoption that could affect long-term adaptation.

SOURCES

American Academy of Child and Adolescent Psychiatry. (2002). *The adopted child, no. 15*. Retrieved March 13, 2008, from www.aacap.org/cs/root/facts_for_families/the_adopted_child
Child Welfare Information Gateway. (2004). *How many children were adopted in 2000 and 2001?* Washington, DC: U.S. Department of Health and Human Services, Administration on Children, Youth and Families Children's Bureau.

PART II • QUESTIONS

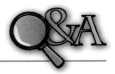

For each of the following questions, choose the **one best** answer.

1. What are genes?
   a. Long strands of deoxyribonucleic acid (DNA)
   b. The sequences in which nucleotide bases are arranged
   c. Multiple combinations of nucleotide bases
   d. The functional units of DNA
2. Skin cells contain
   a. 46 chromosomes.
   b. 23 chromosomes.
   c. 46 autosomes.
   d. 23 sex chromosomes.
3. Which process is responsible for the genetic variability among human organisms?
   a. Mitosis
   b. Meiosis
   c. Fertilization
   d. Capacitation
4. Where does fertilization occur in the female?
   a. Uterus
   b. Vagina
   c. Fallopian tubes
   d. Ovaries
5. The critical period of organogenesis occurs during
   a. the embryonic period.
   b. the germinal period.
   c. the fetal period.
   d. at the time of conception.
6. Research suggests that insufficient folic acid in the mother's diet may contribute to the failure of the neural tube to close, resulting in spina bifida. At which point in prenatal development does the neural tube close?
   a. Fourth week
   b. Eighth week
   c. Fourth month
   d. Sixth month
7. The causes of infertility are
   a. unknown.
   b. male.
   c. female.
   d. male or female.

8. Estimates are that one in every _____ American couples are infertile.
   a. two or three
   b. three or four
   c. five or six
   d. seven or eight

9. A major concern for sperm banks is control of
   a. disease.
   b. donor availability.
   c. confidential information.
   d. technological innovation.

10. For all assisted reproductive technologies (ARTs), _____ is critical.
    a. location
    b. climate
    c. timing
    d. contingency

11. Genes make up _____% of DNA.
    a. 1
    b. 2
    c. 3
    d. 4

12. The Human Genome Project (HGP) is an attempt to map
    a. all human genes.
    b. cellular materials.
    c. nucleotides.
    d. cell divisions.

13. An example of a single-gene genetic disorder is
    a. Down syndrome.
    b. Turner syndrome.
    c. Klinefelter syndrome.
    d. sickle-cell anemia.

14. An example of a chromosomal disorder is
    a. spina bifida.
    b. chronic disease syndrome.
    c. phenylketonuria (PKU).
    d. Turner syndrome.

15. How is prematurity defined?
    a. Infants are premature if born before 37 weeks, regardless of weight.
    b. Infants are premature if they weigh less than 2500 g at birth, regardless of age.
    c. Infants are premature if they weigh less than 1500 g and are born before 37 weeks.
    d. Prematurity is based on the relationship between weight and gestational age.

16. The organ system that is most critical to the premature infant's outcome is
    a. the heart.
    b. the lungs.
    c. the brain.
    d. the nervous system.

17. Which characteristic makes regular use of alcohol during pregnancy a teratogen?
    a. Alcohol interferes with fetal cell division and growth throughout pregnancy.
    b. Alcohol alters the development of the fetus's central nervous system during the last trimester.
    c. Women who abuse alcohol are less likely to be well nourished.
    d. All of the above are correct.

18. What is the best-known cause of deafness in newborns?
    a. Cocaine use by the mother during pregnancy
    b. Mother's contraction of rubella during the first trimester
    c. Mother's exposure to radiation during the last trimester
    d. Mother's exposure to cytomegalovirus (CMV)

19. When a natural mother retains input into the adoption process, it is called _____ adoption.
    a. selected
    b. congruent
    c. accommodated
    d. open

20. Couples considering adoption should think carefully about the _____ of the child.
    a. weight
    b. age
    c. size
    d. cognition

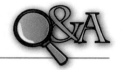

PART II · ANSWERS

1. **The answer is d.** Genes are the functional units of DNA. The DNA molecule consists of chemical compounds called nucleotides, which are linked together in two long chains. These chains coil to form a double helix, which looks like a twisted ladder. The key is the sequence in which the nucleotide bases are arranged along and between the ladder (i.e., on the "sides" and the "rungs"). A code word refers to a specific arrangement of three bases, and multiple combinations of code words along the DNA strand form genes. Where and how in the longer strand of DNA they start and stop, and whether they overlap, depend on the careful placement of specific code words. Genes—sometimes alone, sometimes in combination—contain the coded information that determines particular traits in an individual person.

2. **The answer is a.** Skin cells are somatic cells—that is, the type of cells that make up the major organs and body systems. Genes are arranged in linear order on chromosomes. Somatic cells contain 46 chromosomes arranged in 23 pairs of homologous chromosomes. One member of each pair is inherited from each parent. Of the 23 pairs, 22 pairs are autosomes and 1 pair is the sex chromosomes. Autosomes control most body traits, whereas the sex chromosomes determine gender as well as other traits. Females contain two X chromosomes: XX. Males contain one X chromosome and one Y chromosome: XY.

3. **The answer is b.** Meiosis is the process of cell division by which one diploid somatic cell produces four haploid gamete cells. First, the 46 chromosomes in the diploid somatic cell replicate, so that each of the 46 chromosomes has a doubled structure. Then, rather than separate into two identical cells as in mitosis, the chromosomes literally intertwine. As chromosomes carrying similar genes touch, they exchange genetic material. This exchange is responsible for genetic variability, such as differences in eye color or height. When the original cell divides, it forms two cells, each containing 23 chromosomes that are doubled in structure, but in combinations that are different from those found in the original cell.

4. **The answer is c.** After the ovum is released by the ovaries, it is carried into the fallopian tubes. Fertilization usually takes place in the outer third of the fallopian tubes, called the ampulla. The mature ovum is fertile for only 24 hours after ovulation. Sperm can survive in the female reproductive tract for 72 hours, but are at peak performance during the first 24 hours. Of the 200 to 400 million sperm released during ejaculation, only approximately 200 will reach the ampulla in about 4 hours. Only one sperm fertilizes an ovum.

5. **The answer is a.** *Embryo* is the name given to the fertilized ovum during the first 8 weeks of prenatal development. The first 2 weeks are also called the germinal period, or the period of the ovum. From 3 to 8 weeks is the critical period of organogenesis, during which all of the fetus's major organs develop.

6. **The answer is a.** During the 4th week, the heart begins to beat; limb buds are visible; eyes, ears, nerves, and the skeletomuscular and digestive systems begin to form; and the neural tube closes. The embryo is about 0.5 cm long and weighs 0.4 g. Women who are planning to become pregnant should be sure they have adequate amounts of folic acid in their diets to prevent spina bifida.

7. **The answer is d.** One of the myths concerning infertility is that it is essentially a female problem. Today, research clearly indicates that either the male or the female may be responsible in any given case of infertility.

8. **The answer is c.** These figures testify to the extent of this problem. Research has opened many new possibilities for infertile couples.

9. **The answer is a.** Concern about the possibility of disease has caused sperm banks to exercise extreme caution in their screening procedures.

10. **The answer is c.** Once detailed information about the reproductive process became available, the timing for the union of sperm and egg was seen as a key element in ensuring a successful procedure.

11. **The answer is c.** The small amount of genetic material in each cell illustrates the difficulty of the task facing researchers. The rest of the material is referred to as "evolutionary junk."

12. **The answer is a.** The HGP is an international effort that intends to identify the 50,000 to 100,000 genes in each cell. These discoveries will lead to many medical breakthroughs.

13. **The answer is d.** Single-gene disorders are caused by changes or mutations that occur in the DNA sequence of one recessive gene. In sickle cell anemia, two carriers who each have one recessive gene have a one in four chance of passing two recessive genes to a child, who will then develop the disorder. The other answers are chromosomal disorders.

14. **The answer is d.** Knowledge of chromosomal disorders has increased tremendously. Chromosomal disorders seem to be associated with age.

15. **The answer is d.** According to the World Health Organization, infants are premature if born before 37 weeks, regardless of weight. Low birth weight (LBW) refers to infants weighing less than 2500 g at birth, even if they were born at term. Very-low-birth-weight (VLBW) infants weigh less than 1500 g and are unlikely to be born at term. Although the terms "premature" and "low birth weight" are often used interchangeably, the determination of prematurity is based on the relationship between weight and gestational age. Gestational age is determined through neurological and physical assessment between 2 and 8 hours after birth. Premature infants are considered appropriate for their gestational age (AGA) when their weight at birth is typical of that for a fetus of the same gestational age.

16. **The answer is b.** While many complications of prematurity are possible, the organ system that is most critical to the infant's outcome is the lungs. Surfactant, which begins to form at approximately 28 weeks' gestation, allows the alveoli to expand so that oxygen and carbon dioxide can be exchanged. Poor gas exchange at the cellular level has cascading consequences on all major organ systems. The combination of decreased oxygen perfusion, acid–base imbalances in metabolism and respiration, and related difficulties with regulation of blood flow can adversely affect the developing brain, the retinas of the eyes, and the intestines; it can also complicate the closure of the patent ductus in the heart.

17. **The answer is d.** Regular use interferes with fetal cell division and growth throughout pregnancy. During the third trimester in particular, alcohol adversely alters development of the central nervous system and brain. Alcohol constitutes empty calories; that is, it has no nutritional value but contributes to weight gain. Women who abuse alcohol during pregnancy are less likely to eat well and to seek regular prenatal care. Fetal alcohol syndrome affects approximately 40% of infants born to alcoholics.

18. **The answer is b.** Rubella (German measles) affects fewer than one child per 1000 live births. If a mother is infected during the first trimester, rubella can cause deafness, heart defects, and cataracts in her child.

19. **The answer is d.** Because the number of children available for adoption is far less than the demand, a woman today may exercise considerable control over the adoption process for her child.

20. **The answer is b.** In opting for adoption, parents should be aware of a child's age in light of their own compatibility with a particular age group. Other characteristics, such as weight, usually do not have the same impact on a relationship as age.

III
Infancy

- Reflexes are automatic responses to certain stimuli, such as the eye blink and the knee jerk.
- Reflexes serve a definite purpose: They sustain life's functions by enabling infants to react to threats without thinking.
- Infant reflexes differ from those of later childhood and adulthood in that they change with maturity.
- The rooting reflex is an adaptive behavior that facilitates feeding.
- The sucking reflex , also essential for feeding, is a building block for voluntary mother–child interactions.
- The Moro reflex provokes the infant to believe that it is falling, which then causes it to extend its arms, throw back its head, and spread its fingers.
- With the grasping reflex, the infant curls its fingers around an object placed in its hand, which is a building block for grabbing and letting go.

21

Reflexes

TERMS

- ☐ Grasping
- ☐ Moro reflex
- ☐ Myelin sheath
- ☐ Myelination
- ☐ Peripheral nervous system (PNS)
- ☐ Reflex
- ☐ Reflex arc
- ☐ Rooting
- ☐ Sucking

REFLEXES: AN OVERVIEW

Reflexes are involuntary stimulus–response behaviors of the human nervous system. The sequence of neural events that gives rise to reflexive behaviors is called the **reflex arc**:

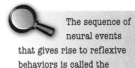

The sequence of neural events that gives rise to reflexive behaviors is called the **reflex arc**.

1. A receptor organ (skin, eye, mouth) receives a stimulus from the external environment (hot touch, bright light, sour taste).
2. Information about the stimulus is transmitted along a sensory—that is, afferent—neuron in the **peripheral nervous system (PNS)**.
3. The information reaches a specialized region of the central nervous system (CNS) where the information is integrated and synapse occurs.
4. The CNS relays the synaptic impulse to a motor neuron in the PNS.
5. The PNS transmits the synaptic impulse to an effector organ (muscles, glands) that produces the observable behavior called a **reflex.**

The conduction of all of this information is facilitated by the **myelin sheaths** that insulate the nerve cells along the reflex arc (**Figure 21-1**). As Rose (2005) notes, the previously unused infant reflexes now must be brought into play and under control. Popular examples include the eye blink and the knee jerk. All of the activities needed to sustain life's functions are present at birth (breathing, sucking, swallowing, elimination). These reflexes serve a definite purpose: The gag reflex enables infants to spit up mucus; the eye blink protects the eyes from excessive light; the anti-smothering reflex facilitates breathing.

The specialized regions that give rise to reflexes are found in the more primitive areas of the CNS, such as the spinal cord, brain stem, and cerebellum. Evolutionary biologists consider reflexes to be built-in mechanisms that sustain life and allow humans to react to threat without thinking. As reviewed in Chapter 25, the CNS is not fully developed at birth, but rather continues to grow, reorganize, and mature. For example, **myelination** of the nerve cells in the cerebellum, which coordinates sensory–motor information, continues for several years.

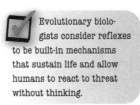

Evolutionary biologists consider reflexes to be built-in mechanisms that sustain life and allow humans to react to threat without thinking.

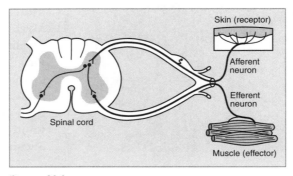

Figure 21-1 Simple Reflex Arc

Because their nervous systems are maturing, infants exhibit reflexive behaviors that are different from those found in older children and adults. Infant reflexes are interesting for several reasons. Some are adaptive behaviors arising from the primitive CNS, which develops early in utero and infancy, before the higher regions of the cortex, which are themselves responsible for thinking and volitional behavior. These reflexes are adaptive because the primitive

> Because their nervous systems are maturing, infants exhibit reflexive behaviors that are different from those found in older children and adults.

CNS also developed early in the evolution of our history as human primates, and it has helped to ensure the survival of our young. Some adaptive infant reflexes are building blocks for voluntary motor behaviors that develop with experience and with maturity of the cortical regions of the brain. Thus reflexes can also provide a window into neurological development because they should change as the nervous system matures (**Figure 21-2** and **Table 21-1**). Finally, some reflexes are permanent and persist throughout life; these reflexes are designed to protect us from potential harm (**Table 21-2**).

REFLEXES THAT ARE ADAPTIVE BEHAVIORS

Rooting

Stroke an infant's cheek, and the head turns to that side, the mouth opens, and the infant attempts to suck your finger. This reflex is adaptive because it facilitates feeding. The touch of the breast against the infant's cheek elicits this response. **Rooting** disappears by 4 months.

Sucking Reflex

Put your finger or a nipple into the infant's mouth. The infant begins **sucking** rhythmically. This reflex is adaptive because it is essential for feeding. Premature infants may not suck, which can threaten their survival. Reflexive sucking disappears by the age of 2 months as infants gain control over a

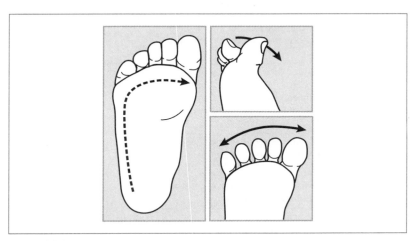

Figure 21-2 Babinski Reflex

> Premature infants may not suck, which can threaten their survival.

"burst–pause" pattern in their sucking. They suck vigorously in short bursts and then pause, breaking the tension at the nipple. As the mouth releases, the infant appears to smile. The mother smiles, and speaks to her infant. The infant attends to this interesting and cozy stimulus, focusing the eyes, and cooing. In this way, reflexive sucking is a building block for voluntary mother–child interactions.

Moro Reflex

Hold an infant horizontally on its back above a dressing table. Suddenly, lower the infant about 6 inches and stop abruptly, simulating a free fall. Alternatively, with the infant lying on the back, raise the head slightly and then release it suddenly, again allowing the infant to feel the force of gravity. In either case, the infant extends the arms, throws back the head, and spreads the fingers. Then the infant brings the arms back to the center of the body with hands clenched, and the spine and legs extended. This reflex is adaptive when you consider our evolutionary roots as primates. The infant feels as if it 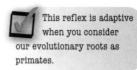 This reflex is adaptive when you consider our evolutionary roots as primates.

is falling, displays alarm to the mother, and then tries to grab on for safety, a mechanism that would serve infant monkeys in tall treetops well. The **Moro reflex** weakens by 5 months, and disappears by 8 months.

Table 21-1 Reflexes that Change or Disappear with Neurological Maturity

Reflex	Stimulus and Response	Comments
Babinski	Stroke the sole of foot as shown in Figure 21-2. Toes fan out and extend; big toe dorsiflexes.	Gone by 1 year of age With maturity toes flex.
Tonic neck	Turn infant's head to one side while lying on back. Arm and let on that side extend; arm and leg on the opposite side flex (looks like a fencer's stance).	Disappears after 3–4 months. Response becomes symmetric.
Stepping	Hold infant upright with feet lightly touching surface. Feet step rhythmically in place. Term infants step on the soles of feet, preterm infants step with toes.	Present for 3–4 years after term, then fades.
Plantar	Apply pressure with finger against ball of foot. All toes plantar flex, grasping the finger.	Lessens by 8 months; gone by 1 year.
Startle	Stimulus is a loud noise. Response is similar to Moro reflex. Arms at first flail out, then pull in; fists clench.	Present for 3–4 weeks.
Crawling	Place newborn on abdomen. Infant makes crawling movement with arms and legs.	Gone by about 6 weeks.

Table 21-2 Permanent Reflexes Designed to Protect Against Harm

Reflex	Stimulus and Response	Comments
Blinking	Flash light in eyes or brush against eyelashes. Eyes close.	Protects eyes.
Gag	Touch back of throat (pharynx). Person gags as throat closes.	Prevents objects in mouth from entering trachea.
Withdrawal	Prick sole of foot with a pin. Person pulls foot away.	Protective reflex. With repeated pricks, response fades.

Grasping

Place an object in the palm of an infant's hand. The infant will curl the fingers around the object strongly enough to hold the infant's weight. **Grasping** on for dear life is adaptive behavior in young primates. It is also a building block for the complex skill of grabbing and letting go that evolves over the first year of life. By 3 to 4 months, the grasping reflex declines, and infants will involuntarily let go of objects placed in their palm. By 4 months, they voluntarily grasp an object by closing their whole palm over it, but cannot let go. By 5 months, they reach and grasp what is in their line of view, but do not have full control over letting go. By 6 months, infants deliberately reach, and grab with their whole hand and thumb like a mitten. Once sitting up at 6 to 8 months, infants transfer objects from hand to hand across the midline of their bodies, and release objects at will. By 9 to 12 months, they control the individual movements of the thumb and forefinger to use a pincer-like grasp to pick up finger foods.

Grasping is a good example of how development evolves. It begins with a behavior that is global and diffuse (grasp reflex), becomes more differentiated (palmar grasp evolves into the mitten grasp, in which the thumb is separate), and is finally hierarchically integrated. Sitting in a high chair using the pincer grasp to pick up food requires the integrated development of hand–eye coordination, spatial relationships, chewing, and swallowing.

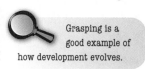

Grasping is a good example of how development evolves.

SOURCE

Rose, S. (2005). *The future of the brain.* New York: Oxford.

- The transition from uterine to extrauterine life happens quickly, thanks to the brain stem's detection of the rise and fall of arterial oxygen and carbon dioxide.
- The Apgar score is an assessment of the infant's ability to adjust to extrauterine life minutes after birth.
- During the first 24 hours after birth, healthy newborns undergo predictable changes in physiological and behavioral processes.
- The New Ballard Scale is used to determine the gestational age of infants who are born prematurely.
- The Brazelton Neonatal Behavioral Assessment Scale is designed to measure newborns' success in organizing their behavior.
- The Newborn Behavioral Observation procedure focuses on both infant behavior and parenting skills.

22

Neonatal Assessment

TERMS
- ☐ **Apgar scores**
- ☐ **First period of reactivity**
- ☐ **Second period of reactivity**
- ☐ **New Ballard Scale**
- ☐ **Competent infant**
- ☐ **Brazelton Neonatal Behavioral Assessment Scale (BNBAS)**
- ☐ **Newborn Behavioral Observation (NBO)**
- ☐ **Self-regulation**

PHYSICAL CHANGES DURING BIRTH

The transition from uterine to extrauterine life happens in moments. The initial breath is probably triggered by changes in pressure on the thorax during birth. Fluid is squeezed from the lungs and replaced by a rush of air. Within 1 minute, the brain stem picks up signals about the rise and fall of arterial oxygen and carbon dioxide, triggering a gasping breath and crying. The child's lungs clear, promoting the conversion from fetal to infant heart–lung circulation. Sensory changes such as air temperature, noise, and light also contribute to the first breath.

 Within 1 minute, the brain stem picks up signals about the rise and fall of arterial oxygen and carbon dioxide, triggering a gasping breath and crying.

Apgar scores are used as a rough assessment of immediate adjustment to extrauterine life. Heart rate, respirations, muscle tone, reflexes, and skin color are assessed at 1 and 5 minutes after birth, with each being given a score of 0, 1, or 2 (**Figure 22-1**). Total scores lower than 3 indicate severe stresses. Scores of 4 to 6 signify moderate difficulty, and scores of 7 to 10 indicate no difficulty in adapting to extrauterine life. Apgar scores are affected by prematurity and maternal medication, but are not indicative of the presence or absence of neurological or physical abnormalities. **Figure 22-2** cites normal vital signs in newborns.

 Heart rate, respirations, muscle tone, reflexes, and skin color are assessed at 1 and 5 minutes after birth, with each being given a score of 0, 1, or 2.

During the first 24 hours after birth, healthy newborns undergo predictable changes in physiological and behavioral processes. The **first period of reactivity** covers the initial 6 to 8 hours. For the first 30 minutes, infants are highly active. They cry, suck their fists, and pass meconium and urine. Mucus secretions, heart rate, and respirations increase. Infants then become attentive to their surroundings, with eyes open, and will nurse vigorously.

During the first 24 hours after birth, healthy newborns undergo predictable changes in physiological and behavioral processes.

During the second stage, which lasts 2 to 4 hours, heart and respiratory rates and body temperature decrease as infants become calm. They sleep deeply, blocking out stimuli. The **second period of reactivity** follows. Infants are alert and responsive, providing an optimal situation for parents and newborns to interact. Heart rate and respirations increase again, and then stabilize.

The **New Ballard Scale** is used to determine gestational age in infants who are born prematurely or who are small or large for their apparent gestational age (Ballard et al., 1991). Maturity is rated on a scale from s1 to r5 in 13 areas, such as flexion of extremities, quality of skin, creases on the soles of the feet, and development of eyes, ears, and genitals. Total scores range from s10 (20 weeks' gestation—extremely premature) to r50 (44 weeks' gestation—postmature). The combination of accurate gestational age and birth weight are good predictors of perinatal morbidity and mortality.

 The **New Ballard Scale** is used to determine gestational age in infants who are born prematurely or who are small or large for their apparent gestational age.

 Total scores lower than 3 indicate severe stresses.

Sign	0	1	2
Heart rate	Absent	Slow (<100)	>100
Respiratory effort	Absent	Slow, irregular	Good cry
Muscle tone	Flaccid	Some flexion of extremities	Active motion
Reflex irritability	No response	Cry	Vigorous cry
Color*	Blue, pale	Body pink, extremities blue	Completely pink

* Blue indicates cyanosis (i.e., poor perfusion of oxygenated blood) pink indicates the skin is well perfused. The colors are not intended to indicate racial characteristics.

Figure 22-1 Apgar Scoring

BEHAVIORAL ASSESSMENT

Newborns arrive preadapted to interact with the physical and social environment. Parents often ask if their baby can see them. The answer is yes. Although visual acuity at birth is between 20/100 and 20/400, newborns can see and fixate on objects within 20 cm of the center of their bodies. They can see their parents' faces clearly while being held or bathed. Babies have an inborn preference for looking at complex patterns rather than solid fields. They prefer light and dark patterns over color, and they visually follow a moving object.

Human faces fit these criteria. Babies gaze at their parents with great interest, a behavior that endears them to parents and enhances survival. Newborns also prefer the sound of human voices, and at birth will turn their heads toward any sound to locate it. At 3 days, newborns can discriminate their mother's voice from the voices of other women. At 5 days, they can use their sense of smell to identify their mother's breast milk.

Newborn behavior has four characteristics:

- In-born physiological mechanisms, such as reflexes, enhance survival.
- Newborns organize their behavior in response to stimuli (e.g., turning their heads in response to a sound).

Heart rate	Respirations	Blood Pressure	Temperature	Neuromuscular
120–140/min apical	30–60/min abdominal breathing	65/41 mm Hg in arm or calf, increases with crying	36.5–37.0°C axillary, increases with crying	Extremities flexed, can extend; arms rest on chest; when prone, holds head in line with back, turns it to side

Figure 22-2 Normal Vital Signs in Newborns (0–28 days)

- They respond selectively to certain stimuli (e.g., patterns of light and dark).
- Newborns demonstrate contingency-seeking behavior—that is, they look for predictability in the environment) for events that go together.

Thus we refer to the preadapted neonate as a **competent infant**.

The **Brazelton Neonatal Behavioral Assessment Scale (BNBAS)**, developed by T. Berry Brazelton, is based on these characteristics. It is designed to assess 28 newborn behaviors, clustered in 7 areas (**Figure 22-3**). A key factor is the newborn's state of consciousness at the time of the assessment. The BNBAS identifies 6 states along a continuum from deep sleep to active and alert (Brazelton & Nugent, 1995).

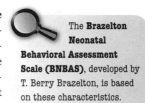

The **Brazelton Neonatal Behavioral Assessment Scale (BNBAS)**, developed by T. Berry Brazelton, is based on these characteristics.

Infants are not easily aroused from *deep sleep*, during which time their breathing is regular. During *light sleep*, breathing is irregular and infants can be awakened by a noise. *Drowsy* infants have their eyes open and are aroused by stimuli; breathing is irregular, and they squirm. *Quiet alert* infants are attentive. Their eyes are open, they orient to stimuli, and they may coo or smile. Breathing is regular. *Active alert* infants are fussy and restless. They respond to stimuli, but may not attend for long. *Crying* ranges from whimpering to howling. Stimuli are shut out. The best time to perform the BNBAS is when infants are quiet and alert.

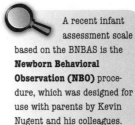

A recent infant assessment scale based on the BNBAS is the **Newborn Behavioral Observation (NBO)** procedure, which was designed for use with parents by Kevin Nugent and his colleagues.

A recent infant assessment scale based on the BNBAS is the **Newborn Behavioral Observation (NBO)** procedure, which was designed for use with parents by Kevin Nugent and his colleagues. The NBO is a brief neurobehavioral assessment intended to examine a newborn's physiological, motor, state, and social capacities and reflects the conceptual content of the NBAS. While the focus of the NBO is on the infant's behaviors, it is also designed to encourage positive parenting, thereby strengthening the relationship between the parents and their newborn baby.

Habituation: baby attends to novel stimuli, gets used to it, inhibits attention

Orientation: baby is alert and attending to stimuli

Motor performance: movement and tone

Range of state: arousal level

Regulation of state: baby responds when aroused

Autonomic stability: homeostatic regulation

Reflexes: inborn neuromotor behaviors

Figure 22-3 Neonatal Behaviors in Brazelton Neonatal Behavioral Assessment Scale

SELF-REGULATION AND INFANT LEARNING

Evidence of infant learning is based on the inborn tendency to seek out contingencies and to build on reflexes. Volitional control over the sucking reflex increases in the first few weeks of life. In a classic experiment, DeCasper and Fifer (1980) demonstrated that infants can learn to adjust their rate of sucking, using the mother's voice as a reward. When they sucked at a fast pace, a tape of the mother's voice was played. They also learned a reverse contingency, wherein the tape played only when they sucked slowly.

Thus we see that infants begin to regulate their own behavior (**self-regulation**) in response to environmental stimuli. Infants have the inborn capacity to self-quiet, to reorganize, and to pay attention to their surroundings. They learn to do so of their own volition in the context of sensitive caretaking by parents. Distressed infants who are firmly but gently held, who hear a soothing voice and smell a familiar smell, and who can predict that a cry will get a caring response learn to use parents as a resource to help them regulate their own behavioral state. That is the beginning of trust.

SOURCES

Ballard, J. L., et al. (1991). New Ballard score, expanded to include extremely premature infants. *Journal of Pediatrics, 119,* 417.

Brazelton, T. B., & Nugent, K. (1995). *Neonatal behavioral assessment scale.* London: Heinemann.

DeCasper, A., & Fifer, W. (1980). Of human bonding. *Science, 208,* 1174.

- Growth during infancy is the most rapid in the human life span.
- By 1 year, birth height has increased by 50%.
- Children's adult height can be estimated by doubling their height at age 2 years.
- Human breast milk is the best diet for infants during the first 6 months of life. It also helps to protect infants from disease.
- The feeding process contributes to many aspects of an infant's development.
- When parents report a sleeping problem, it usually has nothing to do with parenting itself.
- "Failure to thrive" children typically fall below the third percentile for weight and height.

23

Growth and Development I

TERMS
- ☐ **Breast milk**
- ☐ **Breastfeeding**
- ☐ **Failure to thrive (FTT)**
- ☐ **Nonorganic FTT**
- ☐ **Organic FTT**
- ☐ **Sleep pattern**

DEVELOPMENT IN INFANCY

The well-known pediatrician T. Berry Brazelton once said that newborn babies are beautifully programmed to fit their parents' fantasies and to reward the work of pregnancy. His statement seems to describe the growth pattern of the infant years. During the first year, infants grow rapidly. During the second year, the rate of physical growth slows, and there are significant gains in cognition and language.

On average, boys are bigger than girls. The data in **Figure 23-1** and **Figure 23-2** are based on national averages of all U.S.-born children. Separate data for different racial and ethnic groups are available from the National Center for Health Statistics. Tables developed for children who were born prematurely or who have Down syndrome are often used by pediatricians and nurses.

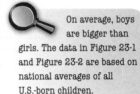 On average, boys are bigger than girls. The data in Figure 23-1 and Figure 23-2 are based on national averages of all U.S.-born children.

HEIGHT, WEIGHT, AND HEAD CIRCUMFERENCE: FIRST YEAR

The average U.S. newborn weighs 3.27 kg. By the second day of life, newborns lose 5% to 10% of their birth weight, but steadily regain it by 14 days. This loss is not a problem for healthy babies, who are born with a reserve of fat that helps them get through the first few days of life until their mother's breast milk supply is established. Infants then gain 680 g each month until 5 to 6 months of life, when their birth weight doubles. Birth weight triples by the end of the first year, to approximately 10 kg.

The average U.S. newborn weighs 3.27 kg. By the second day of life, newborns lose 5% to 10% of their birth weight, but steadily regain it by 14 days.

By age 1 year, birth height has increased by 50%. During the first 6 months after birth, height increases 2.5 cm per month from the average 50 cm at birth, and then slows during the second half of the first year. Most of this growth occurs in the trunk, not the legs. A typical 1-year-old is approximately 76 cm tall. Birth height doubles by age 4 years.

	Height by percentile (cm)			Weight by percentile (kg)		
Age (months)	5th	50th	95th	5th	50th	95th
Birth	46.4	50.5	54.4	2.54	3.27	4.15
3	56.7	61.1	65.4	4.43	5.98	7.37
6	63.4	67.8	72.3	6.20	7.85	9.46
9	68.0	72.3	77.1	7.52	9.18	10.93
12	71.7	76.1	81.2	8.43	10.15	11.99
18	77.5	82.4	88.1	9.59	11.47	13.44
24	82.5	86.8	94.4	10.49	12.34	15.50

Figure 23-1 Height and Weight Measurements: Boys

Height by percentile (cm)				Weight by percentile (kg)			
Age (months)	5th	50th	95th		5th	50th	95th
Birth	45.4	49.9	52.9		2.36	3.23	3.81
3	55.4	59.5	63.4		4.18	5.40	6.74
6	61.8	65.9	70.2		5.79	7.21	8.73
9	66.1	70.4	75.0		7.00	8.56	10.17
12	69.8	74.3	79.1		7.84	9.53	11.24
18	76.0	80.9	86.1		8.92	10.82	12.76
24	81.6	86.8	93.6		9.95	11.8	14.15

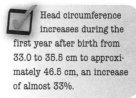

Figure 23-2 Height and Weight Measurements: Girls

Head circumference increases during the first year after birth from 33.0 to 35.5 cm to approximately 46.5 cm, an increase of almost 33%. The weight of the brain has more than doubled at this point. Growth of the head is indicative of brain maturation, which is best seen in the extraordinary motor and sensory achievements of the first year (see Chapter 24).

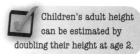 Head circumference increases during the first year after birth from 33.0 to 35.5 cm to approximately 46.5 cm, an increase of almost 33%.

HEIGHT, WEIGHT, AND HEAD CIRCUMFERENCE: SECOND YEAR

The rate of growth slows during the toddler years. At age 2 years, the average toddler weighs about 12 kg and is 86.8 cm tall. During the second year, most of the growth in height occurs in the legs and not the trunk. Children's adult height can be estimated by doubling their height at age 2. Head circumference increases by only 2.5 cm during the second year, to approximately 49 cm. It takes another 16 years to add 7 cm to head circumference to reach adult size.

Children's adult height can be estimated by doubling their height at age 2.

During this time of rapid growth, infants experience changes in shape and body composition, in the distribution of tissues, and in their developing motor skills. Different tissues (muscles, nerves) also grow at different rates, and total growth represents a complex series of changes. These changes then influence cognitive, psychosocial, and emotional development. Underlying this rapidly unfolding and complex process is, of course, proper nutrition.

NUTRITION

Human **breast milk** is the best diet for infants during the first 6 months of life. Milk from a well-nourished mother contains all of the nutrients essential for sustaining newborn life and promoting

The digestive tracts of young infants are not fully mature, so they cannot adequately extract nutrients from fruits, vegetables, and meats, even in pureed form.

infant growth. The digestive tracts of young infants are not fully mature, so they cannot adequately extract nutrients from fruits, vegetables, and meats, even in pureed form. Cow's milk should not be used to feed newborns because it is poorly digested and causes cramping. Breast milk also contains maternal antibodies against common illnesses that help to protect infants while their immune systems are still developing. Commercial infant formulas are an acceptable substitute if a mother does not wish to breastfeed.

Human **breast milk** is the best diet for infants during the first 6 months of life.

Feeding—and especially **breastfeeding**—contributes to development in other ways. Sucking is an inborn reflex, but feeding is a learned behavior that contributes to self-regulation in infants and to sensitive responding in mothers. Mother and infant learn to coordinate supply and demand of milk. This give-and-take requires that mothers learn to read infants' signals of hunger, fatigue, distress, and satisfaction. As infants learn to regulate the flow of milk, they also learn to organize their own behavior. Feeding, especially at the breast, helps them to calm down and focus. An attentive infant in the arms of a responsive mother is ready to interact with her, to focus its eyes on her face and listen to her voice.

These types of interactions—whether with mothers, fathers, or other responsive caretakers—are the foundation of trust. Trust versus mistrust is the first of Erikson's stages of the human life cycle. Viewed in evolutionary terms, eating is a fundamental social event that bonds family members together.

Solid foods in pureed form can be introduced at 5 to 6 months of life, when teeth begin to appear and infants can sit up with support. Finger foods can be introduced toward the end of the first year. By 1 year, infant digestive tracts can handle the usual family diet.

Toddlers develop strong likes and dislikes in foods. They prefer to feed themselves or to just play with the food. Not only is this messy, but parents may worry that toddlers are not adequately nourished. As physical growth slows and gross motor skills improve, busy toddlers typically have decreased appetites. They benefit from frequent snacking throughout the day.

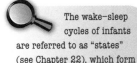

Toddlers develop strong likes and dislikes in foods.

SLEEP

The wake–sleep cycles of infants are referred to as "states" (see Chapter 22), which form a continuum of arousal. Newborns are in deep sleep (i.e., they are not easily aroused) for 4 to 5 hours each day at intervals of 10 to 20 minutes. Light sleep takes up 12 to 15 hours of their day, with longer intervals of 20 to 45 minutes. Breastfed infants usually sleep for somewhat shorter periods of time because they eat more often.

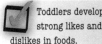

The wake–sleep cycles of infants are referred to as "states" (see Chapter 22), which form a continuum of arousal.

Infants develop a nocturnal **sleep pattern** through a combination of physical and neurological maturity and self-regulation in response to parents' efforts to promote predictable feeding, waking, and sleeping habits. By 3 to 4 months, infants sleep about 9 hours at night and nap about three times per day for an hour or so at a time. By the end of the first year, babies nap twice a day, and then only once a day by 18 months. They extend their nighttime sleep to 11 to 12 hours.

The American Academy of Pediatrics urges parents to follow these guidelines:

- Place infants on their backs on a firm mattress that meets safety standards.
- Remove all pillows, quilts, comforters, and soft toys from the crib.
- If using a blanket, tuck it around the mattress and be sure it reaches only to the baby's chest.

FAILURE TO THRIVE

Failure to thrive (FTT) is usually diagnosed during the first year of life. In FTT, weight falls below the third to fifth percentile, there is deviation from the growth curve, and the characteristic posturing and interactive behaviors of infancy may be absent. There is often a history of feeding and sleeping disturbances and irritability. There are two types of FTT: organic and nonorganic. **Organic FTT** has physical causes (e.g., digestive, endocrine, or enzyme disorders). Infants who have neurological deficits or are fatigued due to heart defects or infections may not feed well. **Nonorganic FTT** is usually caused by psychosocial factors (e.g., poverty, lack of knowledge about infant nutrition, inconsistent and poor quality of infant care, and disturbances in maternal–child attachment). Nonorganic FTT is difficult to diagnose and treat.

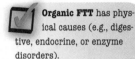

Organic FTT has physical causes (e.g., digestive, endocrine, or enzyme disorders).

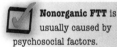

Nonorganic FTT is usually caused by psychosocial factors.

In FTT, weight falls below the third to fifth percentile, there is deviation from the growth curve, and the characteristic posturing and interactive behaviors of infancy may be absent.

QUICK LOOK AT THE CHAPTER AHEAD

- Gross motor development refers to an infant's ability to control large muscle groups.
- Fine motor development refers to the development of manual skills (reaching, grasping).
- Motor development proceeds in a cephalocaudal (head-to-toe) direction.
- Head control is a good indicator of brain maturation.
- Crawling forward commences at about 7 months.
- Creeping on all four limbs begins at about 9 months.
- Infants usually stand holding on to something by 9 months.
- At birth, visual acuity is about 20/100 and steadily improves.
- Binocular vision typically is well established by 4 months.

24

Growth and Development II

TERMS
- ☐ Binocular vision
- ☐ Cephalocaudal
- ☐ Fine motor development
- ☐ Gross motor development
- ☐ Head control
- ☐ Visual acuity
- ☐ Visual cliff

Research into infant locomotion had long been at a standstill because of the belief that neuromuscular maturation was the primary cause of motor development. Current investigators, however, have used high-speed film, computerized video recordings, and infrared emitting diodes to offer rare insights into the coordination, balance, and strength of infants' locomotion.

Gross motor development refers to the infant's ability to control large muscle groups (e.g., lifting the head, crawling). **Fine motor development** refers to manual skills (e.g., reaching, grasping). Motor development is closely tied to sensory development. For example, reaching and grasping require hand–eye coordination.

Sequencing of motor development proceeds in a **cephalocaudal** direction—that is, from head to toe. The brain matures in such a way that babies can control their heads, shoulders, and arms before they can control their legs. Children who persistently lag behind in meeting milestones (**Table 24-1**) need to be assessed for evidence of developmental delay.

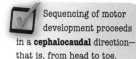 Sequencing of motor development proceeds in a **cephalocaudal** direction—that is, from head to toe.

GROSS MOTOR DEVELOPMENT

Head control is a good indicator of brain maturation. Newborns turn their head to the side to free their nose when lying on their abdomen on a flat surface. They cannot lift their head until they are 6 weeks old, however, and then do so briefly. By 3 to 4 months, they can raise their head, shoulders, and upper body while supporting themselves on their forearms. When newborns are pulled to sit, their head falls back. Head lag decreases and infants have steady head control by 5 to 6 months, when they can sit with support.

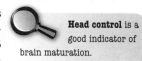 **Head control** is a good indicator of brain maturation.

Infants begin purposely rolling from their back to one side at 4 months of age. As they begin raising their upper body from a flat surface by pushing up with their arms, they learn to flip from their abdomen to their back. Rolling from back to front is accomplished by 6 months.

During the first 2 months after birth, infants need to be in a position of full body support. By 5 months, they can sit up with back support; by 7 months, they can sit alone, leaning forward onto their hands. Infants can sit alone securely by 8 months, with their hands free to manipulate objects.

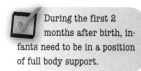 During the first 2 months after birth, infants need to be in a position of full body support.

While many infants begin to propel themselves backward by pushing with their arms when they are lying prone, true locomotion implies bearing body weight. Pushing backward gives way to crawling forward with their abdomen still on the floor at about 7 months of age. Once babies begin creeping on all four limbs by 9 months, they are very mobile.

Infants' legs can hold their weight by 8 months, but they do not pull themselves into a standing position holding onto furniture until 9 months. At first, they sit down by letting go and falling. By 1 year, they ease themselves down. It takes several more months to stand, bend down, and sit without holding on. Pulling to stand gives way to cruising by 10 to 12 months. First steps typically follow around 13 to 15 months.

Infants' legs can hold their weight by 8 months, but they do not pull themselves into a standing position holding onto furniture until 9 months.

Table 24-1 Sensory/Peceptual and Motor Milestones

Age	Gross Motor	Fine Motor	Sensory/Perceptual
1–3 months	When prone, lifts head a little, finally to 45 degrees Head tag when pulled to sit lessens	Grasp reflex strong, then gone by 3 months Hands begin to open, hold rattle, pull at blankets	Visual acuity 20/100 at birth When supine, visually follows light to midline, to side, to 180 degrees
4–6 months	When prone, raises head and shoulders 90 degrees Rolls back to side, belly to back, back to front Sits with support	Plays with hands, toes Inspects clothing, blankets Grasps objects with both hands (e.g., bottle) Brings objects to mouth	Has binocular vision Early hand–eye coordination Visually follows an object when it is dropped Localizes sounds by looking
7–9 months	Sits alone Sits to play Pulls to stand, falls to sit Creeps, starts to crawl	Transfers objects hand to hand, bangs them on table Grabs and releases objects Early pincer grasp	Aware of depth and spatial relationships Responds to own name Has taste preferences
10–12 months	Moves from prone to sitting Stands holding furniture, cruises, may walk Can sit down from standing	Eats using fingers Good pincer grasp Grasps spoon by handle Flips pages in book	Drops objects just to watch them fall Fascinated by "in" and "out"
13–15 months	Walks alone Creeps up stairs	Handedness is apparent Throws things down Scribbles, uses cup	Intense interest in pictures Identifies forms (e.g., circle) Good binocular vision
16–18 months	Runs but falls Walks up stairs with help Jumps in place	Builds tower of 3–4 cubes Manages with spoon Tries to imitate your scribble	
By 24 months	Walks up stairs two feet at a time, runs well Bends down to pick things up without falling	Turns pages in book to "read" Turns doorknobs, unscrews lids	Accommodation of eyes well developed Discriminates pictures of objects

This sequence is a generalization of infant development. Some infants never crawl, but rather are quite content to sit and play. One day, they cruise and the next day they walk. Others are barely walking when suddenly they are climbing stairs. Toddlers have the physical ability and the motivation to be on the move, but lack the judgment their newfound abilities require.

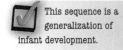

This sequence is a generalization of infant development.

FINE MOTOR DEVELOPMENT

As noted in Chapter 23, the ability to use the hands is built on a primitive grasping reflex. At birth, infants close their entire hand around an object (e.g., a parent's finger) placed in their palm. As the brain matures, the reflex fades (by 3 months) and infants begin to control grasping and letting go.

Over time, they hold something (e.g., a rattle) that is given to them (3 months), hold a bottle with two hands (4 months), grasp using the whole hand (5 months), begin to release objects (6 months), transfer hand to hand (7 months), and finally grasp and release at will (8 months). At the same time, their grip becomes more refined, from using the whole hand, to isolating the thumb (6 to 8 months), and finally developing a pincer grasp, using the thumb and forefinger (9 to 10 months).

SENSORY/PERCEPTUAL DEVELOPMENT

During infancy, the capacity to take in information through the major sensory channels, to make sense of the environment, and to attribute meaning to information improves dramatically. Infants are born ready to process visual and auditory information, movement of objects, and the spatial relationship between their body and the physical space they inhabit. Fine and gross motor development is closely integrated with changes in perceptual development. Infants cannot reach and grab something if they cannot judge how far away it is.

At birth, **visual acuity** is about 20/100 and steadily improves. Objects within close range, such as the mother's face, are perfectly clear. A preference for patterns is evident within hours after birth. Infants do not discern color until 2 months. Patterns that are somewhat complex and that have moving parts are of greatest interest, especially the human face. Infants recognize pictures of their mother by 3 months, and they prefer pictures of children over adults. They discriminate their mother's voice from the voices of other women at 3 days, having heard it since the 4th month of gestation.

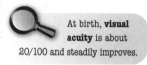

At birth, **visual acuity** is about 20/100 and steadily improves.

Binocular vision, in which the different images taken in by the two eyes are integrated into one picture in the brain, begins to develop at 6 weeks and is well established by 4 months. Binocular vision is related to hand–eye coordination, which first appears at 4 months as infants are learning to grasp voluntarily. Hand–eye coordination continues to mature into childhood.

Binocular vision, in which the different images taken in by the two eyes are integrated into one picture in the brain, begins to develop at 6 weeks and is well established by 4 months.

Depth perception develops, not coincidentally, when infants need to appreciate near and far—that is, when they start to creep, crawl, and cruise during the second half of the first year. About this time, infants become fascinated by falling objects, dropping spoons from their high chair just to watch them fall. In a classic study involving a **visual cliff** (Gibson & Walk, 1960), infants were placed on a level glass surface. On the shallow side, they could see the "floor," a black-and-white tile pattern, a few inches below them. On the deep side, the "floor" was 2 feet or so below them. Infants who appreciated depth would not crawl from the shallow to the deep side.

SOURCE

Gibson, E., & Walk, R. (1960). The "visual cliff." *Scientific American, 202,* 64–72.

QUICK LOOK AT THE CHAPTER AHEAD

- At about the beginning of the third week of pregnancy, the first signs of the fetus's nervous system appear.
- Neural induction causes a portion of the ectoderm to become the neural plate, which leads to the formation of the nervous system.
- The neural plate forms a groove and begins to fold in on itself, leading to the creation of the neural tube.
- Developmental biologists believe that neurons know which part of the brain they will travel to and which type of nerve cell they will become (e.g., motor, vision, hearing).
- The speed of nervous system development is stunning. To produce the 100 billion neurons of the adult brain, nerve cells are produced at the rate of 250,000 per minute during pregnancy.

25

Brain Development

TERMS
- ☐ Brain lateralization
- ☐ Cell migration
- ☐ Frontal lobe
- ☐ Glia
- ☐ Neural induction
- ☐ Neural tube
- ☐ Neurogenesis
- ☐ Neurons
- ☐ Occipital lobe
- ☐ Parietal lobe
- ☐ Temporal lobe

Any aspect of development—physical, emotional, cognitive, or psychosocial—depends on the intricacy of the brain for its optimal development. In spite of today's sophisticated technology, just how many neurons develop in the course of a lifetime is not known. Nevertheless, the rapid development of the nervous system is reflected in the following numbers:

- 200 billion brain cells develop in the fetus's brain by the fifth month.
- 100 billion **neurons** (brain cells) survive in a newborn baby's brain.
- 1 trillion **glia** (support) cells appear in a baby's brain.
- 1000 trillion connections are formed in a baby's brain.

What causes the fetus to lose 100 billion brain cells in the space of the 4 remaining months of pregnancy? The answer lies in nature's overproduction of brain cells or neurons. Those neurons that *do not* make connections simply die. This startling fact recalls Darwin's famous belief in the survival of the fittest: The fittest of our neurons are those that make connections and survive.

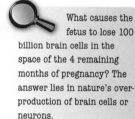

What causes the fetus to lose 100 billion brain cells in the space of the 4 remaining months of pregnancy? The answer lies in nature's overproduction of brain cells or neurons.

These amazing figures testify to an infant's potential for processing information. For example, the appearance of new cognitive abilities is correlated with rapid brain growth, both of which are major features of infancy.

BEGINNINGS OF BRAIN DEVELOPMENT

The beginning of brain development (about the 3rd prenatal week) lies in a process called **neural induction**, when a chemical signal from the mesoderm to the ectoderm triggers the onset of nervous system development (**Figure 25-1**). Nerve cells proliferate rapidly in the **neural tube**, but quickly leave this area and commence a sometimes lengthy, tortuous, and even perilous journey to the region of the brain where they will become functional. This phase, called **cell migration,** begins during the 7th prenatal week. During their passage, the nerve cells may double back, twist, and turn—some will even die. In their migration, the nerve cells continue to grow and develop and acquire their familiar neuronal shape. Those destined for survival reach their point of destination and become functional.

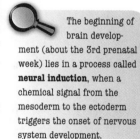

The beginning of brain development (about the 3rd prenatal week) lies in a process called **neural induction,** when a chemical signal from the mesoderm to the ectoderm triggers the onset of nervous system development.

During infancy, connections among the neurons begin to increase notably; as many as 100 to 1000 connections form for each of the billions of neurons. This growth rate translates into a brain size of approximately 0.5 lb at birth to 1.5 lb at the end of the first year and then to 3 lbs by 5 years (adult size). This amazing complexity provides the biological basis for cognitive development.

During infancy, connections among the neurons begin to increase notably; as many as 100 to 1000 connections form for each of the billions of neurons.

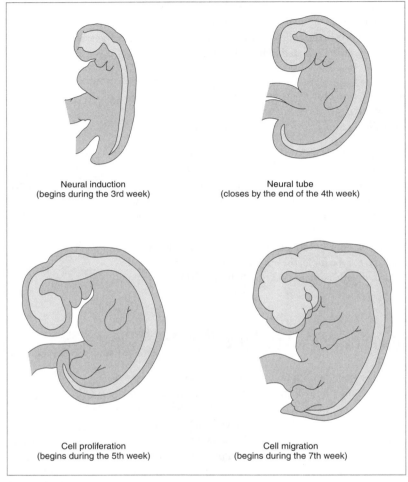

Neural induction
(begins during the 3rd week)

Neural tube
(closes by the end of the 4th week)

Cell proliferation
(begins during the 5th week)

Cell migration
(begins during the 7th week)

Figure 25-1 The Timing of Brain Development

CONTINUATION OF BRAIN DEVELOPMENT

Nervous system development begins during the embryonic period, when neurons reproduce at a rapid rate. The baby's brain at birth is approximately one-fourth of its adult size. It is 50% of its adult weight at 6 months, 60% at 1 year, 75% at 2 years, 90% at 6 years, and 95% at 10 years. In other words, while the brain takes 2½ years to grow to 75% of its adult weight, in another 3½ years growth increases only by 15%.

In the first 2 years following birth, brain development follows a definite pattern. Different parts develop at different rates:

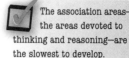

* The motor area is the most advanced (for survival purposes), followed in descending order by the sensory area, the visual area, and the auditory area.
* The association areas—the areas devoted to thinking and reasoning—are the slowest to develop.
* By the age of 2 years, growth in the sensory area slows and the association area shows signs of rapid development.

The association areas— the areas devoted to thinking and reasoning—are the slowest to develop.

Each of the brain's four lobes (frontal, parietal, temporal, and occipital) exercises specialized functions. For example, the **frontal lobe** contains the motor area for control of the skeletal muscles, the **parietal lobe** seems to be the controlling center for the body's sense areas, the **temporal lobe** manages auditory functions, and the **occipital lobe** analyzes visual information.

Each of the brain's four lobes (frontal, parietal, temporal, and occipital) exercises specialized functions.

Another example of startling new breakthroughs in brain research, called **neurogenesis**, is the ability to grow new brain cells to replace damaged brain cells (in mice). It was long thought that brain cells, once damaged, could never be replaced. Recent research has discovered that neural brain cells migrate through the brain, attach to damaged nerves, and transform themselves into the appropriate nerve cells. As a result, the future looks brighter for sufferers of such diseases as Parkinson's disease and amytrophic lateral sclerosis (Lou Gehrig's disease).

BRAIN LATERALIZATION

The stroke unit of any hospital offers powerful evidence of the effects of hemispheric brain damage. A stroke involves a stoppage of blood flow to a certain area of the brain, resulting in damage to that spot. Usually only one side of the brain is affected, and stroke victims are typically paralyzed on either the left or the right side of the body. In patients with right-side paralysis, the stroke damaged the left side of the brain; in patients with left-side paralysis, the damage was done to the right side of the brain.

It was not until the latter part of the 19th century, however, that right-side paralysis plus loss of speech was formally linked to damage to the left hemisphere. It took even longer to recognize the contributions that the right hemisphere makes to human functioning.

Language is an excellent example of **brain lateralization** because language entails the combining of discrete elements—letters, syllables, and words. In 95% to 99% of right-handed people and 70% of left-handed people, language is lateralized to the left side of the brain. Babbling studies suggest that brain lateralization for language is present before children begin to speak and is more than simple motor exercise.

A stroke involves a stoppage of blood flow to a certain area of the brain, resulting in damage to that spot.

IMPLICATIONS FOR HEALTHCARE PROVIDERS

For healthcare providers, it is important to recognize that brain development is not complete at birth. To ensure continued growth, the brain requires appropriate stimulation from the environment. In your work with infants, observe how the parents talk to their child. This interaction is a major stimulator during these early years and has a dynamic, effective influence on nervous system development. Urge parents to vary stimulation—auditory, visual, tactile—in their infant's surroundings, thereby providing a rich texture for brain development.

SOURCES

Andreasen, N. (2001). *Brave new brain*. New York: Oxford University Press.

Campbell, N., & Reece, J. (2005). *Biology*. New York: Pearson/Cummings.

Eliot, L. (2000). *What's going on in there? How the brain and mind develop in the first five years of life*. New York: Bantam.

- "Sensorimotor" refers to infants' ability to interact with the physical environment using their bodies and, as they do, to develop increasingly effective cognitive structures.
- There are six substages of the sensorimotor period.
- Primary circular reactions describes the repetition of motor acts involving infants' own bodies (sucking their fingers).
- Secondary circular reactions mean that infants use their own bodies to act on the environment (shaking a rattle).
- Coordination of secondary circular reactions refers to use of one action to help achieve another action (pushing a toy out of the way to get to a piece of cake).
- Tertiary circular reactions are repetitions, but with a variation as infants explore the environment's possibilities. Dropping a toy on a rug produces a different sound from dropping it on a wood floor.
- Representational thought is the ability to picture objects , places, and events in the mind.
- Object permanence refers to an infant's understanding that an object exists when out of sight.

26

Cognitive Development

TERMS
- ☐ Causality
- ☐ Cognitive structures
- ☐ Coordination of secondary circular reactions
- ☐ Egocentrism
- ☐ Habituate
- ☐ Object permanence
- ☐ Primary circular reactions
- ☐ Recall memory
- ☐ Representational thought
- ☐ Secondary circular reactions
- ☐ Sensorimotor
- ☐ Spatial relationships
- ☐ Tertiary circular reactions
- ☐ Time

The competent infant is born ready to learn, and learning promotes development of the brain. Infants demonstrate learning by organizing their behavior in response to stimuli. To make sense of stimuli and to overcome the limitations of **egocentrism** (seeing the world only from their viewpoint), they coordinate information using their sensory, physical, mental, and perceptual abilities. Did you ever wonder what infants think about as they lie in their cribs? Probably not, but Piaget did—and his research made a lasting impression on studies of cognitive development.

PIAGET'S SENSORIMOTOR PERIOD

By **sensorimotor**, Piaget meant that mental life begins with infants' ability to interact with the physical environment using their bodies and, as they do, to develop increasingly effective **cognitive structures**. (Think of cognitive structures as blueprints that allow us to organize and adapt to our world.) Physical actions are joined by a growing awareness of how behavior affects the environment. There are four accomplishments in this period:

> By **sensorimotor**, Piaget meant that mental life begins with infants' ability to interact with the physical environment using their bodies and, as they do, to develop increasingly effective **cognitive structures**.

- **Spatial relationships**—in and out, up and down, near and far
- **Time**—before and after
- **Causality**—cause and effect, one event leads to another
- **Object permanence**—objects exist when out of sight **(Figure 26-1)**

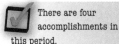

There are four accomplishments in this period.

There are six substages of the sensorimotor period:

Substage 1 (0–6 weeks [neonate]): reflexes. Infants' behavior is based on inborn reflexes, such as sucking, rooting, and grasping.

Substage 2 (1–4 months): **primary circular reactions**. As infants gain more motor control over their own bodies (primary), they repeat movements (circular) just for the sake of doing so (e.g., sucking their fingers, kicking their legs).

Substage 3 (4–8 months): **secondary circular reactions**. Infants use their bodies to act on the physical environment (secondary), repeating actions (circular) because they produce a desired effect. Infants realize they can make things happen. Examples include shaking a rattle, hitting a hanging toy to make it swing, and patting and squeezing toys.

Substage 4 (8–12 months): **coordination of secondary circular reactions**. One action is performed as a means of achieving another action. Babies can think one step ahead, which is highly adaptive when they can crawl or cruise. An example is pushing an object out of the way to get a toy.

Substage 5 (12–18 months): **tertiary circular reactions**. Actions are performed to learn about the possible relationship between different actions and objects. The busy toddler is experimenting with effects. For example, a ball, a block, and a cat bounce differently when you drop them down the stairs. Tossing the same toy with different amounts of force also produces different effects.

Substage 6 (18–24 months): beginning of **representational thought**. Representational thought is the ability to picture objects, places, and events in the mind. It is related to language development. Toddlers think about actions and their consequences based on previous experience, and adjust their behavior accordingly. For example, toddlers may place their cup away from the edge of the table so that it will not fall.

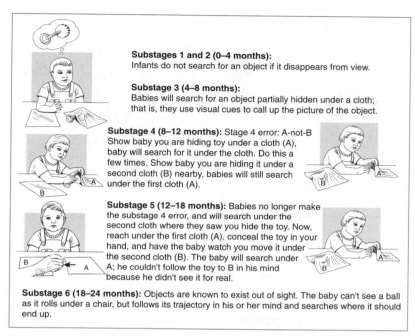

Substages 1 and 2 (0–4 months):
Infants do not search for an object if it disappears from view.

Substage 3 (4–8 months):
Babies will search for an object partially hidden under a cloth; that is, they use visual cues to call up the picture of the object.

Substage 4 (8–12 months): Stage 4 error: A-not-B Show baby you are hiding toy under a cloth (A), baby will search for it under the cloth. Do this a few times. Show baby you are hiding it under a second cloth (B) nearby, babies will still search under the first cloth (A).

Substage 5 (12–18 months): Babies no longer make the substage 4 error, and will search under the second cloth where they saw you hide the toy. Now, reach under the first cloth (A), conceal the toy in your hand, and have the baby watch you move it under the second cloth (B). The baby will search under A; he couldn't follow the toy to B in his mind because he didn't see it for real.

Substage 6 (18–24 months): Objects are known to exist out of sight. The baby can't see a ball as it rolls under a chair, but follows its trajectory in his or her mind and searches where it should end up.

Figure 26-1 Development of Object Permanence According to Piaget

Piaget's theory has been challenged by other researchers, who found that infants develop some cognitive abilities earlier than Piaget thought. Piaget's theory was built on observations of children, especially his own, whereas others tested infants under more structured research conditions. The type of task that is used to measure what infants know shapes the findings.

OTHER RESEARCH

One way to study infant cognition is to rely on infants' inborn tendency to pay attention to a novel stimulus and then to **habituate** to it; that is, infants lose interest when the stimulus is no longer new and renew interest when the stimulus changes again. Studies are also based on contingency-seeking behavior; that is, infants look for events that go together. When infants respond to events based on previous experience, it implies they can organize, store, and retrieve their experience of events cognitively.

Memory

At 3 months, infants can remember a contingency for as long as a week, and as much as a month later if given a visual cue. For example, if taught to make a mobile move by kicking one leg, which is attached to the mobile by a ribbon, infants will kick again a week later.

> At 3 months, infants can remember a contingency for as long as a week, and as much as a month later if given a visual cue.

A month later, if the babies are shown the mobile one day, the next day they begin kicking immediately when the ribbon is attached, indicating they used a visual cue to remind themselves.

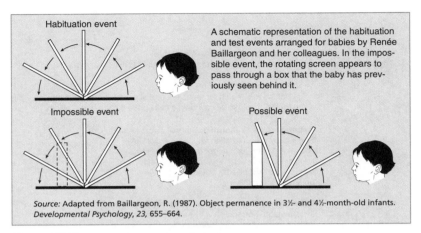

A schematic representation of the habituation and test events arranged for babies by Renée Baillargeon and her colleagues. In the impossible event, the rotating screen appears to pass through a box that the baby has previously seen behind it.

Source: Adapted from Baillargeon, R. (1987). Object permanence in 3½- and 4½-month-old infants. *Developmental Psychology, 23,* 655–664.

Figure 26-2 Object Permanence Experiment

Recall memory, in which visual cues are not used to remember something, improves during the second half of the first year, a period of considerable brain development (see Chapter 25). Short-term memory grows from 2 to 10 seconds. By 9 months, babies' long-term memory for novel events extends to a day. They can imitate a simple action that they witnessed yesterday, such as pressing a button to make a noise. By the time babies are crawling, they make mental maps of their surroundings and remember where furniture should be.

Object Permanence

Piaget thought that infants did not have object permanence until at least 18 months (see Figure 26-1); others disagreed. Try this experiment with a 4-month-old child. Place a block on a table and put a screen in front of it within view of the baby (**Figure 26-2**). If the screen falls forward, the baby can still see the block. If the screen falls backward, its fall is stopped by the block against which it will rest; the baby

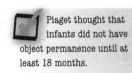

Piaget thought that infants did not have object permanence until at least 18 months.

cannot see the block. Secretly remove the block so that the screen falls backward all the way. The baby will stare at this seemingly impossible event, suggesting knowledge that the block should still be present to stop the screen.

Remember, Piaget's tests for object permanence required infants to physically search for objects he had hidden. Piaget did not consider the roles that neurological development, memory, or infants' impulsiveness to repeat a rewarding contingency might play in the stage 4 error.

SOURCES

Bjorklund, D. (2005). *Children's thinking.* Belmont, CA: Wadsworth.

Dacey, J., Travers, J., & Fiore, L. (2008). *Human development across the lifespan* (7th ed.). New York: McGraw Hill.

Siegler, R., & Alibali, M. (2005). *Children's thinking.* Upper Saddle River, NJ: Prentice Hall.

QUICK LOOK AT THE CHAPTER AHEAD

- The acquisition of language is one of the most stunning achievements of humans.
- With no formal instruction and often exposed to faulty language models, children nevertheless learn words, meanings, and ways to combine them to communicate with others.
- Children throughout the world go through exactly the same process of language development.
- Key signs of language development appear during the infancy period (e.g., cooing, babbling).
- Children begin to speak their first words from 10 to 13 months of age.
- Holophrases refer to children using one word to convey multiple meanings.
- Telegraphic speech refers to sentences of two or three words.

27

Language Development

One of the most amazing accomplishments of infancy is the beginning of actual speech. The sounds, the words, the two- and three-word sentences, and the tremendous explosion of vocabulary are stunning achievements that we still do not fully understand. Infants have no way of knowing what adults are trying to say. Without an understanding of what linguistic symbols are and how they work, speech is just noise. Yet with no formal learning and often exposed to dramatically faulty language models, children nevertheless learn words, meanings, and ways to combine them in a purposeful manner.

ACQUIRING LANGUAGE

Children in all parts of the world go through a process in which they first emit sounds, then single words, then two words, and finally fairly complex sentences (**Table 27-1**). By the time they are approximately 5 years of age, they have acquired the basics of their language, an astonishing accomplishment. Here is an example, using English.

> Children in all parts of the world go through a process in which they first emit sounds, then single words, then two words, and finally fairly complex sentences.

If I said to you, "Will you please *park* your car in the *driveway*?", you would probably know exactly what I mean. When you leave, I tell you that the quickest way home is to *drive* on the *parkway*. Again, you understand exactly what is meant here. Despite the switch in words, children easily master such intricacies of language.

Or consider this: After you finish reading this section, take a break and have dinner. I suggest that you eat some *ghotti*—it's always so tasty and it's good for you. If you follow my advice, what will you be having for dinner? Put it all together: *gh* as in "tough," *o* as in "women," *ti* as in "nation"—you'll have a delicious *fish* dinner.

The well-known commentator on language development, Lois Bloom (2000), has identified several transitions that help to explain children's amazing language achievements:

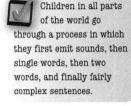

> The well-known commentator on language development, Lois Bloom (2000), has identified several transitions that help to explain children's amazing language achievements.

- The first transition occurs at the end of the first year and continues in the second year with the appearance of words and the acquisition of a basic vocabulary.
- The second transition occurs when children change from saying only one word at a time to combining words into phrases and simple sentences at about the end of the second year.

Table 27-1   Phases in Language Development

Language	Age
Crying	From birth
Cooing	2–5 months
Babbling	5–7 months
Single words	12 months
Two words	18 months
Phrases	2 years

* The final transition occurs when children move beyond using simple sentences to express one idea to complex sentences.

KEY SIGNS OF LANGUAGE DEVELOPMENT

Babies continue to learn the sounds of their language throughout the first year. As the neuropsychologist Steven Pinker (1994) has noted, not much of linguistic interest happens in the first 2 months. Often the coughs, cries, and hiccups during this time disturb the parents of a firstborn, but they are reflective noises indicating the baby's general physical condition.

Too much individual variation exists to say that all children babble at 5 months, or that all children utter their first words at 11 months. Babies begin **cooing** (vowel-like sounds intermingled with consonants) at the end of the second month and into the third. At about 3 or 4 months, infants begin to combine vowels and consonants to produce syllable-like sounds: *mu*, *ba*, and so forth. Between 5 and 7 months, these sounds appear with increasing frequency, marking the beginning of **babbling**. Babbling probably appears initially because of biological maturation. At 7 and 8 months, sound-like syllables appear—*da-da-da*, *ba-ba-ba* (a phenomenon occurring in all languages)—a pattern that continues for the remainder of the first year.

Late in the babbling period (usually by 9 or 10 months), children use consistent and specific sound patterns to refer to objects and events. These **vocables** suggest children's discovery that meaning is associated with sound. For example, a lingering "L" sound may mean that someone is at the door.

 Late in the babbling period (usually by 9 or 10 months), children use consistent and specific sound patterns to refer to objects and events.

 Too much individual variation exists to say that all children babble at 5 months, or that all children utter their first words at 11 months.

First Words

Most children begin to speak their first words from the ages of 10 to 13 months. About half of these words are for objects (food, clothing, toys). This one-word stage may last 2 months to 1 year and has a strong relationship to words used by the mother, such as "bye-bye" or "see da-da."

At 18 months, children acquire words at the rate of one new word every 2 hours, a condition that lasts until about age 3 years and is frequently referred to as the **word spurt**. Vocabulary constantly expands, but estimating the extent of a child's vocabulary is difficult because youngsters know more words (their comprehension) than they say (their production). Estimates are that a 1-year-old child may use from 2 to 6 words, whereas a 2-year-old has a vocabulary ranging from 50 to 250 words. Children at this stage also begin to combine two words.

Most children begin to speak their first words from the ages of 10 to 13 months. About half of these words are for objects (food, clothing, toys). This one-word stage may last 2 months.

At 18 months, children acquire words at the rate of one new word every 2 hours, a condition that lasts until about age 3 years and is frequently referred to as the **word spurt**.

Holophrases

You will notice a subtle change before the two-word stage: Children begin to use one word to convey multiple meanings. For example, youngsters say "ball," meaning "give me the ball," "throw the ball," or "watch the ball roll." They have now gone far beyond merely labeling this round object as a ball. Often called holophrastic speech (use of one word to communicate many meanings and ideas), this phenomenon is difficult to analyze. These

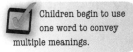

Children begin to use one word to convey multiple meanings.

first words, or **holophrases**, are usually nouns, adjectives, or self-inventive words and often contain multiple meanings.

Telegraphic Speech

At 18 to 24 months, simple two- and three-word sentences appear. Children primarily use nouns and verbs (not adverbs, conjunctions, or prepositions), and their sentences demonstrate grammatical structure. The initial multiple-word utterances (usually two or three words: "Timmy runs fast") are called **telegraphic speech**. Telegraphic speech contains considerably more meaning than what superficially appears in the two or three words.

IMPLICATIONS FOR HEALTHCARE PROVIDERS

If you find yourself working with children of this age, we urge you to consider the following points:

- Be certain that the infant's hearing ability is normal. Children of this age should be able to distinguish speech sounds and turn toward the sound of a voice.
- Have family members help you interpret the infant's gestures and sounds.
- Use the developmental sequence presented here to help you understand the meaning of the infant's babbling and single words.
- If the infant and family are from a different culture with a different language, obtain help with both language and any cultural practices that are important for the child's recovery.

SOURCES

Bloom, L. (2000). Language acquisition in its developmental context. In W. Damon (Series Ed.) & D. Kuhn & R. Siegler (Volume Eds.), *Handbook of child psychology: Volume 2, Cognition, perception, and language.* New York: John Wiley.

Pinker, S. (1994). *The language instinct.* New York: Morrow.

- Children from birth begin to interpret surrounding environmental stimulation such as parental treatment.
- A relationship implies a pattern of interactions between two people over time.
- Parental behaviors have their roots in many sources, a phenomenon frequently referred to as "ghosts in the nursery."
- Temperament refers to a child's behavioral style when interacting with the environment.
- Goodness of fit is linked to the demands and expectations of parents and the child's temperament and abilities.
- Parents and their children develop a style of interacting that is the beginning of social development.

28

First Relationships

TERMS

- ☐ **Difficult children**
- ☐ **Easy children**
- ☐ **Ghosts in the nursery**
- ☐ **Goodness of fit**
- ☐ **Reciprocal interactions**
- ☐ **Relationship**
- ☐ **Slow-to-warm-up children**
- ☐ **Temperament**

Children from birth seek stimulation from their environment and instantly interpret how they are being treated. This process is called **reciprocal interactions (Figure 28-1)**; that is, infants react to the way they are treated and they change accordingly. As a result of the changes in babies, those persons around the infants (usually the parents) also change.

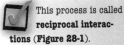 This process is called **reciprocal interactions (Figure 28-1)**.

Infants are ready to respond to social stimulation. It is not just a matter of responding passively, however: Infants in their own way initiate social contacts. Many of their actions (such as turning toward the mother or gesturing in her direction) are forms of communication. Those around infants may try to attract their attention, but the babies actively select from these adult actions. In other words, infants begin to structure their own relationships according to their own unique temperaments.

WHAT IS A RELATIONSHIP?

A **relationship** implies a pattern of interactions between two people over an extended period of time. A child's relationships incorporate many aspects of development:

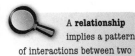 A **relationship** implies a pattern of interactions between two people over an extended period of time.

- *Physical aspects*, such as walking, running, and playing with a peer
- *Language aspects*, which enable youngsters to share their lives
- *Cognitive aspects*, which allow them to understand one another
- *Emotional aspects*, which permit them to make a commitment to another
- *Social aspects*, which reflect both socialization and individuation

In other words, a relationship is a superb example of the influence of biopsychosocial interactions.

There are many dimensions to a relationship: the role that parents see themselves playing, their behavior, their perceptions, and their feelings for their child. What parents say or do is significant, but how their child perceives and judges that behavior is even more important. Children are excellent judges of how they are being treated.

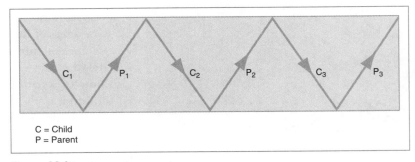

C = Child
P = Parent

Figure 28-1 Reciprocal Interactions

Ghosts in the Nursery

The manner in which parents were treated by their own parents, their observation of those individuals whom they consider good parents, and their reading about parenting strongly influence what they see as their parental role. Selma Fraiberg (1959), a well-known child psychiatrist, referred to the presence of **ghosts in the nursery**, which can have many consequences.

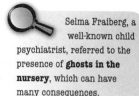

Selma Fraiberg, a well-known child psychiatrist, referred to the presence of **ghosts in the nursery**, which can have many consequences.

For example, some parents feel *their* parents looking over their shoulder and telling them how to bring up their child—ideas that they may well have rejected or even rebelled against. Does their child remind them of someone from the past, and do they begin to react to their child as they did to that other person? Or do the parents tend to imitate a friend whom they admire? Or have they been impressed by the ideas of some "expert" they have read about or seen on television? The encouraging conclusion is that in spite of these findings, when parents are aware that ghosts from the past may influence them, they are able to overcome these relics and move on to form positive relationships with their children.

Children's Temperament

Parental expectations as to role, however, is merely one of many influences on a relationship. **Temperament** refers to a child's unique behavioral style when interacting with the environment. Differences in temperament become obvious in the first days and weeks after birth and have an immediate and decided impact on reciprocal interactions. Even mothers of identical twins report that they can distinguish their babies by the differences in their reactions to faces, voices, various colors, and so on.

Temperament refers to a child's unique behavioral style when interacting with the environment.

Today's acceptance of the importance of inborn temperament reflects the work of two child psychiatrists, Stella Chess and Alexander Thomas (1987).

To test their ideas, Chess and Thomas conducted what came to be called the New York Longitudinal Study (NYLS), a study of 141 middle-class children. They found that they could draw a behavioral profile of the children by age 2 or 3 months. Certain characteristics clustered with sufficient frequency for the authors to identify three general types of temperament:

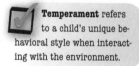

To test their ideas, Chess and Thomas conducted what came to be called the New York Longitudinal Study (NYLS), a study of 141 middle-class children.

- **Easy children**, characterized by regularity of bodily functions, low or moderate intensity of reactions, and acceptance of, rather than withdrawal from, new situations (40% of the children)
  Difficult children, characterized by irregularity in bodily functions, intense reactions, and withdrawal from new stimuli (10% of the children)
- **Slow-to-warm-up children**, characterized by a low intensity of reactions and a somewhat negative mood (15% of the children)

Difficult children, characterized by irregularity in bodily functions, intense reactions, and withdrawal from new stimuli (10% of the children)

The authors were able to classify 65% of the infants, leaving the others with a mixture of traits that defied neat categorization. Chess and Thomas also found that a **goodness of fit** existed when the demands and expectations of parents were compatible with their child's temperament, abilities, and other characteristics.

Today's research testifies to the possibility of changes in the expression of temperament over time. A child's family, the social environment, socioeconomic status, and cultural influences together weave a network of external forces that contribute to the shaping of temperament over the years.

 # CHARACTERISTICS OF DEVELOPING RELATIONSHIPS

Three motives seem to be at work in the development of relationships:

> Three motives seem to be at work in the development of relationships.

- *Bodily needs*—food, for example—lead to a series of interactions that soon become a need for social interaction.
- *Psychological needs* can cause infants to interrupt one of their most important functions, such as feeding. Children, from birth, seem to seek novelty; they require increasingly challenging stimulation. For infants, adults become the source of information as much as the source of bodily need satisfaction.
- *Adult response needs* reflect that adults satisfy needs, provide stimulation, and initiate communication, thereby establishing the basis for future social interactions.

The rhythm of the interactions between parents and their babies marks the beginning of the children's social development. Discussing these initial interactions, the prominent pediatrician ⊠T. Berry Brazelton and the child psychoanalyst Bert Cramer (1990) identified several characteristics that identify a successful relationship (**Figure 28-2**).

Characteristic	Meaning
Synchrony	Refers to parents' ability to adjust their behavior to that of their children
Symmetry	Refers to an infant's capacity for attention and style of responding, which uniquely influence any reciprocal interactions
Contingency	Refers to the effect parents' behavior has on their infant's emotional state
Entrainment	Refers to the rhythm established between parents and infants
Autonomy	Refers to the time when infants realize they have a share in controlling the interactions (about 6 months of age)

Figure 28-2 Parent–Child Interactions

IMPLICATIONS FOR HEALTHCARE PROVIDERS

As a healthcare provider working with infants, be alert to the quality of the relationships that these babies have with their families. Given what we know today about the effects that emotions have on health, you will want to do as much as possible to provide a warm, supportive environment for infants. If you feel your options are limited in working with families, do not hesitate to turn to qualified counseling services.

SOURCES

Brazelton, T. B., & Cramer, B. (1990). *The earliest relationship*. Reading, MA: Addison-Wesley.

Chess, S., & Thomas, A. (1987). *Know your child*. New York: Basic Books.

Fraiberg, S. (1959). *The magic years*. New York: Charles Scribner's & Sons.

- Attachment is the special bond between an infant and another person, usually the mother, which develops in the first 6 months of life.
- Attachment is generally accepted as the foundation of social development.
- John Bowlby is usually regarded as the initial main influence in the attachment movement.
- Mary Salter Ainsworth devised the "strange situation" technique to study attachment.
- The Adult Attachment Interview, created by Mary Main (1996), was designed to assess the relationship of parents with their own parents.

29

Attachment

TERMS

- ☐ Adult Attachment Interview
- ☐ Ambivalently attached infants
- ☐ Attachment
- ☐ Avoidantly attached infants
- ☐ Despair
- ☐ Detachment
- ☐ Disorganized/disoriented
- ☐ Protest
- ☐ Securely attached infants
- ☐ Strange situation

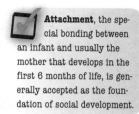

Attachment, the special bonding between an infant and usually the mother that develops in the first 6 months of life, is generally accepted as the foundation of social development. Attachment figures are secure bases that encourage infants to explore their environments but remain reliable retreats when stress and uncertainty appear. Infants who develop a secure attachment to their mother have the willingness and confidence to seek out future relationships. **Table 29-1** presents the developmental stages of attachment.

> **Attachment**, the special bonding between an infant and usually the mother that develops in the first 6 months of life, is generally accepted as the foundation of social development.

THE NATURE OF ATTACHMENT

John Bowlby (1969) and his colleagues observed a number of young children aged 15 to 30 months who not only were separated from their mothers, but also for weeks or months were cared for in hospitals or nurseries where they had no mother substitute. A predictable sequence of behaviors followed:

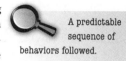

> A predictable sequence of behaviors followed.

1. **Protest**, the first phase, appeared immediately and persisted for about 1 week. Loud crying, extreme restlessness, and rejection of all adult figures marked an infant's distress.

Table 29-1 The Development of Attachment

Age	Characteristics	Behavior
4 months	Perceptual discrimination, visual tracking of mother	Smiles and vocalizes more with mother than anyone else; shows distress at separation
9 months	Separation anxiety; stranger anxiety	Cries when mother leaves; clings at appearance of strangers
2–3 years	Intensity and frequency of attachment behavior remain constant	Notices impending departure, indicating a better understanding of surrounding world
3–4 years	Growing confidence, tendency to feel secure in a strange place with subordinate attachment figures (relatives)	Begins to accept mother's temporary absence; plays with other children
4–10 years	Less-intense attachment behavior, but still strong	May hold parent's hand while walking; anything unexpected causes child to turn to parent
Adolescence	Weakening attachment to parents; peers and other adults become important	Becomes attached to groups and group members
Adult	Attachment bond still discernible	In troubled times, adults turn to trusted friends; elderly direct attention toward younger generation

Source: Adapted from Bowlby, J. (1982). Attachment and loss. *Am J Orthopsychiatry* 52:664-678. Reprinted with permission from the *American Journal of Orthopsychiatry*. Copyright © 1982 by the American Orthopsychiatry Association, Inc.

2. **Despair**, the second phase, followed next. Infants demonstrated a growing hopelessness: monotonous crying, inactivity, and steady withdrawal.

3. **Detachment**, the final phase, materialized when an infant displayed renewed interest in the surroundings, but it was a remote, distant kind of interest.

Bowlby believed that attachment is any form of behavior that results in a person attaining or maintaining proximity to some other clearly identified individual who is perceived as better able to cope with the world. He also thought that while attachment is most obvious in infancy and early childhood, it can be observed throughout the life cycle.

THE STRANGE SITUATION

Mary Salter Ainsworth (1973) devised the **strange situation** technique to study attachment. Ainsworth brought a mother and her infant to an observation room. The child was placed on the floor and allowed to play with toys. A stranger (female) then entered the room and began to talk to the mother. Observers watched to see how the infant reacted to the stranger and to what extent the child used the mother as a secure base. The mother then left the child alone in the room with the stranger; observers then noted how distressed the child became. The mother returned, and the quality of the child's reaction to the mother's return was assessed again. Next the infant was left completely alone, followed by the stranger's entrance, and then the entrance of the mother. These behaviors were used to classify children as follows:

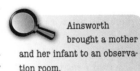

Ainsworth brought a mother and her infant to an observation room.

- **Securely attached infants** were secure and used the mother as a base from which to explore. These mothers were warm and consistently displayed sensitive responsiveness. During separation, the children exhibited considerable distress, ceased their explorations, and at reunion sought contact with their mothers.

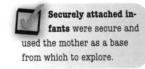

Securely attached infants were secure and used the mother as a base from which to explore.

- **Avoidantly attached infants** rarely cried during separation and avoided their mothers at reunion. The mothers of these babies were casual, almost indifferent, to their babies, while the babies seemed to dislike any physical contact with their mothers.

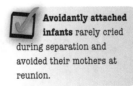

Avoidantly attached infants rarely cried during separation and avoided their mothers at reunion.

- **Ambivalently attached infants** manifested anxiety before separation and were intensely distressed by the separation. These mothers were erratic with their babies, often attentive, but not sensitively responsive. On reunion, the babies displayed ambivalent behavior toward their mothers; they sought contact but simultaneously seemed to resist it.

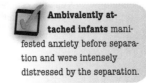

Ambivalently attached infants manifested anxiety before separation and were intensely distressed by the separation.

- **Disorganized/disoriented infants** manifested confused behavior on being reunited with their mothers. They often looked at the mother, then looked away in a disinterested manner.

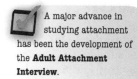

Disorganized/ disoriented infants manifested confused behavior on being reunited with their mothers.

By age 7 or 8 months, when attachment behavior (as defined by Bowlby and Ainsworth) normally appears, infants are attached to both mothers and fathers and prefer either parent to a stranger.

RECENT RESEARCH INTO ATTACHMENT

A major advance in studying attachment has been the development of the **Adult Attachment Interview**. During a 1-hour interview, participants are asked to furnish five adjectives describing their relationship to each of their own parents. Later during the interview, they are asked to give memories of specific incidents supporting these earlier answers. **Table 29-2** illustrates the way in which the answers are categorized.

A major advance in studying attachment has been the development of the **Adult Attachment Interview**.

Researchers are also focusing on the relationship between early attachment and children's drawings and stories in middle childhood. When presented with instances of children who were separated from their mothers, secure 6-year-olds tend to make up positive, constructive responses about the child in the story. By contrast, disorganized children typically give frightened responses: "The mother is going to die" or "The girl will kill herself."

Studies have shown an association between the way a mother recalls her childhood experiences and the present quality of the relationship with her children. Women who had been securely attached have securely attached children. Fathers also contribute substantially to the financial, social, and emotional healthy development of their children, but not by physical presence alone. The effect of a father's role in his child's life—especially a nurturing, caring father to whom the child is attached—cannot be overlooked.

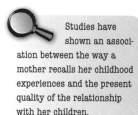

Studies have shown an association between the way a mother recalls her childhood experiences and the present quality of the relationship with her children.

Table 29-2 Adult Attachment Interview

Adult Attachment Interview	Strange Situation Response
Secure, autonomous—Coherent; values attachment; accepts any unpleasant, earlier experience	Secure
Dismissing—Positive statements are unsupported or contradicted; they claim earlier unpleasant experiences have no effect	Avoidant
Preoccupied—Seems angry, confused, passive, or fearful; some responses irrelevant	Resistant-ambivalent
Unfocused, disorganized—Loses train of thought during discussion of loss or abuse; lapses in reasoning (speaks of dead people as alive)	Disorganized/disoriented

Source: Adapted from Dacey, J., & Travers, J. (1999). *Human development across the lifespan* (4th ed.). New York: McGraw-Hill.

IMPLICATIONS FOR HEALTHCARE PROVIDERS

The contacts with mothers and their infants give nurses an opportunity to model desirable behaviors (talking to the baby, nurturing, recognizing clues to a baby's behavior). It is also an ideal time to share ideas with the mother—an exchange of views that many women find both supportive and instructive. These exchanges can be particularly valuable if the infant is preterm or ill. If the attachment process is interrupted by a hospital stay, then considerable care should be taken to explain techniques that parents can adopt to sustain the attachment process, and what to expect with regard to their own feelings and behaviors and those of their baby.

SOURCES

Ainsworth, M. (1973). The development of infant–mother attachment. In B. Caldwell & H. Ricutti (Eds.). *Review of child development research*, (pp. 1–94). Chicago: University of Chicago Press.

Bowlby, J. (1969). *Attachment*. New York: Basic Books.

Main, M. (1996). Introduction to the special section on attachment and psychopathology: Overview of the field of attachment. *Journal of Consulting Clinical Psychology, 64,* 237–242.

QUICK LOOK AT THE CHAPTER AHEAD

- Modern theorists view emotions as a complicated mixture of contributions from the brain, the body, and the environment.
- Emotions appear rapidly at varying intervals following birth.
- The circumstances that elicit the various emotions change with age.
- Emotional development seems to move from the general to the specific.
- Emotions also have a key adaptive function in motivating, organizing, and regulating behavior.
- Two-month-old infants are referred to as "smilers."

30

Emotional Development

TERMS
- ☐ **Adaptive behavior**
- ☐ **Emotion**
- ☐ **Emotional differentiation**

151

Children's emotions were long thought to be an important part of child development and in need of detailed study. Interest waned as investigators realized that neither theories nor research were sufficiently reliable to reach definite conclusions. In the last decade, however, enthusiasm about emotions and their development has returned and sparked renewed studies and speculation. Current views of emotions consider not only the brain's role in emotional development, but also the contributions of body and the environment. As psychiatrist Joseph Ratey (2001) notes, emotion is messy, complicated, primitive, and undefined because it is all over the place, intertwined with cognition and physiology.

In the last decade, however, enthusiasm about emotions and their development has returned and sparked renewed studies and speculation.

THE NATURE OF EMOTIONS

Daniel Goleman (1995, p. 289) defined **emotion** as "a feeling(s) and its distinctive thoughts, psychological and biological states, and range of propensities to act." Goleman also presented several categories of emotions, together with representative members of each family:

Anger: fury, resentment, animosity
Sadness: grief, sorrow, gloom, melancholy
Fear: nervousness, apprehension, dread, fright
Enjoyment: happiness, joy, bliss, delight
Love: acceptance, trust, devotion, adoration
Surprise: shock, astonishment, amazement, wonder
Shame: guilt, embarrassment, mortification, humiliation

Another well-known student of emotional development, Carroll Izard (1991), proposed this definition: "An emotion is experienced as a feeling that motivates, organizes, and guides perception, thought, and action." Careful examination of these definitions shows that emotion consists of three components:

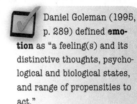

Daniel Goleman (1995, p. 289) defined **emotion** as "a feeling(s) and its distinctive thoughts, psychological and biological states, and range of propensities to act."

Another well-known student of emotional development, Carroll Izard (1991), proposed this definition: "An emotion is experienced as a feeling that motivates, organizes, and guides perception, thought, and action."

1. The *feeling* that the emotion engenders: Feelings may range from pleasant to unpleasant, from enjoyment to rejection. You can induce some of the signs of an emotion—quickened breath, rapid heartbeat—but if pleasure or distress does not accompany these signs, it probably is not emotional behavior.
2. The *internal changes* associated with an emotional reaction (e.g., changes in blood pressure and heart rate).
3. The emotional *behavior* itself: Humans express emotional feelings by definite and specific behavioral reactions, such as laughing, crying, and looking sad.

SIGNS OF EMOTIONAL DEVELOPMENT

What elicits children's emotions changes at different ages (**Table 30-1**). Six-month-old children show amusement when tickled by their mothers, which is far different from a 16-year-old's amuse-

Table 30-1 The Development of Emotions

Age	Emotion
Birth	Ability to express emotions
1–3 months	Distress, rage, beginning of social smile
4–6 months	Sadness, disgust, fear
7–9 months	Joy, anger, fear, separation, and stranger anxiety

ment at a funny story told by a friend. Both may be labeled as "amusement," but the emotion is not the same. As children grow, the circumstances that elicit an emotion change radically.

Emotional development seems to move from the general to the specific. General positive states differentiate into such emotions as joy and interest; general negative states differentiate into fear, disgust, or anger. These primary emotions emerge during the first 6 months of life. Sometime after 18 months, secondary emotions that are associated with a child's growing cognitive capacity for self-awareness appear.

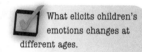
What elicits children's emotions changes at different ages.

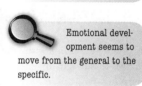
Emotional development seems to move from the general to the specific.

The classic **emotional differentiation** is illustrated in **Table 30-2** (Bridges, 1932). A general state of excitement is the basic emotion at birth, which is followed quickly by a differentiation into pleasant and unpleasant emotions. The various specific emotions continue to develop until they are recognized as responses to specific stimuli (e.g., anger at the removal of a toy). Other research by Izard and Ackerman (2000) suggests that a few discrete emotions appear early in life: joy, interest, sadness, anger, fear, and disgust. Izard also stresses that each of these emotions has a unique adaptive function in motivating, organizing, and regulating behavior (**adaptive behavior**), both alone and in emotion patterns. Izard also points out that each emotion plays a significant role in the development of personality and individual differences.

Emotionally, infants begin to acquire a sense of trust in those around them. This ability reaches a peak between ages 4 and 6 months (Greenspan, 1995). During these months, children who experience upsetting conditions (rough handling, chaotic feeding patterns, overstimulation) learn that they cannot depend on their environment. Mistrust begins to develop.

At about 6 months, children start to react to the facial expressions of those around them, to read body language, and to recognize any tensions in their surroundings. Gradually their nonverbal communication skills sharpen. They begin to understand the basics of human interactions from about 12 to 18 months (Greenspan, 1995).

Table 30-2 Excitement—from Birth

Distress—shortly after birth	Delight—about 3 months
Anger, disgust, fear—about 4–6 months	Elation—about 8 months
Jealousy—about 12 months	Affection for adults—about 10 months
	Affection for children—about 15 months
	Joy—from 18–24 months

THE SMILE

A baby's smile is one of the first signs of emotion. Most parents immediately interpret a smile as a sign of happiness. In reality, early smiles do not have the social significance of the smile that emerges at about 6 weeks. These early smiles are usually designated as "false" smiles because they lack the emotional warmth of the true smile. By the baby's third week, the human female voice elicits a brief, real smile. By the 6th week, the true social smile appears, especially in response to the human face. By 2 months infants are often referred to as "smilers."

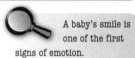

A baby's smile is one of the first signs of emotion.

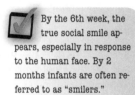

By the 6th week, the true social smile appears, especially in response to the human face. By 2 months infants are often referred to as "smilers."

IMPLICATIONS FOR HEALTHCARE PROVIDERS

In your interactions with your clients, you will encounter a wide range of emotions, from fear and anxiety to outright anger. Recognizing the components of emotion—feelings, internal changes, and behavior—will guide your reactions to a person's behavior. Your analysis of the emotions expressed will help you decide whether support, encouragement, or firmness is needed. By maintaining an open and honest relationship with clients, you will be able to help them not only with their physical problems, but also with any emotional difficulties.

SOURCES

Bridges, K. (1932). Emotional development in early infancy. *Child Development, 3,* 324–334.

Goleman, D. (1995). *Emotional intelligence.* New York: Bantam.

Greenspan, S. (1995). *The challenging child.* Reading, MA: Addison-Wesley.

Izard, C. (1991). *The psychology of emotions.* New York: Plenum.

Izard, C., & Ackerman, B. (2000). Motivational, organizational, and regulatory functions of discrete emotions. In M. Lewis & J. Haviland-Jones (Eds.), *Handbook of emotions* (pp. 253–264). New York: Guilford.

Ratey, J. (2001). *A user's guide to the brain.* New York: Pantheon.

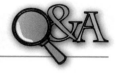

PART III · QUESTIONS

For each of the following questions, choose the **one best** answer.

1. At what point after birth do typical infants double their birth weight?
   a. 3 months
   b. 6 months
   c. 9 months
   d. 12 months

2. You notice that a new mother feeds her baby boy by propping a bottle on a pillow next to him. Why do you want to discourage this practice?
   a. The baby will have difficulty regulating the flow of formula.
   b. The baby is not learning how to organize his behavior.
   c. The mother and the baby are not learning to read each other's signals.
   d. All of the above are correct.

3. You observe a baby lying on her abdomen, raising her head, shoulders, and upper abdomen while supporting herself with her forearms. About how old is this baby?
   a. 6 weeks
   b. 8 weeks
   c. 3 months
   d. 6 months

4. A new mother who is breastfeeding her baby asks you if her baby can see her. What is your answer?
   a. "No. Babies cannot see clearly until they are about 6 weeks old."
   b. "Yes. Babies have 20/20 vision at birth."
   c. "No. Visual acuity is about 20/100 at birth."
   d. "Yes. Objects that are within close range, especially your face, are perfectly clear."

5. Apgar scores are recorded at 1 and 5 minutes after birth. What do they measure?
   a. Heart rate, respiratory effort, muscle tone, reflex irritability, and skin color
   b. First and second periods of reactivity
   c. Behavioral states: sleeping, waking, and crying
   d. Gestational maturity, such as flexion of extremities, quality of skin, and development of eyes, ears, and genitals

6. Which of the following is an example of contingency seeking in newborns?
   a. Infants learn to adjust their rate of sucking by using the mother's voice as a reward.
   b. Infants prefer complex patterns of black and white.
   c. Newborns discriminate their mother's voice from the voices of other women.
   d. Infants turn their head to search for a sound.

7. The final area of the brain to develop is the
   a. occipital lobe.
   b. association area.
   c. sensory area.
   d. auditory area.

8. Nervous system development commences in a process called
   a. neural induction.
   b. tubular processes.
   c. neural migration.
   d. neuronal balance.

9. Human infants exhibit reflexes because
   a. their nervous systems are not fully mature.
   b. some infant reflexes are building blocks for voluntary motor behavior.
   c. some reflexes are designed to protect them from potential harm.
   d. of all of the above.

10. To elicit the Babinski reflex, you stroke the sole of a baby's foot, beginning at the heel and moving toward the toes. The toes flex, as if they are going to grab your finger. Is this normal?
    a. No. If the baby is younger than 1 year, the toes should fan out and extend.
    b. Yes. If the baby is older than 1 year, the toes will flex.
    c. Both A and B are true.
    d. Neither A nor B is true.

11. According to Piaget, what are the four accomplishments of the sensorimotor period?
    a. Rolling over, sitting up, crawling, and walking
    b. Time, spatial relationships, cause and effect, and object permanence
    c. Visual acuity, binocular vision, depth perception, and spatial relationships
    d. Primary circular reactions, secondary circular reactions, coordination of secondary circular reactions, and tertiary circular reactions

12. You are watching a baby who is sitting up in her mother's lap. The baby is playing with a box of animal crackers, by shaking it, hitting it on the arm of the chair, and patting the lid with her hand. What age range and what substage of Piaget's sensorimotor period is this baby in?
    a. Age 1–4 months, primary circular reactions
    b. Age 4–8 months, secondary circular reactions
    c. Age 8–12 months, coordination of secondary circular reactions
    d. Age 18–24 months, beginning of representational thought

13. When parents feel that other adults, including their own parents, are looking over their shoulder and telling them how to bring up their child, this phenomenon is called
    a. ghosts in the nursery.
    b. generational interest.
    c. parental transference.
    d. social sharing.

14. Most children begin to speak their first words at an age of approximately
    a. 6 months.
    b. 12 months.
    c. 18 months.
    d. 24 months.

15. Which of the following statements is incorrect?
    a. Children instantly tune into their environment.
    b. Children give clues to their personalities.
    c. Children, from birth, engage in reciprocal interactions.
    d. All children are temperamentally similar at birth.

16. *Role* refers to _____ about behavior.
    a. observations
    b. insights
    c. expectations
    d. comments

17. The special bonding between an infant and usually the mother is called
    a. detachment.
    b. attachment.
    c. relating.
    d. symmetry.

18. The person most associated with the attachment movement is
    a. Sigmund Freud.
    b. B. F. Skinner.
    c. Jean Piaget.
    d. John Bowlby.

19. The three components of an emotion are feelings, internal changes, and
    a. behavior.
    b. continuity.
    c. congruence.
    d. assimilation.

20. The true social smile appears at an age of approximately
    a. 4 weeks.
    b. 6 weeks.
    c. 8 weeks.
    d. 10 weeks.

PART III • ANSWERS

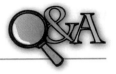

1. **The answer is b.** The average newborn in the United States weighs 3.27 kg. Infants gain 680 g per month until about age 5 to 6 months, by which time their birth weight has doubled. Birth weight triples by the end of the first year, to approximately 10 kg.

2. **The answer is d.** Feeding, especially breastfeeding, is a learned behavior that contributes to self-regulation in infants and to sensitive responding in mothers. Mothers and infants learn to coordinate supply and demand of milk, especially during the first few weeks of life. This give-and-take requires that mothers learn to read infants' signals of hunger, fatigue, distress, and satisfaction. As infants learn to regulate the flow of milk, they also learn to organize their own behavior. Feeding, especially at the breast, helps them to calm down and focus. An attentive infant in the arms of a responsive mother is ready to interact with her, to focus his or her eyes on her face, and to listen to her voice.

3. **The answer is c.** Head control is a good indicator of brain maturation. Newborns cannot lift their heads until they are 6 weeks old, and then do so briefly. By 3 to 4 months, they raise their head, shoulders, and upper abdomen while supporting themselves on their forearms. When newborns are pulled to sit, their head falls back. Head lag decreases and infants have steady head control by 5 to 6 months, when they can sit with support.

4. **The answer is d.** At birth, visual acuity is about 20/100 and steadily improves. Newborns can see and fixate on objects within 20 cm of the center of their bodies. Thus objects within close range, such as the mother's face, are perfectly clear. A preference for patterns is evident within hours after birth. Patterns that are somewhat complex and that have moving parts, especially the human face, are of greatest interest.

5. **The answer is a.** Apgar scores are used as a rough assessment of immediate adjustment to extrauterine life. Heart rate, respirations, muscle tone, reflexes, and skin color are assessed at 1 and 5 minutes after birth, with each being given a score of 0, 1, or 2. Total scores less than 3 indicate severe distress. Scores of 4 to 6 signify moderate difficulty, and scores of 7 to 10 indicate no difficulty adapting to extrauterine life. Apgar scores are affected by prematurity and maternal medication, but are not indicative of the presence or absence of neurological or physical abnormalities.

6. **The answer is a.** Newborn behavior has four characteristics. Inborn physiological mechanisms, such as reflexes, enhance survival. Newborns organize their behavior in response to stimuli (e.g., turning their head in response to a sound). They respond selectively to certain stimuli (e.g., patterns of light and dark). Newborns demonstrate contingency-seeking behavior; that is, they look for predictability in the environment, for events that go together. In a classic experiment, DeCasper and Fifer demonstrated that infants learn to adjust their rate of sucking by using the mother's voice as a reward. That is, infants learned that hearing their mother's voice was contingent on how fast they sucked on a pacifier.

7. **The answer is b.** The complex cognitive activities that slowly appear throughout development are rooted in the association area and testify to the interaction between body and mind.

8. **The answer is a.** Once neural induction begins, the nervous system development process is swift and steady. Any interference with the process (disease, chemicals) can produce serious damage.

9. **The answer is d.** The CNS is not fully developed at birth, but rather continues to grow, re-organize, and mature. The specialized regions that give rise to reflexes are found in the more primitive areas of the CNS, such as the spinal cord, brain stem, and cerebellum. Some adaptive infant reflexes are building blocks for voluntary motor behaviors that develop with experience and with maturity of the cortical regions of the brain. Thus reflexes can also provide a window into neurological development because they should change as the nervous system matures. Finally, some reflexes—such as blinking—are permanent and persist throughout life; these reflexes are designed to protect humans from potential harm.

10. **The answer is c.** The Babinski reflex is an example of how reflexes change as the nervous system matures. In infants, the toes fan out and extend, and there is dorsiflexion of the big toe. By age 1 year, the reflexive fanning out disappears and is replaced by the mature response found in children and adults: The toes flex when the sole of the foot is stroked.

11. **The answer is b.** By "sensorimotor," Piaget meant that mental life begins with infants' ability to interact with the physical environment using their bodies. Physical actions are accompanied by a growing awareness by infants of how their behavior affects the environment. The four accomplishments of this period are (1) spatial relationships—in and out, up and down, near and far; (2) time—before and after; (3) causality—cause and effect, one event inevitably leads to another; and (4) object permanence—objects exist when out of sight.

12. **The answer is b.** During the substage of secondary circular reactions (age 4 to 8 months), infants use their bodies to act on the physical environment (secondary), repeating actions (circular) because they produce a desired effect. Infants realize they can make things happen. Examples include shaking a rattle, hitting a hanging toy to make it swing, and patting and squeezing toys.

13. **The answer is a.** With personal experience and interest generated by television and child-rearing books, many adults unknowingly interfere in parenting. Almost all parents are able to move beyond these unwelcome intrusions and develop healthy relations with their children.

14. **The answer is b.** Although first words usually are spoken at approximately 1 year, parents should not be disturbed if language is delayed. The best advice is to watch this phase of development carefully and seek advice if any delay is worrisome.

15. **The answer is d.** Research has shown that children's personalities are unique from birth. This conclusion offers clues for parents to use in establishing positive interactions with their children.

16. **The answer is c.** People associate certain characteristics with individuals, tasks, occupations, and so forth. They then formulate expectations about these characteristics.

17. **The answer is b.** Most developmental psychologists believe that attachment is the basis for social development. Once again, the importance of the initial interactions between parent and child is emphasized.

18. **The answer is d.** Bowlby's work on children's first relationships made psychologists aware of the significance of the initial interactions for future social development.

19. **The answer is a.** We judge emotional behavior by what we see. Emotions are characterized by specific types of behavior—joy, sadness, and so forth.

20. **The answer is b.** Many developmental features come together at approximately 6 weeks for babies to display a true social smile. In addition, psychosocial and cognitive factors interact to enable a baby to display the smile.

IV

Early Childhood

QUICK LOOK AT THE CHAPTER AHEAD

- During the early childhood years, the rate of physical growth slows.
- Muscles and bones are not fully developed, which has strong implications for participation in athletic activities.
- Hand–eye coordination improves noticeably, and fine motor ability continues to progress.
- Growth and organization of the brain leads to an increase in the number of dendrites and synapses.
- As children come to the end of the early childhood period (about 6 years of age), their brains are approximately 90% of the final adult weight.
- The great task of the brain during the early childhood years is to form connections.
- Developmental delay is a problem for some children.

31

Growth and Motor Development

TERMS

- ☐ Dendrites
- ☐ Developmental delay
- ☐ Handedness
- ☐ Neocortex
- ☐ Neurons
- ☐ Synapses
- ☐ Visuomotor development

The rate of growth slows during the preschool years. Children gain about 2.3 kg (5 lb) each year and grow taller by 6.0 to 7.5 cm (2 to 3 inches) per year (**Table 31-1**). Although few physical differences between boys and girls are evident during this time, there is increasing variability among individual children.

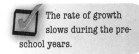

The rate of growth slows during the preschool years.

While most of the increase in height occurs in the legs, the chubby pot-bellied body of the toddler gives way to a more slender and posturally erect profile. Preschoolers are better coordinated than their younger selves. By age 3, children are walking, running, jumping, and climbing well. Their sense of balance improves markedly. A 3-year-old can stand on one foot for a few seconds; by age 4, the same child is hopping around on one foot. At 3 years, most children are riding a tricycle; by 6 years, many have mastered riding a two-wheel bike. At 3 years, children can go upstairs using alternating feet, but still descend placing both feet on each step. By age 4, they descend using alternating feet, holding the railing. At age 6, they are running up and down stairs easily (**Table 31-2**).

Muscles and bones are not yet fully developed, however. While most preschoolers appear sturdy, able, and motivated, they are not physically ready for athletic activities that require endurance and coordination for sustained periods of time. This age group is also reckless owing to a lack of judgment and impulsiveness. Injuries are the leading cause of death between ages 1 and 4.

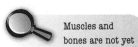

Muscles and bones are not yet fully developed, however. While most preschoolers appear sturdy, able, and motivated, they are not physically ready for athletic activities that require endurance and coordination for sustained periods of time.

Fine motor skills also improve markedly as preschoolers use their hands as tools. They enjoy projects that involve finger painting, working with Play-Doh, pasting, and coloring. They build with blocks, put together large-piece puzzles, and zoom little cars around toy villages. They button and zip, although tying shoelaces takes much practice.

VISUOMOTOR DEVELOPMENT: HAND-EYE COORDINATION AND DRAWING

Vision is 20/20 by age 4. Children also become more efficient and proficient in how they move their eyes to scan a page, an ability essential for reading readiness. At age 3, when asked to find an object

Table 31-1 Height and Weight Measurements: 50th Percentiles

| | Boys | | Girls | |
Age (yr)	Height (cm)	Weight (kg)	Height (cm)	Weight (kg)
2½	90.4	13.53	90	13.03
3	94.9	14.62	94.1	14.1
3½	99.1	15.68	97.9	15.07
4	102.9	16.69	101.6	15.96
4½	106.6	17.69	105	16.81
5	109.9	18.67	108.4	17.66
6	116.1	20.69	114.6	19.52

Table 31-2 Motor Development

Age	Gross Motor	Fine Motor	General Physical
3	Rides tricycle Jumps, climbs, kicks Stands on one foot for a few seconds Goes up stairs alternating feet, down using two feet	Builds tower of nine cubes Adept at placing pellet into a narrow-necked bottle In drawing, copies strokes Draws a face using a circle Uses fork	Average weight 14.6 kg (32 lb) Average height 95 cm (37.2 in) May have achieved night-time control of bowel and bladder Vision is 20/30
4	Skips, hops on one foot Catches a ball with two hands Walks down stairs alternating feet	Uses kiddie scissors Can lace shoes, cannot tie In drawing, copies square Adds three parts to stick figure	Average weight 16.7 kg (37 lb) Average height 103 cm (40.5 in) Length at birth is doubled Vision is 20/20
5	Skips, hops alternating feet Jumps rope Ice skates with balance Throws, catches ball well	Uses scissors, pencil well Ties shoelaces, buttons Draws stick figure Prints some letters/numbers	Average weight 18.7 kg (41 lb) Average height 110 cm (43 in) Handedness is established May start to lose baby teeth
6	Very active physically Runs up and down stairs May ride bicycle Throws ball overhand	Cuts, folds, pastes Uses knife to spread jam Knows right from left Likes to draw, color	Weight 16–23 kg (35–58 lb) Height 106–123 cm (42–48 in) Permanent teeth erupting, can brush them

or the page of a book, children initially scan haphazardly, looking here and there. Systematic scanning side to side and up and down develops between ages 3 and 6.

 Vision is 20/20 by age 4.

The combination of perceptual development and fine motor development (**visuomotor development**) produces the ability to hold a pencil or crayon for the purposes of drawing, tracing, and copying pictures, letters, and numbers. Three-year-old children can copy a picture of a circle and will draw crude facial features in it; left to themselves, however, they scribble. By age 4, they will copy a square and are more adept at tracing shapes, such as a cross or diamond. While not adept at drawing human stick figures, they can add a few parts, such as arms and legs, to one partially drawn for them. At age 5, they add more detail to stick figures, such as fingers, hair, and earrings. In kindergarten, children can copy most basic shapes, and trace and print numbers and letters.

 # BRAIN DEVELOPMENT

Developmental psychologists agree that brain development begins within weeks of conception and continues through adolescence, displaying a pattern of nonlinear changes that commence in the early childhood period. Changes in brain development during the early childhood period show an increase in the number of **dendrites**, accompanied by growth in the number of **synapses** formed, which helps to explain the increasing cognitive ability of children of this age. Thus the neural foundation is being formed for children to develop more connections, providing a network to facilitate further cognition and learning.

> Developmental psychologists agree that brain development begins within weeks of conception and continues through adolescence, displaying a pattern of nonlinear changes that commence in the early childhood period.

For example, **handedness**, improvement in fine and gross motor skills, and advances in cognitive development (see Chapter 32) are related to maturational changes in the brain and spinal cord. Neural development is of two kinds: growth and organization. The number of synapses and amount of myelin increase in several major areas of the brain simultaneously between ages 2 and 5, with a spurt occurring between 5 and 7 years. At age 3, the brain is 50% of its adult weight; by age 6, it has reached 90% of the final adult weight. How the different areas communicate with one another and coordinate activity accounts for behavioral changes.

Consider the example of riding a bike. Improvement in balance is attributed not just to growth of the cerebellum (more synapses), but also to its ability to organize information about where the body is in space and how it is moving based on signals from the muscles, the joints, the semicircular canals of the inner ear, and the perceptual systems (vision, hearing, sensation). The ability to regain balance rests in the thalamus, which in coordination with the **neocortex** regulates arousal by calling attention to relevant information, such as changes in road surface. This development means a 6-year-old can learn to ride a two-wheel bike, whereas a 3-year-old cannot.

The neocortex is the last part of the human brain to evolve but accounts for 75% of its **neurons**. It is responsible for higher-level functions, such as thought and emotion. The neocortex is divided into right and left hemispheres. The great task of the early childhood years is to form connections. During these years, children absorb information from the outside world through their eyes, ears, nose, hands, and so on, and translate this information into nerve impulses. These impulses then travel along neural pathways and make connections with other neurons. The brain cells that receive this information survive; those that do not die.

> The neocortex is the last part of the human brain to evolve but accounts for 75% of its **neurons**.

> The brain cells that receive this information survive; those that do not die.

DEVELOPMENTAL DELAY

Developmental delay refers to a significant lag in one or more of four areas: gross motor coordination, fine motor and visuomotor coordination, language, and social skills. Delays in fine motor and visuomotor skills may not become apparent until the preschool years, but can complicate developmental progress in other areas. Children who have difficulty building with blocks or cutting and pasting typically also have trouble playing with peers, which can lead to frustration and inappropriate behaviors. Developmental screening is routinely done as part of well-child visits during the preschool years.

> **Developmental delay** refers to a significant lag in one or more of four areas: gross motor coordination, fine motor and visuomotor coordination, language, and social skills.

SOURCES

Ratey, J. (2001). *A user's guide to the brain.* New York: Pantheon.

Springer, S., & Deutsch, G. (1997). *Left brain, right brain: Perspective from cognitive neuroscience.* New York: Freeman.

QUICK LOOK AT THE CHAPTER AHEAD

- The early childhood years are synonymous with Piaget's preoperational period.
- Children's mental lives expand noticeably during these years.
- The outstanding mental achievement of these years is the growing ability to represent people, things, objects, and events.
- Children of these years tend to focus on only one aspect of something, a characteristic known as centration.
- Conservation remains a problem for children at this cognitive level.
- Early-childhood youngsters begin to master the notion of classification.
- Explanations of causality are linked to association without distinguishing cause and effect.

32

Cognitive Development I

TERMS
- ☐ **Causality**
- ☐ **Centration**
- ☐ **Classification**
- ☐ **Conservation**
- ☐ **Preoperational**
- ☐ **Representation**

The physical changes discussed in Chapter 31 are not the only significant developmental advances occurring during the early childhood years. The mental lives of these children expand considerably as they extend their formation and use of ideas and demonstrate startling growth in their language development and usage. To help us better understand what is happening in the cognitive world of these children, we turn once again to Piaget.

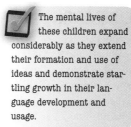

The mental lives of these children expand considerably as they extend their formation and use of ideas and demonstrate startling growth in their language development and usage.

PREOPERATIONAL PERIOD

Piaget referred to the period from ages 2½ to 6 as **preoperational** (or "prelogical") because it precedes the period of concrete operations that is associated with the school-age years, roughly ages 7 to 11. Preschoolers think about things in ways that infants and toddlers do not: They represent ideas in their minds (**representation**). They recognize that physical events have explanations, although their explanations may not make sense. Preschool-aged children try to figure things out, but there are limitations in their ability to reason logically.

Preoperational thinking is referred to as "magical," meaning that children's ideas about how the world works can be quite fanciful and are not grounded in the principles of physics (**Table 32-1**). A young child truly believes he or she can disappear down the bathtub drain.

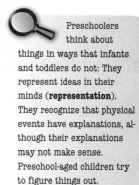

Preschoolers think about things in ways that infants and toddlers do not: They represent ideas in their minds (**representation**). They recognize that physical events have explanations, although their explanations may not make sense. Preschool-aged children try to figure things out.

Table 32-1 Preoperational Period

Characteristics	Examples
Centration	Focus on one aspect of something at a time (e.g., how much juice in a glass depends on either width or height, but not both).
Perceptually bound	Deal with appearances, cannot work out a problem in their minds; not impressed by magic tricks because they do not appreciate the trick.
Cause by association	If two events happen close together, one is assumed to have caused the other.
Lack of conservation: mass	Thinks a ball of clay gets bigger when it is rolled into a snake.
Lack of conservation: number	Given two rows of 10 M&Ms each, will say the row that is more spread out contains more.
Lack of conservation: quantity	Says the glass with the most juice is the taller one, even if the child just saw it poured from a shorter to wider glass.
Classification	Classify objects based on only one aspect (e.g., color, size).

CENTRATION

Preschool children focus on only one aspect of something at a time—often the most obvious aspect—and fail to consider how several aspects might interact to produce the event. This characteristic is termed **centration.** When pouring juice between a tall skinny glass and a short wide glass, for example, they focus on only the height of the tall skinny glass in concluding that it is "bigger" and so contains more juice. They cannot account for height and width simultaneously.

 Preschool children focus on only one aspect of something at a time—often the most obvious aspect—and fail to consider how several aspects might interact to produce the event.

 ## APPEARANCE-REALITY PROBLEM

Preschool children are perceptually bound; that is, they deal with what appears to be true. "What you see is what you get." Santa can be in the mall and on the sidewalk at the same time because they saw him in both places. The sun truly goes down into the ground at night.

 Preschool children are perceptually bound; that is, they deal with what appears to be true.

 ## CAUSE BY ASSOCIATION

Causality is explained in a circular fashion, without distinguishing between cause and effect. If two events appear to happen at the same time, one is believed to have caused the other, although children cannot explain how. Children believe they catch cold from being outside in winter. Cause by association also explains why some adults think AIDS can be transmitted by shaking hands—it can just happen.

 Causality is explained in a circular fashion. If two events appear to happen at the same time, one is believed to have caused the other, although children cannot explain how.

 ## DIFFICULTY WITH CONSERVATION

Conservation refers to the ability to understand that something remains the same even if its appearance is altered and nothing was seen to be taken away or added. Because preschool children are swayed by appearances, focus on one aspect of something at a time, and have difficulty working out events in their minds, they have difficulty with conservation tasks.

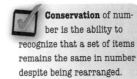 **Conservation** of number is the ability to recognize that a set of items remains the same in number despite being rearranged.

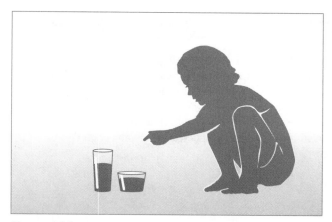

Figure 32-1 Conservation of Quantity Experiment

Conservation of number is the ability to recognize that a set of items remains the same in number despite being rearranged. Preschoolers are not so sure. For example, in an experiment to test for perceptually bound thinking and lack of conservation of number, present a child with two rows of M&Ms, with 10 candies in each row. In one row, bunch the M&Ms closely together. In the second row, spread them apart so that when side by side the second row extends beyond the first. Ask the child which row has more M&Ms. Why? The child will focus on the length of a row, deciding that the longer of two rows has "more." If small numbers of items—three or four items—are used, the child demonstrates conservation skills.

Conservation of quantity is recognizing that liquids take the form of their containers; a cup of water is a cup of water regardless of whether it is in a tall or short glass. Again, preschoolers will focus on the height of the tall glass in concluding it contains "more," even if children pour the water back and forth between the two glasses themselves (**Figure 32-1**). They cannot mentally reverse this action and conceptualize that the quantity of water stays the same. They also cannot compensate height for width.

Conservation of mass and/or length is the ability to understand that the appearance of solid objects can be altered, even though their mass and/or length remains the same. Preschoolers think that a ball of Play-Doh gets bigger when it is rolled into a snake. They are sure that a ball of string pulled out to its full length grows longer.

Conservation refers to the ability to understand that something remains the same even if its appearance is altered and nothing was seen to be taken away or added. Because preschool children are swayed by appearances, focus on one aspect of something at a time, and have difficulty working out events in their minds, they have difficulty with conservation tasks.

 Conservation of quantity is recognizing that liquids take the form of their containers; a cup of water is a cup of water regardless of whether it is in a tall or short glass.

Conservation of mass and/or length is the ability to understand that the appearance of solid objects can be altered, even though their mass and/or length remains the same.

CLASSIFICATION

If preschoolers were asked to help sort belongings from a closet, they might put a shoe and shirt together because they are both red, then add a blue belt because it has a buckle like the shoe. **Classification** is initially based on saliency—that is, what is obvious, what appeals at the time. By kindergarten, children begin to understand class inclusion. For example, shoes, sneakers, and boots are footwear; a shirt does not belong.

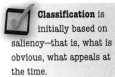

Classification is initially based on saliency—that is, what is obvious, what appeals at the time.

- Piaget's theory, which has been in existence for more than 70 years, has been constantly evaluated and found wanting in several respects.
- Studies have shown that children can achieve many cognitive tasks earlier than Piaget believed.
- As children move through Piaget's preoperational period, their cognitive skills steadily sharpen.
- Early-childhood youngsters begin to develop different types of memory strategies.
- Attention becomes more focused during these years.
- Early-childhood youngsters begin to develop a theory of mind.

33

Cognitive Development II

TERMS
- ☐ Encoding
- ☐ Information processing
- ☐ Neocortex
- ☐ Theory of mind

Piaget's theory, which has been in existence for more than 70 years, has been constantly evaluated and found wanting in several respects. Studies have repeatedly shown that early-childhood children possess greater intellectual competence than Piaget believed.

 Studies have repeatedly shown that early-childhood children possess greater intellectual competence than Piaget believed.

ALTERNATIVES TO PIAGET'S THEORY

Piaget's reliance on a verbal explanation of events is a major weakness in his theory. As noted in Chapter 26 on infant cognition, the nature of the task used to investigate how children think can influence the results. For example, compare two seriation tasks: ordering sticks according to length and stacking measuring cups inside of one another. For the sticks, children use trial and error, and cannot focus on two things at once—length of stick and its relationship to what is before and after it. Thus they tend to "complete" the task incorrectly. For the cups, there is only

 As noted in Chapter 27 on infant cognition, the nature of the task used to investigate how children think can influence the results.

one correct solution. The task tells them when they are wrong, and encourages children to "reverse" the results of incorrect trials—if not in their minds then with their hands. Children successfully seriate the cups because the task provides "error information"—that is, the big cup cannot fit into the little cup. Seriating sticks does not provide that kind of feedback.

During the preschool years, improvements occur in both how much children remember and how they remember it. Capacity improves because of maturation of the **neocortex** and the explosion in language skills. Words help children to construct a useful network of associations about things, a process called **encoding**. They store this network in long-term memory, which appears to be unlimited over their lifetimes. Short-term memory lengthens to 30 seconds but is limited to three to five pieces of information. The short-term capacity of an older child or adult is seven to nine pieces of information.

INFORMATION PROCESSING THEORY

As one example of alternative explanations, **information processing** theorists believe that cognitive development occurs by the improvement of cognitive processes such as attention and memory. Consequently, researchers examine which types of information children represent, how they process it, how these cognitive changes affect their behavior, and which psychological mechanisms are responsible for these changes.

 As one example of alternative explanations, **information processing** theorists believe that cognitive development occurs by the improvement of cognitive processes such as attention and memory.

For example, attention becomes increasingly important for early-childhood youngsters as they become more expert in focusing on pertinent information. As Siegler and Alibali (2005) note, the selectivity with which children focus their attention on relevant items increases substantially between 3 and 8 years of age.

Much the same holds true for memory. During the preschool years, children begin to develop efficient memory strategies such as rehearsal, organization, and retrieval, which improve markedly, but still are not as efficient as those in older children. Ask young children to remember a phone number: 555-1234. Seven digits exceeds their short-term capacity, and they have trouble chunking the number into two pieces of information—555 and 1234—which older children can do. To overcome these problems, they might rehearse it out loud. But a clue—the number starts with 555—will jog their memory. However, if the phone number is set to a familiar tune, children will remember it better because songs and music are stored whole in a different area of the brain.

Adults are often amazed by young children's memory. Keep in mind that preschoolers remember what they pay attention to and they pay attention to what is salient. Their network of associations can be fanciful. A 4-year-old girl will remember what you wore to a family wedding, but may forget whose wedding it was.

 Much the same holds true for memory. During the preschool years, children begin to develop efficient memory strategies such as rehearsal, organization, and retrieval, which improve markedly, but still are not as efficient as those in older children.

Keep in mind that preschoolers remember what they pay attention to and they pay attention to what is salient.

THEORY OF MIND

Clearly, their rapidly improving cognitive processes such as attention and memory help children to acquire a theory of mind. Many developmental psychologists believe that today's cognitive psychology is actually the psychology of children's **theory of mind**—that is, the beliefs, desires, knowledge, and thoughts of children's mental states. In other words, theory of mind describes children's understanding of other people's thoughts, desires, and emotional states, an ability that begins to emerge at about 2 to 3 years of age.

The noted cognitive psychologist John Flavell (1998) summarizes children's knowledge about mind as follows:

 Many developmental psychologists believe that today's cognitive psychology is actually the psychology of children's **theory of mind**—that is, the beliefs, desires, knowledge, and thoughts of children's mental states.

- Early-childhood youngsters come to realize that only people are capable of thinking.
- Thinking is an internal, "in-the-head" process.
- People can think about objects not present to them.
- Other people are also capable of thinking.

IMPLICATIONS FOR HEALTHCARE PROVIDERS

A preoperational explanation of illness is based on association of events. Bibace and Walsh (1981) note that an illness is described as its symptoms: A cold is when the nose runs; an external cause may be identified, but children cannot explain how cause leads to effect; a cold is from being outside in the winter; illness can "just happen," out of the child's control. Use associations to manage the treatment regimen: Take medicine at bedtime. Take their fears seriously.

SOURCES

Bibace, R., & Walsh, M. E. (1981). Development of children's concepts of illness. In R. Bibace & M. E. Walsh (Eds.), *New directions for child development: Children's concepts of health, illness, and bodily functions.* San Francisco: Jossey-Bass.

Flavell, J. (1998). Social Cognition. In D. Kuhn & R. Siegler (Eds.), *Handbook of Child Psychology: Volume 2. Cognition, perception, and language.* New York: John Wiley.

Siegler, R., & Alibali, M. (2005). *Children's Thinking.* Upper Saddle River, NJ: Prentice Hall.

 QUICK LOOK AT THE CHAPTER AHEAD

- Demand has grown for well-run early-education programs.
- Modern programs are a blend of both cognitive and social elements.
- The goals of these programs reflect today's realization of the importance of biopsychosocial interactions.
- Among the early proponents of early education programs was Maria Montessori.
- Piaget's ideas of cognitive development—particularly those of the preoperational period—have been widely adopted in preschool programs.
- Project Head Start originated from the federal government's attempt to eliminate poverty in the 1960s.

34

Early Childhood Education

TERMS

- ☐ Absorbent mind
- ☐ Biopsychosocial model
- ☐ Constructivism
- ☐ Developmentally appropriate
- ☐ Prepared environment
- ☐ Project Head Start
- ☐ Sensitive periods

The U.S. Department of Education has identified the "three Rs" of early childhood education:

1. *Relationships*, which refers to the need for loving relationships during the early childhood years to help develop children's sense of confidence and security
2. *Resilience*, which refers to a child's ability to meet challenges successfully
3. *Readiness*, which combines good health, positive schooling, and good schools

The growing demand for early education (preschool and kindergarten programs) is testimony to the critical importance of education during the early years. The National Association for the Education of Young Children (NAEYC) has defined an early childhood education program as any group program in a center, school, or other facility that serves children from birth through age 8 (Bredekamp & Copple, 1997).

Today's programs are not exclusively social or cognitive; typically elements of both occur in all programs (Dacey, Travers, & Fiore, 2008). **Developmentally appropriate** practices are based on data from three sources: child development and learning, the characteristics of individual children, and the contexts in which children develop.

The U.S. Department of Education has identified the "three Rs" of early childhood education:
1. *Relationships*, which refers to the need for loving relationships during the early childhood years to help develop children's sense of confidence and security
2. *Resilience*, which refers to a child's ability to meet challenges successfully
3. *Readiness*, which combines good health, positive schooling, and good schools

Developmentally appropriate practices are based on data from three sources: child development and learning, the characteristics of individual children, and the contexts in which children develop.

THE IMPORTANCE OF BIOPSYCHOSOCIAL INTERACTIONS

In today's early-childhood education programs, children are encouraged to learn through interacting with their environments and to be active participants in constructing knowledge. To help children achieve this goal, developmental psychologists have adopted a **biopsychosocial model** (**Table 34-1**).

Several important biological, psychological, and social characteristics affect growth during early childhood. Even more importantly, the interactions that occur among the three categories are crucial. To give a simple example, genetic damage (biological) may negatively affect cognitive development (psychological) and lead to poor peer relationships (social).

Among those who have contributed to the knowledge of developmentally appropriate practices for early childhood programs are Montessori and Piaget.

Even more importantly, the interactions that occur among the three categories are crucial.

MONTESSORI AND THE ABSORBENT MIND

Maria Montessori (1967) was a strong proponent of early childhood programs. Montessori believed that developing children pass through different physical and mental growth phases that al-

Table 34-1 Biopsychosocial Interactions

Bio	Psycho	Social
Genetics	Cognitive development	Attachment
Fertilization	Information processing	Relationships
Pregnancy	Problem solving	Reciprocal interactions
Birth	Perceptual development	School
Physical development	Language development	Peers
Motor development	Moral development	Television
Puberty	Self-efficacy	Stress
Menstruation	Personality	Marriage
Disease	Body image	Family

Source: Reprinted with permission from Dacey, J., & Travers, J. (1999). *Human development across the life-span* (4th ed.). New York: McGraw-Hill.

ternate with periods of transition. These phases, called **sensitive periods**, signify when children are especially ready for certain types of learning.

Montessori described three major periods of development: the absorbent mind phase, the uniform growth phase, and the adolescent phase. The **absorbent mind** phase, extending from birth to age 6, indicates a child's tremendous ability to absorb, rapidly and effortlessly, experiences from the environment.

From about 3 to 6 years, children mainly learn by doing. As they play with their Lego sets, for example, they manipulate the individual parts and begin to understand how things go together and how one series of actions becomes the basis for another.

Montessori, who worked with the poor children of Rome, suggested that a **prepared environment** was necessary because most children do not live in ideal surroundings. Children love order, and they receive satisfaction and develop feelings of security from perceiving and interacting with an ordered environment.

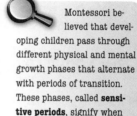 Montessori believed that developing children pass through different physical and mental growth phases that alternate with periods of transition. These phases, called **sensitive periods**, signify when children are especially ready for certain types of learning.

The **absorbent mind** phase, extending from birth to age 6, indicates a child's tremendous ability to absorb, rapidly and effortlessly, experiences from the environment.

 ## PIAGET AND PRESCHOOL PROGRAMS

Perhaps Piaget's main contribution to the development of early childhood programs was his recognition that children are quite different from adults in several important ways, especially their views of reality and their use of language. Because a child's world is qualitatively different from an adult's world the notion of developmentally appropriate practices takes on special meaning. Touching, feeling, and tasting are critical to cognitive development as children construct their own worlds (which is the meaning of **constructivism**).

Children who delight in swinging, in building castles in the sand, or in using the parallel bars are learning more than the muscular coordination needed to perform the exercise. They are also learning about the needed momentum to swing higher, about the texture of sand, or about the smoothness of the bar's metal. In a Piagetian-oriented preschool program, play and games are devised to promote physical, cognitive, and social development.

PROJECT HEAD START

During the 1960s, **Project Head Start** was begun with the intention of improving children's health, both physical and mental, and providing positive schooling. Today, approximately 50,000 Head Start classrooms in the United States serve 1 million children. These programs are designed with the goal of providing good preschool education: low teacher–child ratios, well-trained teachers, abundant resources, and child-centered activities. These goals are sought with the active help of parents and with the intent of meeting the social needs of both parents and children.

During the 1960s, **Project Head Start** was begun with the intention of improving children's health, both physical and mental, and providing positive schooling. Today, approximately 50,000 Head Start classrooms in the United States serve 1 million children.

IMPLICATIONS FOR HEALTHCARE PROVIDERS

The following guidelines offer a blueprint for working with early-childhood youngsters (Bredekamp & Copple, 1997):

- Create a caring community of learners. Developmentally appropriate practices support the development of relationships among children, adults, and families.
- Provide an interactive environment, one that encourages children to construct their own understanding of their world.
- Remember that children's development requires multiple, ongoing assessments that are directed at specific goals and reflect children's individual differences.
- If an early education program is to be successful, then detailed knowledge of children is vital. Parents are obviously a vital source of data, and a family-centered orientation with parents and professionals working together to achieve shared goals offers the most promising means of ensuring children's maximum growth.

SOURCES

Bredekamp, S., & Copple, C. (Eds.). (1997). *Develop mentally appropriate practice in early childhood programs.* Washington, DC: National Association for the Education of Young Children.

Dacey, J., Travers, J., & Fiore, L. (2008). *Human development across the lifespan.* (7th ed.). New York: McGraw-Hill.

Montessori, M. (1967). *The absorbent mind.* New York: Dell.

QUICK LOOK AT THE CHAPTER AHEAD

- Children are adept at using both receptive and expressive language.
- Learning language is an exercise in rule learning.
- Language development seems to follow a predictable pattern.
- In the course of acquiring their language, children experience several language irregularities.
- Children may determine the meaning of a word by a process called fastmapping.
- They also use a procedure called syntactic bootstrapping for word meaning.
- A process known as TESOL is used to help immigrant children learn English.

35

Language Development

TERMS

- ☐ **Expressive language**
- ☐ **Fastmapping**
- ☐ **Overextensions**
- ☐ **Overregularities**
- ☐ **Receptive language**
- ☐ **Syntactic bootstrapping**
- ☐ **Telegraphic speech**
- ☐ **TESOL**

From about ages 2 to 6 years, children's language undergoes a tremendous word spurt. This steady progression in vocabulary development is evident in **Table 35-1**. Children of 5 years seem to know about 2000 words, but that is not the limit of their vocabulary. These same children *understand* many more words than they use. From the first year, children demonstrate **receptive language** (i.e., they receive and understand the words). In early childhood, they produce language themselves, called **expressive language**.

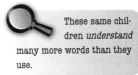

These same children *understand* many more words than they use.

Today, many schools in the United States are enrolling children of immigrant parents. In an effort to help with the inevitable language problems, a technique known as **TESOL** is being widely used to facilitate language development. TESOL refers to Teaching English to Speakers of Other Languages. Teachers are urged to use children's families and communities as resources when using the TESOL model.

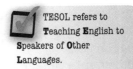

TESOL refers to **T**eaching **E**nglish to **S**peakers of **O**ther **L**anguages.

THE PROCESS OF LANGUAGE ACQUISITION

By the time they are ready to enter kindergarten, most children have a vocabulary of almost 10,000 words. They use questions, negative statements, and dependent clauses, and they have learned to use language in a variety of social situations. Children of this age detect the meaning of new words by using such techniques as **fastmapping**, which enables them to use the context of a sentence to discover a word's meaning, and **syntactic bootstrapping**, which means they use the grammatical structure of the entire sentence to determine a word's meaning.

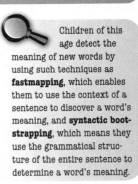

Children of this age detect the meaning of new words by using such techniques as **fastmapping**, which enables them to use the context of a sentence to discover a word's meaning, and **syntactic bootstrapping**, which means they use the grammatical structure of the entire sentence to determine a word's meaning.

Table 35-1 Pattern of Vocabulary Development

Age (years)	Number of Words
2	250+
2½	500+
3	1000
3½	1250
4	1600
4½	1900
5	2000
5½	2500
6	3000

LANGUAGE AS RULE LEARNING

Children deduce the rules they must follow to use words and put words together to make sentences. While this is going on, they are also learning the correct way to combine words—that is, the rules or grammar of their language. The rules describe the relationships between sounds, between words, between words and meaning, and between words and the purpose of communication. These rules (**Table 35-2**) make language a powerful human tool.

The number of sentences that can be generated from English, with its thousands of nouns, verbs, adjectives, adverbs, prepositions, and conjunctions, staggers the imagination.

THE PATTERN OF LANGUAGE DEVELOPMENT

During early childhood, children develop their language as follows:

- *Two years old:* Children's vocabularies expand rapidly, and simple two- and three-word sentences begin to appear: "Me go, Timmy eat." These sentences are referred to as **telegraphic speech**, and may contain multiple meanings. Children primarily use nouns and verbs, and their sentences show grammatical structure. They use the same organizational principles as adults.
- *Three years old:* Children are reaching the end of their word spurt. Although their sentences may sound ungrammatical, they are actually obeying the rules with astonishing regularity. They use correct word order and inflections where required. Three-year-olds, for example, master most constructions; they consistently obey language rules, and even their mistakes occur because they follow the rules *too* strictly ("Janey runned to the door").
- *Four years old:* Children have acquired the complicated structure of their native tongue, are using more complex sentences (four or five words), and ask ceaseless questions. (How many times have you been asked, "Why?" by a child of this age?)
- *Five to six years old:* As children come to the end of early childhood, they speak and understand sentences that they have never previously used or heard. They have become sophisticated language users—which is not to say that their language is flawless.

Table 35-2 Rules for Language

Rules	Meaning
Phonology	How to put sounds together to form words
Syntax	How to put words together to form sentences
Semantics	How to interpret the meaning of words
Pragmatics	How to take part in a conversation

LANGUAGE IRREGULARITIES

Certain irregularities are to be expected during these years. For example, **overextensions** mark children's beginning words. Assume that a child has learned the name of the house pet, "doggy." Think what that label means: an animal with a head, tail, body, and four legs. Now consider what other animals "fit" this label: cats, horses, donkeys, and cows. Consequently, children may briefly apply "doggy" to all four-legged creatures, but they quickly eliminate overextensions.

Overregularities are a similarly fleeting phenomenon. As youngsters begin to use two- and three-word sentences, they struggle to convey more precise meanings by mastering the grammatical rules of their language. For example, for many English verbs, the suffix *-ed* is added to indicate past tense: "I *want* to play ball." "I *wanted* to play ball." But for other verbs, the form is changed much more radically: "Did Daddy *come* home?" "Daddy *came* home." Most children, even after they have mastered the correct form of such verbs as come, see, and run, still add *-ed* to the original form. That is, youngsters who know that the past tense of *come* is *came* will still say, "Daddy *comed* home."

IMPLICATIONS FOR HEALTHCARE PROVIDERS

In working with children of this age, you should be alert to the possibility of hearing problems. Children use their hearing to learn the language and speech skills necessary for social interaction and academic success. Hearing-impaired children possess the same potential for acquiring language as other children, but they lack linguistic input, the raw material of language.

Estimates are that approximately 8% of Americans (more than 17 million children and adults) experience some form of hearing difficulty. Within this group, approximately 100,000 are preschool youngsters.

QUICK LOOK AT THE CHAPTER AHEAD

- Family life consists of complex interactions among several individuals.
- Different styles of parenting have been identified by Diane Baumrind.
- Authoritarian parents exercise absolute control over their children.
- Authoritative parents expect much from their children, but have more reasonable expectations.
- Permissive parents have a tolerant, accepting attitude toward their children's behavior and respond to their children's needs.
- Growing up with siblings creates a different type of family environment.
- Certain characteristics of both parents and children act as determinants of parental behavior.

36

Role of the Family

TERMS
- ☐ **Authoritarian parents**
- ☐ **Authoritative parents**
- ☐ **Context of parenting**
- ☐ **Permissive parents**
- ☐ **Siblings**

Analyzing and understanding today's families became a difficult task once researchers began to study developmental data from a systems perspective. Careful evaluation has led to a realization that family life reflects a complex interaction over time between the effects of the family environment, the personality and temperamental characteristics of children, genetic influences, and resilience factors of children, all of which have differential effects on individual children. When we consider the relationships that exist among these many variables, we realize that a family cannot be viewed merely as a collection of individuals, but rather must be seen as a system whose patterns of interactions become relatively stable.

> Careful evaluation has led to a realization that family life reflects a complex interaction over time between the effects of the family environment, the personality and temperamental characteristics of children, genetic influences, and resilience factors of children, all of which have differential effects on individual children.

Despite the many changes that have occurred in any definition of "family," the vast majority of individuals live in some type of "family." This testifies to the widely held belief in the strength of the family as the basic social structure.

PARENTING BEHAVIORS

Diane Baumrind's (1971) pioneering work on parenting styles has led to many insights into family life (**Table 36-1**).

Authoritarian parents aim to control their children's behavior by enforcing absolute standards for behavior. They value unquestioned respect for and compliance with authority, and they discourage verbal give-and-take with their children. Authoritarian parents resolve conflicts through power assertion; that is, they lay down the law "or else." They may be warm, but not responsive. Their children lack spontaneity, are overly polite, and develop an external locus of control, meaning that they perceive powerful others to be responsible for events. Thus personal initiative and prosocial behaviors are neither valued nor exhibited. Boys, in particular, have lower self-esteem. They experience power assertion as punishment, and are aggressive outside of the home but not necessarily within the family.

> **Authoritarian parents** aim to control their children's behavior by enforcing absolute standards for behavior.

> Authoritarian parents resolve conflicts through power assertion; that is, they lay down the law "or else."

Authoritative parents also make high demands on their children but they are more responsive. They expect mature behavior from their children and actively guide them toward that end. Standards are clear and enforced through contingencies; that is, children are held responsible for the foreseeable consequences of their decisions. This requires some verbal give-and-take, during which parents use inductive reasoning to help children think through their actions. Discipline meted out in this way is

> **Authoritative parents** also make high demands on their children but they are more responsive.

Their children lack spontaneity, are overly polite, and develop an external locus of control, meaning that they perceive powerful others to be responsible for events.

Table 36-1 Parenting Styles

	Warm, Nurturing	Responsive?	Maturity Demands	Discipline	Child: Self-control	Child: Social
Authoritarian	Maybe	No	High, clearly stated	Power assertive	External locus, aggressive	Polite, not prosocial
Authoritative	Yes	Yes	High, clearly negotiated	Inductive reasoning	Internal locus, self-control	Competent, prosocial
Permission/ neglectful	No	No	None, unclear	None	Poor, very aggressive	Poor or no social skills
Permissive/ indulgent	Maybe	Maybe	Low, inconsistent	Avoids	Low, aggressive at home	Not prosocial responsible

not experienced as punitive. Children grow up to be socially competent, friendly, with good self-esteem. Their internal locus of control allows them to believe they are responsible for events, so they take initiative and are achievement oriented. They are more prosocial than other children, and less aggressive.

Permissive parents are either indulgent or neglectful. They have few rules, which are unclear and not consistently enforced, and they make few demands on their children regarding mature behavior. Neglectful parents avoid interactions with their children, whereas indulgent parents avoid circumstances in which they might have to discipline them. Indulgent parents may be warm and responsive but resolve conflicts by letting the children do as they want. These children are immature, have low self-control and a diminished sense of responsibility, and cannot rely on their own judgment. Children who have been indulged exhibit aggressive behavior at home but not in the community. Children who have been neglected are aggressive in both places, have poor self-control, and have difficulty functioning in society.

While parenting style is usually consistent within a family over time, individual parents occasionally deviate from their own style. Circumstances outside of the family also contribute to parenting style. In hostile environments that threaten children's well-being, such as inner cities or civil unrest, an authoritarian style of parenting can be more adaptive.

Permissive parents are either indulgent or neglectful.

Neglectful parents avoid interactions with their children, whereas indulgent parents avoid circumstances in which they might have to discipline them. Indulgent parents may be warm and responsive but resolve conflicts by letting the children do as they want.

SIBLINGS

Growing up with **siblings** (brothers and sisters) is quite different from growing up without them. Brothers and sisters, because of their behavior toward one another, create a different family environment. Siblings play a critical role in the socialization of children. For example, older siblings often act as caregivers for their younger brothers

Growing up with **siblings** (brothers and sisters) is quite different from growing up without them.

and sisters, which provides opportunities for them to learn about the needs of others. Consequently, experience with siblings provides a setting in which the pattern of interactions that has been established transfers to relationships with others.

> Consequently, experience with siblings provides a setting in which the pattern of interactions that has been established transfers to relationships with others.

The interactions between siblings differ from the interactions between children and parents. Whereas conversations between parents and children focus on caregiving and discipline, siblings talk about feelings and their own wants in a playful way. When conflict arises, they lobby for their own point of view. Taking another's viewpoint into consideration while resolving conflict to their mutual benefit is a key task in children's moral and social development.

Older siblings provide more effective scaffolding for younger siblings than do peers. When asked to help a younger sibling with a hands-on project, for example, older siblings provide more explanations and encouragement, and let the younger child have more control. The younger child asks more questions of and demands more control from an older sibling than a peer. Older siblings feel a sense of pride when their younger siblings succeed under their tutelage.

Warm parenting and secure parent–child attachments foster positive sibling interactions, whereas cold and intrusive parenting promotes sibling antagonism. Parents who are hostile and use power-assertive discipline promote aggression between their offspring.

DETERMINANTS OF PARENTING

Certain characteristics seem to be particularly influential in the parent–child relationship. Among them are the following:

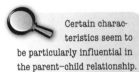

> Certain characteristics seem to be particularly influential in the parent–child relationship.

- Characteristics of parents. For example, personality, age, and stage of life are all important considerations.
- Characteristics of children. For example, health, age, gender, and responsiveness affect the bidirectional nature of parenting.
- The **context of parenting**. For example, social structure, socioeconomic status, culture, and family configuration are important determinants of the quality of parenting.

Three factors determine how people parent their children.

- How parents were raised shapes their beliefs and values about families, and their responsiveness to the needs of others.
- Children's own characteristics contribute to how they are parented. An infant with a difficult temperament may strain the internal resources of immature parents, who may become hostile toward their baby.
- Parents' sources of support and stress in relationships with family, friends, and work affect their parenting. A mutually supportive marital relationship is the foundation for raising a healthy child, whereas a troubled marriage undermines child development. Family and friends can provide child care, advice, and emotional support, but they can also be intrusive.

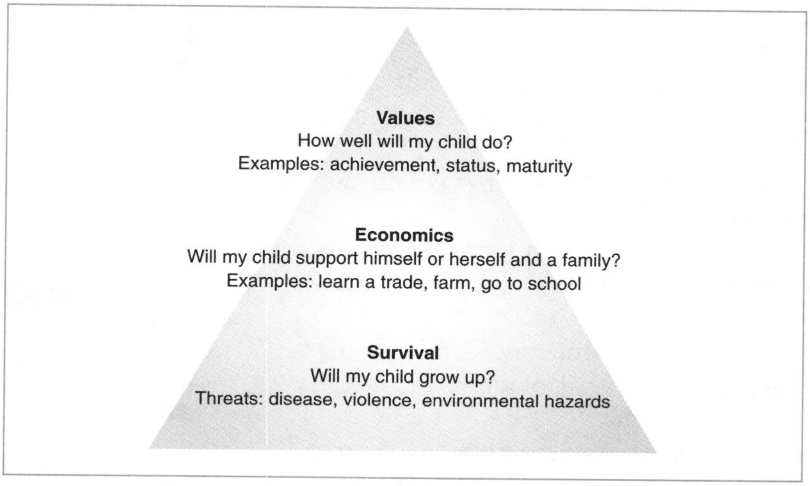

Figure 36-1   Parents' Hierarchy of Goals for Their Children

Around the world, parents have the same hierarchy of goals for their children. They want them to be safe and healthy, to grow up to support themselves and their own families, and to share the values of the family and community (**Figure 36-1**).

SOURCES

Baumrind, D. (1971). Current patterns of parental authority. *Developmental Psychology Monographs, 4,* 1–103.

Bornstein, M. (2006). Parenting science and practice. In W. Damon & R. Lerner (Series Eds.) & K. Renninger & I. Sigel (Volume Eds.), *Handbook of child psychology: Volume 4. Child psychology in practice* (pp. 893–949). New York: John Wiley.

Eisler, I. (2002). Family interviewing: Issues of theory and practice. In M. Rutter & E. Taylor (Eds.), *Child and adolescent psychiatry* (pp. 128–140). London: Blackwell.

Parke, R., & Buriel, R. (2006). Socialization in the family. In W. Damon & R. Lerner (Series Eds.) & N. Eisenberg (Volume Ed.), *Handbook of child psychology: Volume 3. Social, emotional, and personality/development.* New York: John Wiley.

QUICK LOOK AT THE CHAPTER AHEAD

- Definitions of "homeless" are difficult to formulate because of the changing nature of the population.
- A growing share of the homeless population is made up of young families.
- Estimates of the number of homeless are vague and imprecise because of the difficulties in accurately identifying them.
- The homeless population faces a staggering array of problems, many of which affect a child's development.
- The problems the homeless population faces encompass physical, mental, and social adversities.

37

Homeless Children

TERMS
☐ Developmental delays
☐ Homeless

The U.S. Department of Housing and Urban Development (HUD) defines the term **homeless** or "homeless individual or homeless person" as (1) an individual who lacks a fixed, regular, and adequate nighttime residence; and (2) an individual who has a primary nighttime residence that is (a) a supervised publicly or privately operated shelter designed to provide temporary living accommodations (including welfare hotels, congregate shelters, and transitional housing for the mentally ill); (b) an institution that provides a temporary residence for individuals intended to be institutionalized; or (c) a public or private place not designed for, or ordinarily used as, a regular sleeping accommodation for human beings.

In recent years, the homeless population in the United States has changed in important ways (**Table 37-1**). The "new" homeless population is younger and much more mixed: more single women, more families, and more minorities. Lower economic levels affect parents because of the effect on their psychological well-being. Distressed parents state they feel less effective and capable and are less affectionate in their interactions with their children.

> The "new" homeless population is younger and much more mixed: more single women, more families, and more minorities.

It is difficult to estimate the number of homeless in the United States, but reports have ranged from 300,000 to 800,000. In 2006, the Associated Press reported that there were more than 700,00 homeless in the United States.

WHO ARE THE HOMELESS?

Families with young children may be the fastest-growing segment of today's poor and homeless. Today we realize the powerful role that poverty plays in development because of the multiple stresses that it causes. In a penetrating analysis of the environment of childhood poverty, Studies have shown that the children of poverty face more

> Families with young children may be the fastest-growing segment of today's poor and homeless.

family turmoil, violence, instability, and separation, and less social support, less access to books and computers, and less parental involvement in school activities.

Table 37-1 Homeless Children

The typical homeless person in the United States is a child.
Children and families make up the fastest-growing segment of the homeless population.
The typical homeless family is a single, 20-year-old mother with two children younger than age 6.
More than one-third of homeless families have an open case for child abuse or neglect. One out of five has lost at least one child to foster care.
Nearly half of homeless children either have witnessed or have been subjected to violence in their homes.
More than half of all homeless children never have lived in their own home. More than 40% have been homeless more than once.

Estimates are that 30% of U.S. children will experience poverty at some time in their lives. Among the problems associated with poverty are these:

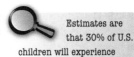

Estimates are that 30% of U.S. children will experience poverty at some time in their lives.

- More poor children die in the neonatal and infancy periods.
- Children of poverty experience more health problems owing to a lack of medical care.
- A larger number of disadvantaged children die from accidents than do more fortunate children.
- These children are subject to greater and longer periods of stress.
- Children of poverty are more frequently the targets of violence (e.g., assault, rape, shootings).

Consequently, children of poverty tend to be characterized by few social contacts, poor health, a high level of contact with the criminal justice system, and ongoing poverty. The typical homeless family of modern U.S. society consists of an unmarried 20-year-old mother with one or two children younger than age 6 years, probably fathered by different men.

Homeless families are forced to move frequently: Length-of-stay restrictions in shelters, short stays with relatives and friends, and relocation to seek employment make it difficult for children to have any sense of stability. Their health suffers, any sense of security is minimal, and schooling is almost nonexistent. Even when school is available, children often lack the means to attend because of a lack of transportation.

Homeless families are forced to move frequently: Length-of-stay restrictions in shelters, short stays with relatives and friends, and relocation to seek employment make it difficult for children to have any sense of stability.

Consequently, it would be a mistake to think of homelessness as merely a housing problem. It is an educational issue, a children's issue, and a family issue. If all of these issues are not addressed, remedial efforts are destined to fail.

THE IMPACT OF HOMELESSNESS ON DEVELOPMENT

Homeless children, like all people, have different levels of stress tolerance. The causes of homelessness, the length of time without a home, the availability of (or lack of) support systems, and the age, sex, and temperament of children all produce different reactions. Feelings of depression, anxiety, and low self-esteem are frequent accompaniments and often lead to either aggression or withdrawal. Truancy, hyperactivity, and underachievement are no strangers to these children. Several specific difficulties associated with the homeless experience are described here.

Health

Homeless individuals experience illness and injury much more often than members of the general population do. Health care is lacking because they do not have health insurance; thus homeless children have much higher rates of both acute and chronic health problems. Homeless women have significantly more low-birth-weight babies and higher levels of infant mortality. Homeless children are more susceptible to asthma, ear infections, and diarrhea and are less likely to receive recommended immunizations on schedule.

Homeless individuals experience illness and injury much more often than members of the general population do.

Hunger and Poor Nutrition

Homeless families struggle to maintain an adequate and nutritionally balanced diet in the setting of no refrigerator, no stove, poor food, and lack of food. Homeless children and their families often depend on emergency food assistance. Many times the facilities themselves suffer from a lack of resources, with the result that the children, and their families, go hungry.

 Homeless families struggle to maintain an adequate and nutritionally balanced diet in the setting of no refrigerator, no stove, poor food, and lack of food.

Developmental Delays

Homeless children experience, to a significantly higher degree than typical children, **developmental delays**—that is, motor coordination difficulties, language delays, cognitive delays, social inadequacies, and a lack of personal skills (e.g., do not know how to eat at a table). The instability of their lives, the disruptions in child care, an erratic pattern of schooling, and how parents adapt to these conditions also impede development.

 Homeless children experience, to a significantly higher degree than typical children, **developmental delays**—that is, motor coordination difficulties, language delays, cognitive delays, social inadequacies, and a lack of personal skills (e.g., do not know how to eat at a table).

Psychological Problems

Homeless children seem to suffer more than other children from depression, anxiety, and behavioral problems. Data that might enable identification of the particular aspect of homelessness that causes a child's anxiety or depression are lacking. It is clear, however, that parental depression affects children, and their children's problems may reflect the parents' own feeling of helplessness.

 Homeless children seem to suffer more than other children from depression, anxiety, and behavioral problems.

Educational Underachievement

Homeless children do poorly in reading and mathematics. This finding should come as no surprise, given that these children have difficulty in finding and maintaining free public education for substantial periods. These children also miss the remedial work they so urgently need.

Homeless children do poorly in reading and mathematics.

Schools are now mandated to provide school services to homeless children that are comparable to those services that other children receive. The act ensures that all homeless children are provided adequate transportation to school, are placed on an immunization schedule, and are furnished their school and health records and that guardianship requirements are met.

IMPLICATIONS FOR HEALTHCARE PROVIDERS

You may encounter homeless children in a number of ways—often in the emergency room, where homeless families go for their primary care. These children frequently come to the attention of school nurses, who may discover mental or physical disabilities. Today, nurses are more active in shelters and other agencies that serve the homeless, doing health teaching and routine screenings to identify health problems.

SOURCES

Dacey, J., Travers, J., & Fiore, L. (2008). *Human development across the lifespan* (7th ed.). New York: McGraw-Hill.

Evans, G. (2004). The environment of childhood poverty. *American Psychologist, 59*(2), 77–92.

NICHD Early Child Care Research Network. (2005). Duration and developmental timing of poverty and children's cognitive and social development from birth through third grade. *Child Development, 76*(4), 795–810.

- Children of divorced parents face multiple transitions in their lives and many adjustments in their reaction to parental divorce.
- In their adjustment to their parents' divorce, children frequently encounter a range of problems.
- The divorce rate has remained stable but high in the United States.
- Divorce encompasses a range of problems, many of which involve children.

38

Divorce

The changes and stresses associated with divorce typically cause multiple problems for all concerned —children, mothers, and fathers. Today, approximately 50% of all first marriages and 62% of remarriages in the United States end in divorce. Sixty percent of the divorces in the United States involve children, which has serious consequences for the children's developmental change: Childhood is different, adolescence is different, and adulthood is different. As a result, there has slowly emerged an agreement that divorce has long-term effects.

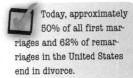

Today, approximately 50% of all first marriages and 62% of remarriages in the United States end in divorce.

CHILDREN AND DIVORCE

Children of divorce and separation face multiple transitions in their lives. They experience the shock of the initial separation and often a move to new living conditions —new housing, new school, new friends. Simultaneously, they typically are involved in a visitation schedule, perhaps one weekend per month, with the separated parent. Given that most divorced adults remarry, this cycle is then repeated: the transition to another new home, a strange adult, any children of the new adult, and new adjustments to schools, teachers, and friends. Children from divorced and remarried families tend to exhibit more behavioral problems and are less academically, socially, and psychologically well adjusted than those in nondivorced families. Nevertheless, 70% to 80% of children from divorced families do not show severe or enduring problems in their reactions to their parents' marital changes and develop as reasonably competent and well-adjusted individuals. **Table 38-1** provides data on the living arrangements of children younger than 18 years old.

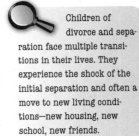

Children of divorce and separation face multiple transitions in their lives. They experience the shock of the initial separation and often a move to new living conditions—new housing, new school, new friends.

Children from divorced and remarried families tend to exhibit more behavioral problems and are less academically, socially, and psychologically well adjusted than those in nondivorced families.

Table 38-1 Living Arrangements of Children Under 18

Children living with	Children under 18*	Percent below the poverty level
All types	73,523	18%
Two parents	49,573	9%
Single parent	20,658	37%
Mother only	17,172	41%
Father only	3,486	18%
Neither parent**	3,293	45%

*Data are in thousands.
**Includes children living with other relatives and those living with nonrelatives.
Source: U.S. Census Bureau, Current Population Survey, America's Families and Living Arrangements, 2005.

CHILDREN'S REACTIONS TO DIVORCE

We think of divorce today as a sequence of experiences. The conflict and disagreements that lead to divorce undoubtedly begin before the divorce itself, and all too often children witness displays of hostility, anger, and arguments. Viewing angry adults is emotionally disturbing for children and may lead to childhood and adolescent problems such as aggression and poor psychological adjustment—problems that have proven to be long-lasting. Thus marital conflict is associated with a wide range of both internalizing problems, such as depression, and externalizing difficulties, such as aggression.

After about 2 years, family arrangements usually stabilize, a remarriage may have occurred, and both children and parents are on the road to adjustment (although boys may still be more aggressive and disobedient). Of course, the divorce itself—that is, the actual separation—may *not* be the major cause of any problem behavior. Too many other factors have intervened (e.g., exposure to conflict, economic decline, erratic parenting) to attribute problem behavior solely to the parents' separation. But how do early-childhood youngsters react to divorce?

We think of divorce today as a sequence of experiences. The conflict and disagreements that lead to divorce undoubtedly begin before the divorce itself, and all too often children witness displays of hostility, anger, and arguments.

Of course, the divorce itself—that is, the actual separation—may *not* be the major cause of any problem behavior.

CHILDREN'S ADJUSTMENT TO DIVORCE

Following the divorce, it takes most children 2 or 3 years to adjust to living in a single-parent home. This adjustment, however, can once again be shaken when a parent remarries. This kind of **marriage transition** means losing one parent in the divorce, adapting to life with the remaining parent, and the addition of at least one new member in a remarriage (**Figure 38-1**).

The transition period in the first year following a divorce is stressful economically, socially, and emotionally. Conditions then seem to improve, and children in a stable, smoothly functioning home are better adjusted than children in a nuclear family that remains riddled with conflict. Nevertheless, school achievement may suffer and impulsivity may increase.

A well-known student of the effects of divorce on children, Judith Wallerstein, identified several psychological tasks that children face in adjusting to their parents' divorce:

1. *Facing the reality of the divorce.* This task relates to a child's cognitive level. Young children simply cannot understand the complexities surrounding their parents' marital rupture, and even older children may at first deny it. Although children come to accept the fact of the split, some still dream about their parents reuniting. For example, a condition called **reconciliation**

Following the divorce, it takes most children 2 or 3 years to adjust to living in a single-parent home.

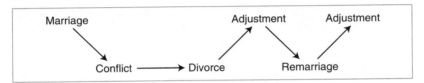

Figure 38-1 Transitions in Marriage

fantasies may continue to exist. Ten years after their parents' divorce, and even after remarriage, some children continue to hope their parents can get together again.

2. *Resuming their own daily lives.* Initially, children may be overwhelmed by what is happening around them. Their schoolwork, their play, and their relationships may all reflect the fallout from their concern about their parents. They gradually adjust and immerse themselves in their daily lives.

 Initially, children may be overwhelmed by what is happening around them.

3. *Reconciling themselves to loss.* A way of life changes and, with the separation of their parents, children frequently experience a loss of security. Their world has been severely shaken. Some children eventually adjust to their new reality, whereas others find it difficult to fully regain their equilibrium.

 A way of life changes and, with the separation of their parents, children frequently experience a loss of security.

4. *Dealing with their emotions.* Some children never really forgive their parents (or parent) and build a reservoir of anger that affects their lives for years. Many of their actions as adolescents, and even adults, reflect the anger that they have carried with them from the time of the divorce. Resolving these feelings is a critical task for healthy adult adjustment.

 Some children never really forgive their parents (or parent) and build a reservoir of anger that affects their lives for years.

5. *Developing a positive outlook for the future.* Children of divorce often avoid forming any close relationships because of their fear of desertion. Most children regain their sense of trust in others, but some experience continuing problems in maintaining relationships.

IMPLICATIONS FOR HEALTHCARE PROVIDERS

In your work with children, you will inevitably find those who are experiencing the shock of family conflict. The behavioral and emotional repercussions affect every aspect of their lives—friendships, schoolwork, and even health. When you contact these children, be alert to emotional issues, such as illness, aggression (or withdrawal), and irritability. Try to attain a comfortable closeness with them so that they realize you are a trusted "secure base."

If possible, work with parents and encourage them to keep their children's needs in focus—not an easy task given their personal emotional crisis. Most parents recognize that they themselves must be, as much as possible, a source of consistent support for their children. Your task, then, is to help parents reach this conclusion, while you offer as much warmth and security as possible for the children.

SOURCES

Dacey, J., Travers, J., & Fiore, L. (2008). *Human development across the lifespan* (7th ed.). New York: McGraw-Hill.

Wallerstein, J., Lewis, J., & Blakeslee, S. (2000). *The unexpected legacy of divorce.* New York: Hyperion.

 QUICK LOOK AT THE CHAPTER AHEAD

- Today more than two-thirds of mothers with children younger than age 6 years work.
- Day care can occur in a variety of settings
- There are more than 116,000 licensed daycare centers in the United States and more than 250,000 licensed childcare homes.
- The developmental outcomes of daycare attendance are closely tied to the quality of care in the center.
- The maternal relationship with the child is the key to understanding the quality of attachment between mother and child.

39

Day Care

After World War II, middle-class families could afford to have one parent at home on a full-time basis—an unprecedented economic luxury. By 1968, 35% of mothers with children ages 3 to 5 years were working. Today, two-thirds of mothers with children younger than age 6 work outside of the home, leaving their children in someone else's care. Parents' choice of a daycare setting for their children is limited by availability, cost, and quality.

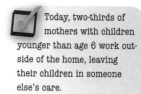

Today, two-thirds of mothers with children younger than age 6 work outside of the home, leaving their children in someone else's care.

DAYCARE SETTINGS

Some children are cared for in their own homes by either a relative or nonrelative. Family **day care** is provided in someone else's home. **Daycare centers** are located in churches, parents' workplaces, and the community. Many children are cared for in more than one setting; for example, they may spend the morning at a center and the afternoon with a grandparent.

In their thoughtful analysis of nonparental child care, the developmental psychologists, Lamb and Ahne (2006) pose two questions intended to help researchers reshape their evaluation of modern child care:

In their thoughtful analysis of nonparental child care, the developmental psychologists, Lamb and Ahne (2006) pose two questions intended to help researchers reshape their evaluation of modern child care.

- What type and how much care do young children receive from adults other than their parents?
- What effects do such care arrangements have on their development?

These questions help us to realize that it is useless to ask simply whether day care is good or bad for children. Rather researchers must examine the nature, extent, quality, and age at onset of care in combination with the characteristics of children from different backgrounds and needs.

Reliable facts about day care are hard to come by, chiefly because of the lack of any U. S. national policy that would provide hard data. There are believed to be more than 116,000 **licensed childcare centers** in the United States and 254,000 **licensed child care homes**. The types of childcare arrangement vary dramatically: One mother may charge another mother several dollars to take care of her child; a relative may care for several family children; churches, businesses, and charities may run large operations; some centers may be sponsored by local or state government as an aid to the less affluent; other centers are run on a pay-as-you-go basis. In 2003, the average cost of child care for one child in a childcare center ranged from $4000 to $6000 per year. Almost everyone agrees that the best centers are staffed by teachers who specialize in daycare services (about 25% of daycare personnel).

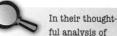

There are believed to be more than 116,000 **licensed childcare centers** in the United States and 254,000 **licensed child care homes**.

DEVELOPMENTAL EFFECTS OF DAY CARE

There has been considerable concern that nonparent child care can disrupt the attachment between mother and child, or have negative effects on the child's social development. Opponents of this view counter that for disadvantaged children, day care can be a form of early intervention, providing an enriching environment when one does not exist at home.

The implications of day care for development include many factors: the number of daycare settings the child has experienced, the number of hours the child is in day care, the quality and stability of the care, the type of setting, and the child's age at entry. A child's daycare experience must also be examined in light of characteristics of the individual child, such as gender and temperament, as well as characteristics of the family, especially socioeconomic status and parenting behaviors.

> The implications of day care for development include many factors: the number of day-care settings the child has experienced, the number of hours the child is in day care, the quality and stability of the care, the type of setting, and the child's age at entry. A child's daycare experience must also be examined in light of characteristics of the individual child, such as gender and temperament, as well as characteristics of the family, especially socioeconomic status and parenting behaviors.

Day Care and Attachment

The National Institute of Child Health and Development (NICHD) has examined the effects of day care on more than 1000 children at 10 different sites. Results indicate that children who have been in day care are no different from those who are cared for by their mothers in regard to mother–child **attachment**, as measured using the "strange situation" technique (see Chapter 29).

The best direct predictors of attachment are not the type, quality, or amount of daycare, but rather the psychological adjustment of the mother and her mothering behavior. The more sensitive and responsive the mother is, the more likely a secure attachment will develop, regardless of whether a child has been in day care.

> The more sensitive and responsive the mother is, the more likely a secure attachment will develop, regardless of whether a child has been in day care.

When low maternal sensitivity is combined with long hours of poor-quality day care, children—especially boys—are more likely to be insecurely attached or avoidant. These children have a "dual risk"; that is, poor-quality care at home and at day care undermines the development of secure attachment. For some children, high-quality day care may compensate for less-sensitive mothering. Poor-quality care does not necessarily undermine the development of a secure attachment, however, if the mother is sensitive and responsive in her interactions with her child (NICHD, 1997).

Table 39-1 Federal Agency Requirements for Day Care

1. Planned activities that are developmentally appropriate and that promote children's intellectual, social, emotional, and physical development
2. Caregivers with specialized training, especially regarding heath and safety standards
3. Nutritious meals
4. A health record for each child
5. Opportunities for parents to observe and to discuss their child's needs
6. Small group sizes and low child–staff ratios

Day Care and Social Development

Follow-up with the NICHD study of children at age 3 years indicates that the incidence of behavior problems is also not related to whether a child is in daycare or how long a child has been in daycare (NICHD, in press). Once again, mothering behaviors and characteristics are stronger predictors of child outcomes than is a child's daycare experience per se. Nevertheless, the quality of day care does matter. Children who have experienced higher-quality day care during their first 2 years have fewer behavioral problems and are more compliant with adult direction (e.g., to help clean up) than are children who were cared for in lower-quality settings.

Quality of Care

The NICHD studies noted that the quality of day care is frequently higher for children who come from families with more economic advantages. Working mothers who are well adjusted, like their jobs, and have choices regarding day care are more likely to be sensitive and responsive when interacting with their children.

The United States lags far behind Western Europe in its attitude and policies regarding day care. Although there are federal requirements for day care (**Table 39-1**) (Clarke-Stewart & Allhusen, 2005), state requirements vary widely. NICHD found that quality of care seems to be improving since the first studies were done 15 to 20 years ago, perhaps because parents are more attuned to the issues involved. **Table 39-2** lists characteristics of high-quality daycare settings (National Association for the Education of Young Children, 1991).

Table 39-2 Characteristics of High-Quality Daycare for Preschool Children

Program Characteristics	Signs of Quality
Physical setting	Indoor environment is clean, in good repair, well ventilated. Classroom space is divided into richly equipped activity areas: make-believe play, blocks, science, math, games, puzzles, art, books, music. Fenced outdoor play area has swings, climbing equipment, tricycles, sandbox.
Group size	No more than 18–20 students with 2 teachers.
Child–caregiver ratio	Ratio of 8 children to 1 caregiver in centers; 6 to 6 in family day care.
Daily activities	Children work individually and/or in small groups, selecting their own activities. Caregivers facilitate children's involvement, adjusting expectations to fit the child.
Teacher qualifications	Caregivers have college-level sepcialized preparation in early childhood development, education, or related field.
Relationships with parents	Parents are encouraged to be involved, to observe, and to meet with caregivers to discuss child's development.
Licensing/accreditation	Program is licensed by state. Centers and preschool programs are accredited by National Academy of Early Childhood Programs. Family day care is accredited by National Association for Family Day Care.

SOURCES

Clarke-Stewart, A., & Allhusen, V. (2005). *What we know about childcare*. Cambridge, MA: Harvard University Press.

Lamb, M., & Ahne, L. (2006). Nonparental child care: Context, concepts, correlates, and consequences. In W. Damon & R. Lerner (Series Eds.) & K. Ann Renninger & Irving Sigel (Volume Eds.), *Handbook of child psychology: Volume 4, Child psychology in practice* (pp. 950–1016). New York: John Wiley.

National Association for the Education of Young Children. (1991). *Characteristics of high-quality day care programs*. Washington, DC: Author.

NICHD. (1997). The effects of infant child care on infant–mother attachment security: Results of the NICHD study of early child care. *Child Development, 68*, 860–879.

NICHD. (in press). Early child care and self-control, compliance and problem behavior at 24 and 36 months. *Early Child Care*.

- The self is a complicated mixture of characteristics and abilities.
- William James identified the dichotomy between the "I" self and the "me" self.
- As children pass through the early childhood years, their ideas of themselves begin to take on a more abstract dimension as their cognitive abilities mature.
- Between 15 and 24 months of age, children begin to display clear signs of self-recognition.
- Children of these years develop a sense of agency: "I did it."
- The development of self-control is an important phase of self-development.
- The acquisition of self-esteem is a significant aspect of the developing self.

40

Development of Self

TERMS
- ☐ Agency
- ☐ "I" self
- ☐ "Me" self
- ☐ Self
- ☐ Self-control
- ☐ Self-esteem
- ☐ Self-regulation

A sense of **self** is a multifaceted composite of one's characteristics and abilities. Self-concept develops as children mature physically, cognitively, and socially, and is subject to influence from parents, peers, and society at large. But what do we mean by "self"?

A sense of **self** is a multifaceted composite of one's characteristics and abilities.

The next time you look into a mirror think of this question: What do you see? Of course, *you* see *you*. But what exactly do you see? When you look in the mirror, you see yourself. But there are two sides to this vision of yourself. The first is referred to as the **"I" self**, that part of you that is doing the actual looking. The second part of what you see is the **"me" self**; that is, the "me" is the person observed, a dichotomy that remains alive and well today.

The first vision of the self is referred to as the **"I" self**, that part of you that is doing the actual looking. The second is the **"me" self**; that is, the "me" is the person observed, a dichotomy that remains alive and well today.

William James proposed this division of the self into two distinct parts. James believed that the "I" part of the self was the knower—that is, the "I" that thinks, makes judgments, recognizes it is separate from everything it sees, and controls the surrounding world. The "me," by contrast, is the object of the "I"'s thinking, judging, and so on. Think of the "me" as your self-image, which helps you to understand how the "I" develops feelings of self-esteem. As a result of the "I" evaluating the "me"'s activities, the self is judged good or bad, competent or incompetent, masterful or fumbling.

During the early childhood years, children change from identifying themselves by physical characteristics (hair or eye color) to more social and emotional characteristics (feeling good or bad about themselves). As children grow, their sense of self is not limited to their reflections in a mirror; they have acquired language and are able to tell us what they think of themselves. Their self-judgments reflect their changing cognitive and social maturity.

During early childhood, children change from identifying themselves by physical characteristics to more social and emotional characteristics. As children grow, their sense of self is not limited to their reflections in a mirror; they have acquired language and are able to tell us what they think of themselves. Their self-judgments reflect their changing cognitive and social maturity.

SELF-RECOGNITION

A clever study by the developmental psychologists Lewis and Brooks-Gunn (1979) suggested that children recognize themselves in a mirror by age 15 months. While wiping a child's nose, researchers smudged it with rouge. Younger infants reached out to touch the nose in the mirror, whereas toddlers between 15 and 24 months responded to the image by wiping their own noses. Between ages 2 and 3, the growth of language and representational thought enables children to identify themselves in a picture and refer to themselves by name. They classify themselves using salient features—for example, boy, girl, big, little.

Lewis and Brooks-Gunn (1979) suggested that children recognize themselves in a mirror by age 15 months.

AGENCY AND SELF-REGULATION

As toddlers explore the world on their own terms, they develop a sense of **agency**: "I did it!" Parental expectations about what they should and should not do conflict with toddlers' desires. As a result, an emerging sense of agency is tempered by regulating one's own behavior in response to parental cues. Whereas a parent may need to physically remove a sharp object from a young toddler's reach, a word of caution about picking it up should suffice with a 3-year-old. Agency and **self-regulation** contribute to self-concept as children identify who they are by what they do.

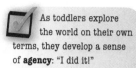

As toddlers explore the world on their own terms, they develop a sense of **agency**: "I did it!"

SELF-CONTROL

Self-regulation in response to parental cues must give way to **self-control** in the absence of authority figures. Children must understand the requirements of social situations, monitor their own behavior, and be motivated to exercise self-control. They also must understand the consequences of their behavior.

Self-regulation in response to parental cues must give way to **self-control** in the absence of authority figures. Children must understand the requirements of social situations, monitor their own behavior, and be motivated to exercise self-control. They also must understand the consequences of their behavior.

Many processes, such as cognitive and emotional development, contribute to the development of self-control. Preschoolers get better at regulating their verbal and physical impulses, especially when parents provide explanations ("We're here to listen"), reminders (a disapproving look), or diversions (a book to read), and when they model the desired behavior. Children internalize these processes, and remind themselves either out loud or in their heads about what is expected when parents are absent. Children do not learn self-control by themselves, and it develops over time.

MASTERY OVER AGGRESSIVE IMPULSES

Children must learn to control their feelings and impulses. When toddlers experience overwhelming arousal, they throw a tantrum. Instrumental aggression appears as they push, pull, and grab to get their way. Young children have difficulty differentiating between "sad," "mad," and "bad" because they experience all of these when their in-

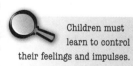

Children must learn to control their feelings and impulses.

tentions are thwarted by disapproving parents. They cry and strike out and try to hide, all at the same time. Hostile aggression, which is meant to hurt, increases between ages 4 and 7. At first it is physical, but as children hone their language skills, verbal insults and taunts increase. The goal is domination, but children learn that victory does not win friends.

Physical punishment such as slapping may stop aggressive behavior immediately, but the behavior may escalate later. This kind of strategy also does not teach children the acceptable alternative to their misbehavior.

Parents employ a variety of disciplinary strategies to teach children to control their aggressive impulses (**Table 40-1**). Verbal instruction encourages children to take the perspective of others and offers alternative behaviors: "It hurts when you push her. How would you feel if she did that to you? If you want the toy, you need to ask for it, not push." Role modeling provides long-term effects when combined with verbal instruction: "I'm so angry right now that I need to leave the room to calm down." Time-out can be an effective way of helping children regain self-control, but works especially well with verbal instruction: "Are you ready to play nicely?" Remember that young children cannot tell time, and parents should set a timer. Physical punishment such as slapping may stop aggressive behavior immediately, but the behavior may escalate later. This kind of strategy also does not teach children the acceptable alternative to their misbehavior.

SELF-ESTEEM AND SELF-CONCEPT

Self-esteem is an evaluation of one's self-concept and inherent worth. During the preschool years, children's self-concept is categorical. It includes descriptions of clothing, hair color, and names of siblings and pets. Toddlers refer to abilities, likes and dislikes, and emotions: "I can swim." "I like to play house." "I get mad." Preschool children can distinguish how well others like them (social acceptance) from how well they can do something (competence): "Sara likes me; she's my friend." "I'm good at coloring."

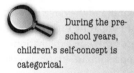

During the preschool years, children's self-concept is categorical.

By age 8, children have a general sense of self-esteem that is subdivided into academic, social, and physical components. With maturity, these become more complex: math versus English, sports

Table 40-1 Disciplinary Strategies That Support Development of Self-Control

Strategy	Description	Example
Verbal instruction	Explain behavior.	"You can't just grab what you want. Next time, ask nicely."
Perspective taking	Provide other's point of view.	"It hurts when you hit her. You wouldn't want her to do that to you."
Role modeling	Adults demonstrate behavior.	Being quiet in church, talking through conflicts.
Time-out	Remove child to quiet area. Set timer. Set contingency for return.	"Sit here for 5 minutes. When you're ready to play nicely, you join us. Nicely means no grabbing."
Positive attribution	Verbally reward child.	"You were a big help. Thanks!"

$$\text{Self-esteem} = \frac{\text{Success}}{\text{Pretense}}$$

Source: James, 1890.

Figure 40-1 Classic Definition of Self-Esteem

versus appearance, and so on. School-age children are better judges of their abilities compared to peers than are preschool-age children. Ask a nursery school class who is the fastest runner, and all hands may go up. Ask a group of third graders, and there is a pause: Do you mean girl or boy? Do you mean in soccer or baseball?

Preschool children do not have either a general or a subdivided sense of self-esteem like their older siblings. Rather, they have an array of self-esteems depending on their experiences. For a 4-year-old, feeling good is the measure of success. Older children look at effort and outcome, and use information from several sources to evaluate themselves.

William James (1890), an American psychologist and philosopher, defined self-esteem as success divided by pretense (**Figure 40-1**). He conceptualized success as being fully human and real, as experiencing oneself as capable and as influencing events. Pretense means a self based on appearances, and lacking substance.

SOURCES

Harter, S. (2006). The self. In W. Damon & R. Lerner (Series Eds.) & N. Eisenberg (Volume Ed.), *Handbook of child psychology: Volume 3. Social, emotional, and personality/development* (pp. 505–570). New York: John Wiley.

James, W. (1890). *Principles of psychology.* Boston: Houghton Mifflin.

Lewis, M., & Brooks-Gunn, J. (1979). *Social cognition and the acquisition of self.* New York: Plenum.

- Children quickly discern differences between male and female.
- An acceptable sense of gender is a changing concept in a modern society.
- Gender development is influenced by physical, psychological, and social factors.
- Several theoretical explanations of gender development have been proposed.
- In spite of a theoretical belief that boys and girls should be treated similarly, parents still tend to respond differently to boys and girls.
- Gender identity refers to the belief that males and females have that they belong to the sex of birth.
- Knowledge of gender roles and gender stereotypes increases with growing cognitive maturity.

41

Gender Development I

TERMS
- ☐ **Cognitive-developmental theory**
- ☐ **Gender**
- ☐ **Gender identity**
- ☐ **Gender role**
- ☐ **Gender schema theory**
- ☐ **Gender stereotype**
- ☐ **Social learning theory**

One of the first categories that children recognize is sex-related; there is a neat division in their minds between male and female. For example, children first indicate their ability to label their own sex and the sex of others between 2 and 3 years of age. By 4 years of age, children are aware that sex identity is stable over time. They then come to the realization that sex identity remains the same despite any changes in clothing, hair style, or activities.

Children first indicate their ability to label their own sex and the sex of others between 2 and 3 years of age. By 4 years of age, children are aware that sex identity is stable over time.

How children acquire their sense of **gender** in a way that they themselves and their society find acceptable remains a central issue in development. "Acceptable" means many things to many people. Although gender roles for boys and girls, men and women are slowly—even grudgingly—changing, sharp differences of opinion are still evident. For example, many parents want their children to follow traditional gender roles (sports for boys, dolls for girls), whereas other parents want to break down what they consider rigid gender role stereotypes. In discussing these issues, we first clarify the meaning of several terms used in any analysis of gender and development.

How children acquire their sense of **gender** in a way that they themselves and their society find acceptable remains a central issue in development.

Gender development is multifaceted, occurs over a period of time, and is influenced by biological, social, and psychological factors (**Table 41-1**). It includes the ability to label oneself and others as male or female (gender identity), knowledge of gender roles, adoption of gender roles, and gender constancy, (i.e., recognizing that one's own gender is permanent). Proponents of **cognitive-developmental theory** take the view that changes in cognitive ability and language com-

Gender development is multifaceted, occurs over a period of time, and is influenced by biological, social, and psychological factors (**Table 41-1**).

Table 41-1 Gender Development

Gender identity	Categorizing oneself as either male or female (ages 2–3)
Gender constancy	Understanding that one will always be the gender one is at present (ages 5–6)
Gender role	Culturally accepted behavior based on gender (e.g., "mother") (appears by age 4 and evolves throughout life)
Gender stereotype	Behavior that reflects characteristics commonly associated with being male or female (e.g., being aggressive vs being passive) (by age 4)
Gender schema	Theory that maintains gender is a social construction by which people organize information about what it means to be male or female in a given social order
Ambiguous genitals	Genitalia that at birth are not clearly differentiated or fully developed as male or female due to chromosomal or hormonal aberrations
Oedipus complex	Freud's explanation of sexual identity in boys
Relational self	Explanation by the Stone Center theorists of how girls develop a self
Rough-and-tumble play	Interactions among peers involving friendly chasing, wrestling, and fighting that children recognize as pretend fun
Aggression	Behavior that is intended to harm another person

bined with children's innate tendency to search the environment for cues about how to behave account for the development of gender knowledge and constancy. **Social learning theory** is associated with adoption of gender roles—that is, developing a preference for clothing and activities appropriate for one's own gender based on social experiences.

Gender schema theory attempts to reconcile the two theories. It maintains that gender is a social construction. That is, as a schema, gender is a way to organize information about the association between culture and gender. Gender schema includes what is considered masculine and feminine, the functional importance of gender in the social order, and the implications for concept of self as male or female.

AGES 2 TO 3: GENDER LABELING AND KNOWLEDGE

Beginning at birth, adults respond differently to male and female infants; men and women treat infants differently as well. Men play more vigorously with babies, especially boys; women talk to infants more, especially girls. By the age of 12 months, infants respond differently to pictures of male and female faces, suggesting they expect different types of interactions from men and women.

Toddlers begin to recognize themselves as individuals separate from their parents during the second year of life. Initially, concepts of self and gender are almost inseparable. A young toddler does not appreciate the anatomical differences between male and female, or that gender is one aspect of self.

> ✓ Beginning at birth, adults respond differently to male and female infants; men and women treat infants differently as well. Men play more vigorously with babies, especially boys; women talk to infants more, especially girls.

By age 2½, children identify themselves as "boy" or "girl." After the second birthday, there is an increased expectation on the part of adults that young children will learn to control their bodily functions. Because toilet training occurs at the same time as representational thinking and advances in language development, children can name body parts and their functions, communicate bodily urges to parents, and begin to anticipate their needs. Adults typically reward young children using gender-based language: "What a big boy you are!" "Aren't you a good girl!"

Gender identity is more than recognizing body parts. Between ages 2 and 3, children get better at labeling strangers as boys or girls, or mommies or daddies, despite the fact that these individuals are fully clothed. Clearly, children use social information about appearance and behavior to develop and label two categories of human beings.

AGES 3 TO 5: GENDER CONSTANCY AND ROLE

Between ages 3 and 5, children's knowledge about **gender roles** and **gender stereotypes** becomes more complete and complex. They still may have difficulty with gender constancy. Cognitive-developmental theorists explain this challenge as an inability to conserve gender—that is, to recognize that gender remains the same despite alterations in outward appearances.

Bem (1985) attributes this difficulty to gender schema. She relates the story of the day her son Jeremy decided to wear barrettes to nursery school. Another boy insisted that Jeremy was a girl because "Only girls wear barrettes." When Jeremy pulled down his pants as proof, the other boy dis-

Also, parenting styles, cultural influences, and children's emotional investment in gender roles contribute to their adoption of stereotyped behaviors.

missed the physical evidence by proclaiming that "Everybody has a penis but only girls wear barrettes." According to Bem, the social construction of gender is more powerful than anatomy.

During the preschool period, children recognize that to fit the category "male" or "female," they have to look and behave the part. Sex-typed behavior increases by age 4 as children become very rigid in their views of gender roles. It is as if by adhering to stereotyped behavior, they can assure themselves of gender identity and constancy: "Boys do this; I do this, so I am a boy." By ages 5 to 6, most children appreciate that gender is a permanent aspect of one's self-identity.

Rigidity regarding gender roles is, in part, attributable to a lack of cognitive flexibility. Recall that preschoolers focus on one aspect of something at a time, and are unable to coordinate multiple pieces of information. Also, parenting styles, cultural influences, and children's emotional investment in gender roles contribute to their adoption of stereotyped behaviors. Children, especially boys, value the gender role of their own sex more highly.

SOURCE

Bem, S. (1985). Gender schema theory: A cognitive account of sex typing. *Psychological Review, 88* (4), 354–364.

QUICK LOOK AT THE CHAPTER AHEAD

- In Freud's Oedipus complex, boys must separate from their mothers to achieve a satisfactory gender identity.
- Among the important influences on a child's gender development are family, peers, and media.
- Regardless of attempts at sexual similarity, parents typically treat boys and girls differently.
- Peers and adults—especially parents—criticize sex-inappropriate play.
- During the early childhood years, children of the same sex tend to play together, a pattern called sex cleavage.
- Television is a powerful influence in fostering stereotypical gender development.
- Children, from an early age, form ideas of what male and female behavior should be.

42

Gender Development II

PSYCHODYNAMIC EXPLANATIONS OF GENDER DEVELOPMENT

Freud's **Oedipus complex** refers to the small boy's need to separate "male self" from "female mother" and yet still retain "female" as an object of sexual desire. Freud thought that boys could accomplish this separation by competing with the father for the mother's affection. By defeating the father with whom they identified, boys secured their sexual identity. Cross-cultural research reveals the competition can be with a father figure (e.g., an uncle or older brother), suggesting that a boy is testing himself against the cultural power structure into which he is being socialized.

Freud's attempts to explain the corollary **Electra complex** in girls were inadequate. While little girls may express a desire to marry their father and get rid of their mother, they must continue to identify with their mother's gender role. That is, in Freud's view, girls are left to identify with the vanquished. Researchers at the Stone Center at Wellesley College, unlike Freud, believe that women's sense of self is based on their relationships with others, not on being separate from them. In forming a self, a young girl differentiates—rather than separates—her femaleness from that of her mother.

> ☑ Freud's **Oedipus complex** refers to the small boy's need to separate "male self" from "female mother" and yet still retain "female" as an object of sexual desire.

> ☑ While little girls may express a desire to marry their father and get rid of their mother, they must continue to identify with their mother's gender role.

INFLUENCES ON GENDER DEVELOPMENT

Children first notice physical differences between the sexes and then begin to understand the behavior expected of male and female. What influences this process?

Family

Evidence clearly suggests that parents treat boy and girl babies differently from birth by the toys they supply, by their room furnishings, and by the type of gender behavior they engage in. Adults tend to engage in rougher play with boys, give them stereotypical toys (cars and trucks), and speak differently to them. By the end of the second year, parents respond favorably to what they consider appropriate sexual behavior (i.e., stereotypical) and negatively to cross-sex play (boys engaging in typical girl's play, and vice versa).

> ☑ Evidence clearly suggests that parents treat boy and girl babies differently from birth by the toys they supply, by their room furnishings, and by the type of gender behavior they engage in.

Parents usually are unaware of the extent to which they engage in this type of reinforcement. In a famous study conducted by Will, Self, and Data (1976), 11 mothers were observed interacting with a 6-month-old infant. Five of the mothers played with the infant when it was dressed in blue pants and called "Adam." Six mothers later played with the same infant when it wore a pink dress and was called "Beth." The mothers offered a doll to "Beth" and a toy train to "Adam." They also smiled more at Beth and held her more closely. The baby was actually a boy. Interviewed later, all of the mothers said that boys and girls were alike at this age and *should be treated identically*.

Parents usually are unaware of the extent to which they engage in this type of reinforcement.

Peers

When children start to make friends and play, these activities foster and maintain **sex-typed play**. When they engage in **sex-inappropriate play** (boys with dolls, girls with footballs), their peers immediately criticize them and tend to isolate them ("sissy," "tomboy"). Although increasing inroads have been made in eroding these stereotypes (girls in Little League and youth hockey, for example), stereotypical behavior increases with age.

When children start to make friends and play, these activities foster and maintain **sex-typed play**. When they engage in **sex-inappropriate play** (boys with dolls, girls with footballs), their peers immediately criticize them and tend to isolate them ("sissy," "tomboy").

During development, youngsters of the same sex tend to play together, a custom called **sex cleavage**. If you think back on your own experiences, you can remember your friends at this age—either all male or female. You can understand, then, how imitation, reinforcement, and cognitive development come together to intensify what a boy thinks is masculine and a girl thinks is feminine. Even in adolescence, despite dating and opposite sex attraction, both males and females want to live up to the most rigid interpretations of what their group thinks is ideally male or female.

During development, youngsters of the same sex tend to play together, a custom called **sex cleavage**.

Media

Television has assumed such a powerful place in the socialization of children that it is safe to say that television is almost as significant as family and peers. What is particularly bothersome is the stereotypical behavior that it presents as both positive and desirable. The more television children watch, the more stereotypical their behavior is.

Television has assumed such a powerful place in the socialization of children that it is safe to say that television is almost as significant as family and peers. What is particularly bothersome is the stereotypical behavior that it presents as both positive and desirable. The more television children watch, the more stereotypical their behavior is.

The central characters of television shows are much more likely to be male than female, the theme will be action oriented for males, and the characters typically engage in stereotypical behavior (men are the executives and leaders, women are the housewives and secretaries). Much the same holds true for television commercials. When asked to rate the behavior of males and females, children aged 8 to 13 responded in a rigidly stereotypical manner: Males were brave, adventurous, and intelligent, and make good decisions; females cried easily and needed to be protected. In other words, gender stereotyping is alive and well.

Problems arise, however, when the characteristics associated with a label create a negative image.

 ## GENDER STEREOTYPING

Gender stereotyping is the beliefs that groups hold about the characteristics and behavior associated with male and female. In other words, from an early age we form an idea of what a male and a female should be, begin to accumulate characteristics about male and female, and assign a label to each category. Gender stereotyping appears between 3 and 5 years of age and peaks at about the time of entrance to first grade.

Problems arise, however, when the characteristics associated with a label create a negative image. "Oh, girls can't do math; girls can't do science; girls are always crying; girls can't be leaders." At this point, we start to treat the individual according to the stereotypes we associate with male or female. Although sexual equality is widely accepted today—legally, professionally, and personally—gender stereotyping is alive and well. Acceptance by the same-sex peer group has a powerful effect on preadolescent children, with all that implies for happy, healthy development.

 Gender stereotyping is the beliefs that groups hold about the characteristics and behavior associated with male and female. In other words, from an early age we form an idea of what a male and a female should be, begin to accumulate characteristics about male and female, and assign a label to each category. Gender stereotyping appears between 3 and 5 years of age and peaks at about the time of entrance to first grade.

SOURCES

Lips, H. (2007). *Sex and gender*. New York: McGraw-Hill.

Ruble, D., Martin, C., & Berenbaum, S. (2006). Gender development. In W. Damon & R. Lerner (Series Eds.) & N. Eisenberg (Volume Ed.), *Handbook of child psychology*: *Volume 3. Social, emotional, and personality development* (pp. 858–932). New York: John Wiley.

Yunger, J., Carver, P., & Perry, D. (2004). Does gender identity influence children's psychological well-being? *Developmental Psychology, 40*(4), 572–582.

Will, J., Self, P., & Data, N. (1976). Maternal behavior and perceived sex of infant. *American Journal of Orthopsychiatry, 46*, 135–139.

QUICK LOOK AT THE CHAPTER AHEAD

- During early childhood, children engage their world symbolically.
- Pretend play is a major characteristic of this developmental period.
- Play is an activity that children enjoy and one that contributes to all aspects of development: physical, intellectual, and psychosocial.
- Piaget believed that children engage in three types of games: practice, symbolic, and games with rules.
- Freud believed that play allowed children to overcome the traumatic events in their lives.
- Erikson interpreted play to be a means of coping with the different psychosocial issues of childhood.

43

Play Behavior

TERMS
- ☐ **Games with rules**
- ☐ **Play**
- ☐ **Practice games**
- ☐ **Repetition compulsion**
- ☐ **Symbolic games**

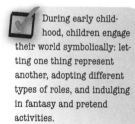

Children cherish their play. Shouting, running, chasing each other, enjoying games, engaging in make-believe, and exploring their worlds—children love to have fun.

During early childhood, children engage their world symbolically: letting one thing represent another, adopting different types of roles, and indulging in fantasy and pretend activities. Children may pretend to drink from play cups, or feed a doll with a spoon, or pretend a box is a truck. Pretend play is a major characteristic of this developmental period. Play also becomes more social, with interactions with other children becoming more important.

> During early childhood, children engage their world symbolically: letting one thing represent another, adopting different types of roles, and indulging in fantasy and pretend activities.

DEFINING PLAY

Several key elements of play contribute to its definition:

> Several key elements of play contribute to its definition.

- Play must be enjoyable and valued by the player.
- Play has no extrinsic goals; that is, play is intrinsically motivated.
- Play is spontaneous and voluntary. No one forces children to play; they freely choose it.
- Play demands that children be actively engaged.
- Play has systematic relations to other behavior that is not play.

Here we define **play** as an activity that children engage in because they enjoy it for its own sake. Children play in a wide variety of situations: alone or with others, with objects, and with ideas. Children's play may be simple, but it also demonstrates great skill and dexterity in complicated patterns (**Table 43-1**).

> Here we define **play** as an activity that children engage in because they enjoy it for its own sake.

EXPLANATIONS OF PLAY

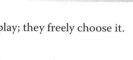

In his book *Play, Dreams, and Imitation in Childhood* (1962), Piaget stated that children initially use their physical activities to build their cognitive structures (see Chapter 3). When children continue these physical acts for the amusement in them, however, Piaget believed they were playing. Sooner or later, children grasp for the pleasure of grasping, and swing for the sake of swinging.

> In his book *Play, Dreams, and Imitation in Childhood* (1962), Piaget stated that children initially use their physical activities to build their cognitive structures.

Piaget next turned his attention to the games children play, identifying three types: **practice games, symbolic games,** and **games with rules**. Each of these games matches a major stage of cognitive development. During early childhood, for example, symbolic games aid children's development by reproducing their world.

> Piaget next turned his attention to the games children play, identifying three types: **practice games, symbolic games,** and **games with rules**.

Another, quite different explanation of play can be found in psychoanalytic theory (see Chapter 1). Freud believed that play provides children with a means for wish fulfillment and a way to overcome

Table 43-1 Play

Play Type	Age (years)	Definition	Examples
Sensorimotor play	0–2	Plays using body	Kicking crib
Pretend play	0–6	Play shifts from solitary to social	Pretend gestures; imitating parents' roles
Functional play	1–2	Simple, repetitive motor movement with or without objects	Running around, rolling a toy car back and forth
Constructive play	3–6	Creating or constructing something	Making a house out of toy blocks, drawing a picture, putting a puzzle together
Make-believe play	3–7	Acting out roles	Playing house, school, or doctor; acting as a television character
Games with rules	6–11	Understanding and following rules in games	Playing board games, cards, baseball

Source: Adapted from Berk, 1997; Rubin, Fein, & Vandenberg, 1983; and Dacey & Travers, 1999.

the traumatic events in their lives. It allows children to escape the restrictions of reality and permits them to rid themselves of dangerous, aggressive impulses. Play also supports children's desire to imitate those whom they love and admire, thus fulfilling the wish to be like these models.

Mastery of the traumatic events of their lives occurs through **repetition compulsion**. Inevitably, children will have experiences that they find too intense to assimilate psychologically. In their play, then, children repeat elements of the disturbing event and gradually diminish the intensity of the initial experience, leading to feelings of mastery.

Erikson (see Chapter 2) believed that the form play takes changes as a child's psychosocial issues change. For the most part, children struggle to make sense of their world and bring it under control. For Erikson, games can be just fun, but they can also be an occasion of social sharing as well as a means of working out an emotional problem.

Freud believed that play provides children with a means for wish fulfillment and a way to overcome the traumatic events in their lives. It allows children to escape the restrictions of reality and permits them to rid themselves of dangerous, aggressive impulses.

Erikson (see Chapter 2) believed that the form play takes changes as a child's psychosocial issues change.

PLAY'S CONTRIBUTIONS TO DEVELOPMENT

Physical Development

Children play for the sheer exuberance of it; play enables them to exercise their bodies and improve their motor skills. The physical activities of running, throwing, and kicking, for example, contribute to children's health, strength, and endurance. When they start to throw and catch a ball, the benefits of muscular coordination and hand-eye coordination are obvious, and children continue to develop feelings of mastery of their environment.

Cognitive Development

Beginning with the notion that play has widespread consequences, we can say that play allows children to explore their environment on their own terms and to take in any meaningful experiences at their own rate and on their own level (e.g., running through a field and stopping to look at rocks or insects). Consequently, play aids cognitive development, and cognitive development aids play.

Social Development

Play helps social development during early childhood because the involvement of others demands a give-and-take that teaches young children the basics of forming relationships. Social skills demand the same building processes as cognitive skills. These social skills do not simply appear, but rather are learned. Much of this learning comes through play (Dacey, Travers, & Fiore, 2008).

IMPLICATIONS FOR HEALTHCARE PROVIDERS

When you come in contact with children, they are probably uncertain, frightened, and anxious, which is one reason why healthcare settings have become more child friendly. The use of playrooms in hospitals—where examinations, shots, and changing of dressings are not permitted—reflects the attempt to reduce children's anxiety. One way of easing their anxiety is to engage in some type of familiar game, such as playing with toys, pretend, or a board game. Let them choose whatever they want, and use the opportunity to ease them into a more accepting attitude.

SOURCES

Berk, L. (2007). *Child development* (4th ed.). Needham Heights, MA: Allyn & Bacon.

Dacey, J., Travers, J., & Fiore, L. (2008). *Human development across the lifespan* (7th ed.). New York: McGraw-Hill.

Ginsburg, K. (2007). The importance of play in promoting healthy child development and maintaining strong parent–child bonds. *Pediatrics, 119*(1), 182–190.

Piaget, J. (1962). *Play, dreams, and imitation in childhood.* New York: W. W. Norton.

Rubin, K., Fein, G., & Vandenberg, K. (1988). Play. In E. M. Hetherington (Ed.), *Handbook of child psychology: Socialization, personality, and social development* (4th ed., pp. 693–744). New York: Wiley.

PART IV • QUESTIONS

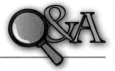

For each of the following questions, choose the **one best** answer.

1. You are going down the stairs behind a little boy who is placing both feet on each step as he goes while holding the railing. About how old is he?
   a. 3 years old
   b. 4 years old
   c. 5 years old
   d. 6 years old

2. Which skill that is essential for reading readiness develops between ages 3 and 6?
   a. Using hands as tools
   b. Coping and tracing figures
   c. Visuomotor scanning
   d. Recognizing the letters of the alphabet

3. You are pouring juice for a 4-year-old and 10-year-old into two different glasses: one short and wide, the other tall and narrow. The 4-year-old insists on having the tall narrow glass despite assurances from the 10-year-old that the two glasses have the same amount of juice. Which term is used to describe the 4-year-old's understanding of this situation?
   a. Centration
   b. Appearance reality
   c. Cause by association
   d. Difficulty with conservation

4. Which of the following is an example of a child's difficulty with conservation during the pre-school period?
   a. Thinks a ball of clay gets bigger when it is rolled into a snake
   b. Given two rows of M&Ms with 10 candies in each row, will say the row more spread out has more
   c. Says the glass with the most juice is the taller one, even if child just saw the juice poured from a shorter but wider glass
   d. All of the above

5. Montessori's ideas concerning _____ periods are important in planning preschool programs.
   a. lengthy
   b. class
   c. sensitive
   d. daily

6. Preschool educators are alert to match materials and methods to appropriate ages because of the theory put forth by
   a. Piaget.
   b. Freud.
   c. Skinner.
   d. Pavlov.

7. The rules of _____ describe how to put words together to form sentences.
   a. phonology
   b. semantics
   c. grammar
   d. pragmatics

8. "Daddy *camed* home" is an example of
   a. overextension.
   b. mispronunciation.
   c. overregulation.
   d. delayed language.

9. Parents who value compliance with their authority and set nonnegotiable standards for their children's behavior are examples of _____ parenting, according to Baumrind.
   a. authoritative
   b. authoritarian
   c. permissive
   d. neglectful

10. Which of the following factors contribute to how parents parent?
    a. Childhood experiences of parents
    b. Personality characteristics of children being parented
    c. Work environment of parents, especially fathers
    d. All of the above

11. Which of the following conditions is not necessarily associated with homelessness?
    a. Health problems
    b. Hunger
    c. Poor nutrition
    d. Low intelligence

12. Recent additions to the number of homeless are
    a. mothers and young children.
    b. single fathers.
    c. individuals with alcohol problems.
    d. individuals with drug problems.

13. One of the major adjustments a child may experience following the divorce of parents is to
    a. siblings.
    b. transitions.
    c. relatives.
    d. synchronicity.

14. Even after their divorced parents remarry, some children still believe their natural parents will reunite. This belief is called
    a. hopeful planning.
    b. wishful thinking.
    c. reconciliation fantasies.
    d. psychic cognition.

15. Erikson called it the period of initiative versus guilt; that is, children recognize that they make choices and are responsible for their behavior. Plato referred to it as "a constitutional government within them." Freud thought that the superego, as "a garrison in the conquered city of the id," is similar. To which developmental task of the preschool years are they referring?
    a. Agency
    b. Sense of self
    c. Mastery of aggression
    d. Self-control

16. Which of the following is an example of a 4-year-old's concept of self?
    a. "I am a better swimmer than my brother."
    b. "People like me because I play fair."
    c. "I like to swim."
    d. "I am better at drawing than at coloring."

17. By what age do children typically develop gender identity?
    a. 18 months
    b. 2 years
    c. 3 years
    d. 5 years

18. Preschoolers tend to engage in sex-typed behaviors, such as boys playing with trucks and girls playing with dolls. How do developmentalists explain this phenomenon?
    a. Males and females have inborn sex-typed tendencies.
    b. Preschoolers are rewarded for exhibiting sex-typed behaviors.
    c. Girls are more rigidly socialized to exhibit certain behaviors than are boys.
    d. Preschoolers are developing concepts of gender constancy and role.

19. The most common type of play during early childhood is _____ play.
    a. physical
    b. unrestricted
    c. social
    d. pretend

20. Children play for fun, learning, and
    a. emotional release.
    b. cognitive dissonance.
    c. physical alignment.
    d. social graces.

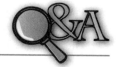

PART IV · ANSWERS

1. **The answer is a.** At age 3, children can go up stairs using alternating feet, but still descend placing both feet on each step. By age 4, they descend using alternating feet and holding the railing. At age 6, they run up and down stairs easily.

2. **The answer is c.** Vision is 20/20 by age 4. Children also become more efficient and proficient in how they move their eyes to scan a page, an ability essential for reading readiness. At age 3, when asked to find the little mouse on the page of a favorite book, children initially scan haphazardly, looking here and there. Systematic scanning from side to side and up and down develops between ages 3 and 6.

3. **The answer is a.** They focus on only one aspect of something at a time—often the most obvious aspect—and fail to consider how several aspects might interact to produce the event. When pouring juice between a tall skinny glass and a short wide glass, they focus on only the height of the tall skinny glass in concluding that it is "bigger" and so contains more juice. They cannot account for height and width simultaneously.

4. **The answer is d.** Conservation refers to the ability to understand that something remains the same even if its appearance is altered and nothing was seen to be taken away or added. Because preschool children are swayed by appearances, focus on one aspect of something at a time, and have difficulty working out events in their minds, they have difficulty with conservation tasks, such as those related to number, quantity, mass, and length.

5. **The answer is c.** Montessori believed that at certain ages in children's lives, they are more attuned or ready (sensitive) for certain experiences.

6. **The answer is a.** Piaget's identification of cognitive stages contributed to a desire to "match the mix"—that is, to make sure that appropriate material would be available for certain ages and stages.

7. **The answer is c.** Syntax is how words are put together to make sentences. In their acquisition of language, children quickly learn the rules of language that enable them to express themselves in a sensible manner to other members of their culture.

8. **The answer is c.** Because children are rule learners, they frequently stay with the rule, even when they know the correct form, which is the meaning of overregulation. This phase of language development is commonly encountered and nothing to worry about.

9. **The answer is b.** Authoritarian parents aim to control their children's behavior by enforcing absolute standards for behavior. They value unquestioned respect for and compliance with authority, and they discourage verbal give-and-take with their children. Authoritarian parents resolve conflicts through power assertion; that is, they lay down the law "or else."

10. **The answer is d.** Research has identified three factors that determine how people parent their children. First, how parents were raised during their own childhood shapes their beliefs and values about families. Second, children's own characteristics contribute to how they are parented. For example, an infant with a difficult temperament may strain the internal resources of immature parents, who may become hostile toward their baby. Third, parents have sources of support and stress in relationships with family, friends, and work. For example, fathers employed in subordinate positions in organizations with a hierarchical power structure tend to have an authoritarian style of parenting at home.

11. **The answer is d.** A person's intelligence is not linked to conditions such as homelessness. This question points out how easily we may jump to conclusions about surface features.

12. **The answer is a.** An alarming statistic is the rising number of single mothers with young children in homeless shelters. There has long been a tendency to view those persons in shelters as having problems with alcohol, but the change in this population necessitates a change in strategies for dealing with this new group.

13. **The answer is b.** Given the current divorce rate, and the rate of divorce following second marriages, children are often shifted from home to home, school to school, and so forth. These transitions require considerable parental sensitivity, which many parents, given their emotional state, find difficult to provide.

14. **The answer is c.** Research has shown that some children hold on to these fantasies for many years, testifying to the effects of divorce on children.

15. **The answer is d.** Self-regulation in response to parental cues must give way to self-control in the absence of authority figures. Children must understand the requirements of social situations, monitor their own behavior, and be motivated to exercise self-control. They also must understand the consequences of their behavior. A moral conscience develops during these years.

16. **The answer is c.** During the preschool years, children's self-concept is categorical. It includes descriptions of clothing, hair color, names of siblings and pets, their school, and prized possessions. They refer to abilities, likes and dislikes, and emotions: "I can swim." "I like to play house." "I get mad." Preschool children can distinguish how well others like them (social acceptance) from how well they can do something (competence): "Sara likes me; she's my friend." "I'm good at coloring."

17. **The answer is b.** By age 2½, children identify themselves as "boy" or "girl." Because toilet training occurs at the same time as representational thinking and advances in language development, children can name body parts and their functions, communicate bodily urges to parents, and begin to anticipate their needs. Gender identity is more than recognizing body parts. Between ages 2 and 3, children get better at labeling strangers as boys or girls, or mommies or daddies, despite the fact that these individuals are fully clothed. Clearly, children use social information about appearance and behavior to develop and label two categories of human beings.

18. **The answer is d.** During the preschool period, children recognize that to fit the category "male" or "female," they have to look and behave the part. Sex-typed behavior increases by age 4 as children become very rigid in their views of gender roles. It is as if by adhering to stereotyped behavior, they can assure themselves of gender identity and constancy: "Boys do this; I do this, so I am a boy." By ages 5 to 6, most children appreciate that gender is a permanent aspect of one's self-identity. Rigidity regarding gender roles is, in part, attributable to a lack of cognitive flexibility. Recall that preschoolers focus on one aspect of something at a time, and are unable to coordinate multiple pieces of information. Also, parenting style, cultural influences, and children's emotional investment in gender roles contribute to their adoption of stereotyped behaviors.

19. **The answer is d.** Pretend play fits well with the growing cognitive ability during early childhood. Although all types of play are attractive, pretend play is particularly prominent during these years.

20. **The answer is a.** Play allows children to release emotional tensions that they may not be allowed to express in school or home, a form of childhood therapy that furthers development.

V

Middle Childhood

QUICK LOOK AT THE CHAPTER AHEAD

- Growth in height and weight is slower and steadier during middle childhood.
- Organ systems become more efficient and adult-like.
- There are significant changes in the organization of the brain, kown as the "5–7 shift."
- Nutritional needs change, requiring less fat and cholesterol and more whole grains.
- The pulse rate is between 65–100 beats per minute, and blood pressure ranges 100–110/60–70.
- As body proportions change, and children become more active, the risk for physical injury increases.

44

Physical Growth and Development

TERMS
☐ **Brain development**
☐ **Nutrition**
☐ **Obesity**

Growth in height and weight is slower and steadier during middle childhood (ages 7 to 12) than the preschool years. Differences between boys and girls are minimal until ages 10 to 12, when girls grow taller than boys, and boys put on extra weight but not height (**Figure 44-1** and **Figure 44-2**). When assessing growth of children with Down syndrome and children adopted from overseas, special growth charts should be used with these populations. Girls also begin to experience pubertal changes (see Chapter 55); the average age of menarche for U.S. girls is 12 years. For boys, puberty arrives at about age 14.

During middle childhood, organ systems become more efficient and adult-like. As the gastrointestinal system matures and grows in capacity, children experience fewer stomachaches, can go longer between meals, and require fewer calories. Heart and respiratory rates decline as blood pressure increases between ages 6 and 12. Vital signs between ages 6 and 12 are as follows: pulse ranges between 65 and 100 beats per minute (average 90), there are 20 to 30 respirations per minute, and blood pressure is in the range 100–110/60–70.

The organization of the central nervous system (CNS) is like an adult's, there are significant changes in the organization of the brain (**brain development**). A neurological shift in the brain occurs between the ages of 5 and 7, as increased myelination of the connections between the right and left hemispheres results in increased lateralization and specialization of areas of the brain. Also, better connections between the frontal and posterior lobes and increases in working memory prepare a child for the educational and behavioral challenges of formal schooling.

Body proportions also change. Children ages 6 to 12 have a lower center of gravity. There is an increase in leg length, a decrease in head size, and a decrease in waist size relative to height. These slender proportions contribute to physical agility, so that riding a bike or hiking a mountain trail is better coordinated. There is an increase in muscle mass relative to body weight, although muscles are still immature and remain vulnerable to injuries from overuse. Bones continue to ossify. If they are broken, bones will heal more quickly than during adolescence because they are still growing.

Children start losing deciduous teeth around age 6. These lost teeth are replaced by permanent teeth by about age 12, with the exception of wisdom teeth, which erupt later in adolescence. As the jaw grows to accommodate permanent adult-sized teeth, the mouth appears disproportionately large. As the eustachian tubes of the ears lengthen, they angle downward, allowing better drainage. Children experience fewer ear infections.

Middle childhood is often idealized as a period of rugged good health. Relatively secure in their agile bodies, children turn their attention outward. This is Erikson's period of industry, when children are busy developing physical, academic, and social skills.

When assessing growth of children with Down syndrome and children adopted from overseas, special growth charts should be used with these populations.

Vital signs between ages 6 and 12 are as follows: pulse ranges between 65 and 100 beats per minute (average 90), there are 20 to 30 respirations per minute, and blood pressure is in the range 100–110/60–70.

A neurological shift in the brain occurs between the ages of 5 and 7, as increased myelination of the connections between the right and left hemispheres results in increased lateralization and specialization of areas of the brain. Also, better connections between the frontal and posterior lobes and increases in working memory prepare a child for the educational and behavioral challenges of formal schooling.

Children start losing deciduous teeth around age 6.

IMPLICATIONS FOR HEALTHCARE PROVIDERS

There are two key areas of health promotion for this age group: **nutrition** and injury prevention.

Nutrition and Obesity

Although caloric needs relative to body mass decrease during middle childhood, an average intake of 2000 kcal/day is needed to sustain slow and steady growth. While very young children need fat and cholesterol in their diets to promote growth of the brain, school-age children do not; fat intake should account for no more than 25% to 35% of calories for members of this age group. Their nutritional needs are best met through whole grains, fresh fruits and vegetables, two to three servings of low-fat milk products per day, and lean meat and fish. Breakfast is the most important meal.

Unfortunately, many U.S. children consume too much fat and sugar, mostly in the form of junk foods that are heavy in carbohydrates (e.g., potato chips, packaged cookies). Soft drinks not only contain sugar and caffeine, but the phosphorus in the carbonation also interferes with the uptake of calcium needed for bone growth. High-fat, low-cost packaged foods, such as macaroni and cheese, may be favored by families with limited income. Fresh fruits and vegetables are more expensive and may be harder to obtain in inner cities or in isolated rural communities.

Malnourished U.S. children tend to be obese, not thin. Obese for ages 2 to 19 is defined as a body mass index (BMI) at or above the 95th percentile for children of the same age and sex. In 2004, 18.8% of U.S. children ages 6 to 11 were obese, almost three times the prevalence in 1980. According to a 2007 report by the Trust for America's Health, 25 million American children are now obese.

Factors contributing to obesity include physical inactivity and family feeding practices. The average child who watches 4 hours of television per day is not playing outside, strengthening muscles and bones, and increasing aerobic capacity. Parents who overfeed children because they use food as reward and as solace, and who rush through meals, are more likely to raise obese children and to be obese themselves. The pattern of inactivity and family habits that leads to obesity may appear as early as 18 months after a child is born.

Obesity represents a complex cycle of cause and consequence. Glucose metabolism in people who are obese favors the storage of fat but not its expenditure for energy. Children who are obese have more trouble sustaining physical activity and so avoid it, further isolating them socially. They soothe emotions using food, which adds to their weight and inactivity. Children who are fat report more depression

Fat intake should account for no more than 25% to 35% of calories for members of this age group.

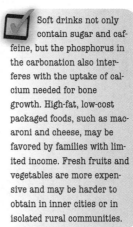
Soft drinks not only contain sugar and caffeine, but the phosphorus in the carbonation also interferes with the uptake of calcium needed for bone growth. High-fat, low-cost packaged foods, such as macaroni and cheese, may be favored by families with limited income. Fresh fruits and vegetables are more expensive and may be harder to obtain in inner cities or in isolated rural communities.

Obese for ages 2 to 19 is defined as a body mass index (BMI) at or above the 95th percentile for children of the same age and sex.

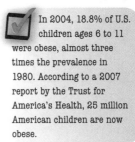
In 2004, 18.8% of U.S. children ages 6 to 11 were obese, almost three times the prevalence in 1980. According to a 2007 report by the Trust for America's Health, 25 million American children are now obese.

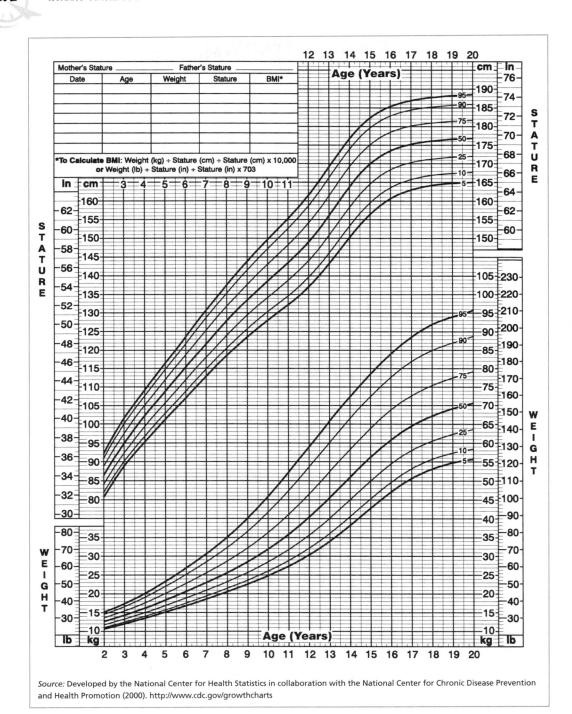

Source: Developed by the National Center for Health Statistics in collaboration with the National Center for Chronic Disease Prevention and Health Promotion (2000). http://www.cdc.gov/growthcharts

Figure 44-1 2 to 20 Years: Boys' Stature-for-Age and Weight-for-Age Percentiles

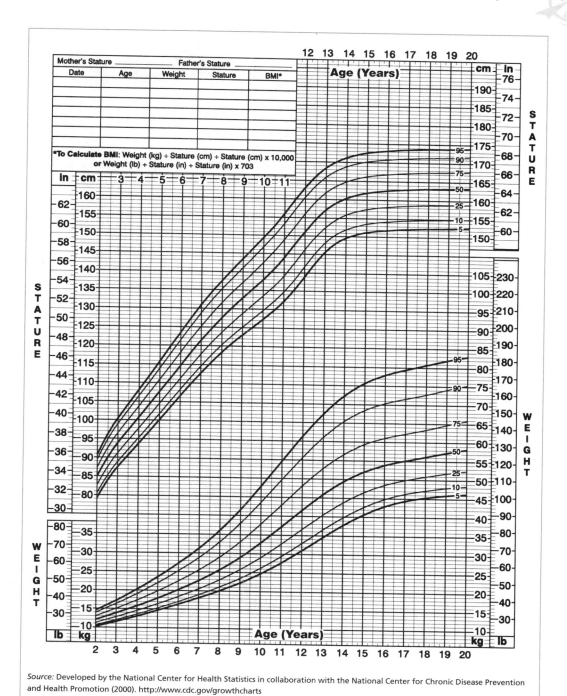

Figure 44-2 2 to 20 Years: Girls' Stature-for-Age and Weight-for-Age Percentiles

and lower self-esteem than their healthier peers. Obese children become obese teenagers; 80% then become obese adults.

The best treatment involves the family and focuses on changing behaviors. Promoting healthy nutritional habits, exercise, and mutual support among family members is key.

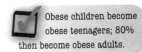

Obese children become obese teenagers; 80% then become obese adults.

Injury Prevention

The increased agility of school-age children, combined with their maturing cognitive abilities (see Chapter 45), contributes to the decreased incidence of some unintentional injuries between ages 6 and 12 compared to the preschool years. While younger children are more likely to drown, fall from high places, and be scalded by hot water, among school-aged children falls, being hit by or hitting up against objects (e.g., hit by a ball, crashing into a goal post), cuts, and bicycle accidents are most likely to result in a visit to the emergency room. Unintentional injuries remain the leading cause of death between ages 1 and 19, with malignant neoplasms in second place for school-aged children. Boys have more frequent and more serious injuries than girls, probably because boys engage in more risk-taking behavior.

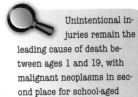

Unintentional injuries remain the leading cause of death between ages 1 and 19, with malignant neoplasms in second place for school-aged children.

Two types of injury are especially prevalent among school-age children: bicycle accidents and sports injuries. Health education programs promote bike safety, encouraging students to use helmets, learn the rules of the road, and keep their bikes in good working condition. In sports, demands on young athletes to train earlier, longer, and harder have increased the incidence of overuse injuries. While an acute blow does obvious damage, the more common and subtle damage is from repetitive microtrauma to muscles and joints that are not fully developed. Stress fractures and Little Leaguer's elbow are examples. It is the responsibility of adults to help children be healthy and safe.

SOURCES

Centers for Disease Control and Prevention. (2007). *Childhood overweight*. Retrieved February 5, 2008, from http://www.cdc.gov/nccdphp/dnpa/obesity/childhood/index.htm

Centers for Disease Control and Prevention. (2007). *Inuuries among children and adolescents*. Retrieved February 5, 2008, from http://www.cdc.gov/ncipc/factsheets/children.htm

Johnson, M. (2000). Functional brain development in infants: Elements of an interactive specialization framework. *Child Development, 71*(1), 75–81.

Trust for America's Health. (2007). *F as in fat: How obesity policies are failing in America*. Retrieved February 5, 2008, from http://healthyamericans.org/reports/obesity/

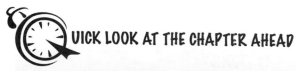

Concrete thinkers are able to:

- Consider two or more pieces of information at one time, for example, height and width (decreasing centration).
- Reverse a sequence of actions in the mind, for example, subtraction (reversibility of a sequence).
- Understand that the identity of a set remains the same despite appearance to the contrary), for example, 10 dots arranged closely together or far apart (set identity).
- Understand that some of the properties of an object remain the same despite appearance to the contrary, for example, the same ball of clay molded into different shapes (conservation of physical properties).
- Understand the relationship between superordinate and subordinate classes, for example, the class of dogs includes beagles and poodles (hierarchical classification), and between categories along two dimensions, for example, a deck of cards can be arranged by suit (spades, hearts, diamonds, clubs) and/or by face (ace through king) (matrix classification).

45

Cognitive Development

TERMS
- ☐ Classification skills
- ☐ Concrete thought
- ☐ Decreasing centration
- ☐ Hierarchical classification
- ☐ Matrix classification

CHARACTERISTICS OF CONCRETE OPERATIONS

Between the ages of 5 and 7, an important shift takes place in how children organize information. Whereas the thinking of preschoolers is shaped by capricious influences, thinking in school-age children is determined by a logical internal organization. The shift is from associative to logical responding, from preoperational to concrete operational thinking. Logical thinkers love rules because rules organize experience and make life orderly.

In school-age children, concrete operational thinking consists of mental operations that allow children to do mentally what had to be experienced physically before. Actions can be played out in their minds, giving them more flexibility in solving problems. **Concrete thought** is characterized by decreasing centration, reversibility of a mental sequence, set identity, conservation of physical properties, classification skills, and an inability to think abstractly (**Table 45-1**).

Decreasing Centration

Decreasing centration refers to children's ability to consider two or more pieces of information at one time when solving a problem. Information can be held in and worked on in their minds. Concrete thinkers still need perceptual supports, however: They need to see the problem and to handle it physically in some way. A concrete thinker pouring juice into two different-sized glasses understands that how much juice a glass can hold depends on both its height and its width.

Reversibility of a Sequence

Concrete thinkers can think through a sequence of actions in their minds, and then reverse it to arrive back where they started. If 5 minus 2 equals 3, the operation can be reversed: 3 plus 2 equals 5. If you eat too much, you gain weight. If you eat less, you lose it. You can roll a ball of clay into a snake and then ball it up again.

Set Identity

In middle childhood, children understand that the identity of a set remains the same despite the fact that its physical properties are rearranged. They are not easily fooled by appearances. Ten M&Ms are still 10 M&Ms, whether they are arranged in one row or two rows. One piece of bread is still one piece of bread whether it is folded or cut up to make a sandwich.

Conservation of Physical Properties

Decreasing centration, reversibility of a sequence, and set identity contribute to a concrete thinker's ability to conserve physical properties. Children understand that some properties of an object remain the same even if they have acted on that object to alter its appearance. This understanding is the basis for science curricula.

When children understand that the 10 M&Ms are still 10 M&Ms, they are able to conserve number. Recognizing that the piece of clay is the same piece of clay no matter its shape is an example of conservation of mass and length. Compensating for glasses of different heights and widths when pouring juice is an example of conservation of quantity (**Figure 45-1**). Knowing that a ton of feathers is the same as a ton of bricks is an example of conservation of weight.

Table 45-1 Characteristics of Concrete Operations

Characteristics	Examples
Decreasing centration	How much juice a glass holds depends on both its height and its width.
Reversibility of a mental sequence	If 5 minus 2 equals 3, then 3 plus 2 equals 5.
Set identity	If you have not added or subtracted anything, the set remains the same.
Conservation of mass	A piece of clay remains the same mass whether it is rolled in a snake or clumped together.
Conservation of number	Ten M&Ms are 10 M&Ms whether they are arranged in one row or two rows.
Hierarchical classification	If you have three spaniels and two retrievers, you have more dogs than spaniels.
Matrix classification	Baseball cards are sorted by team and field position.

Classification Skills

Classification skills expand with the ability to engage in mental operations. **Hierarchical classification** refers to the ability to understand the relationship between subordinate and superordinate classes. Spaniels and retrievers are dogs. If the family has three spaniels and two retrievers, it has more dogs than spaniels. This understanding is the basis for addition and subtraction.

Matrix classification skills are more complex. Children can categorize things along two dimensions simultaneously—for example, color by type. A 2-by-2 matrix would consist of two rows of color (red and blue) and two columns of types (cars and blocks). Given a red car, school-age children will place it correctly in the matrix. This ability is needed to understand multiplication and division in math—and to sort baseball cards.

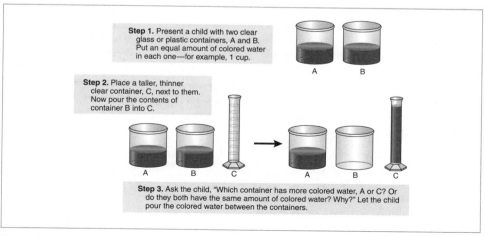

Figure 45-1 An Experiment to Test for Conservation of Liquid

LIMITATIONS OF CONCRETE OPERATIONS

Children are limited by their lack of experience in life. They are constantly adding to their knowledge base of factual information, which they then use to solve problems. Thinking concretely takes practice. Math and science problems, sorting stamps, building cities of Legos, and reading—all exercise the mind.

School-age children have difficulty with abstract reasoning, which involves using symbols that can be manipulated mentally to represent reality. For example, in algebra the symbol x represents different numbers in different problems. In literature, the Grim Reaper symbolizes death. Such abstractions typically are difficult for concrete thinkers to grasp. Abstract thinking develops later, during adolescence.

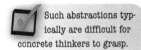

Such abstractions typically are difficult for concrete thinkers to grasp.

IMPLICATIONS FOR HEALTHCARE PROVIDERS

Concrete thinkers conceptualize illness in terms of external cause and internal effect. Something outside, such as cold water or germs, comes in contact with or enters the body, causing the body to malfunction, much like a machine that is broken (Bibace & Walsh, 1981). Germs get into the nose and lungs and clog them up so that breathing is difficult. To fix it, reverse the sequence. Breathe warm air from a humidifier to push the germs out.

To concrete thinkers, a medical procedure is a sequence of predetermined steps. For example, they want to change a dressing the same way each time. Without the benefits of abstract thinking, they do not appreciate the principles of asepsis and wound healing that underlie the procedure, and they have difficulty understanding that there may be more than one right way to do it. Using matrix classification skills, older children with diabetes can learn to sort food groups and exchanges for their diets.

When teaching concrete thinkers about upcoming procedures, use simple diagrams, list the steps in the procedure (e.g., start an IV), and indicate how long each step will take (e.g., 30 seconds) and what the children are likely to experience (e.g., a sharp prick). Tell them when the procedure is halfway completed. For children who worry, tell them that they are allowed to worry for as along as the procedure itself will take—for example, 30 seconds for a needle stick. This helps to put concrete limits on the procedure.

When teaching concrete thinkers about upcoming procedures, use simple diagrams, list the steps in the procedure (e.g., start an IV), and indicate how long each step will take (e.g., 30 seconds) and what the children are likely to experience (e.g., a sharp prick). Tell them when the procedure is halfway completed. For children who worry, tell them that they are allowed to worry for as along as the procedure itself will take—for example, 30 seconds for a needle stick. This helps to put concrete limits on the procedure.

SOURCES

Bibace, R., & Walsh, M. E. (1981). Development of children's concepts of illness. In M. E. Walsh (Ed.), *Children's concepts of health, illness, and bodily functions*. San Francisco: Jossey-Bass.

Siegler, R., & Alibali, M. (Eds.). (2005). *Children's thinking* (4th ed.). Upper Saddle River, NJ: Prentice Hall.

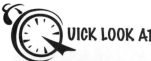

There are newer theories of intelligence that help us understand how people learn to think:

- Gardner's theory of multiple intelligences identifies eight kinds of intelligence: linquistic, musical, logical-mathematical, spatial, kinesthetic, interpersonal and intrapersonal, and naturalistic.
- Sternberg's triarchic model of intelligence proposes three primary aspects to human intelligence: analytical, creative, and practical.

46

Intelligence

TERMS

- ☐ **Theory of multiple intelligences**
- ☐ **Triarchic model of intelligence**

RECENT THEORIES OF INTELLIGENCE

Several recent theories have been proposed to explain intelligence and cognitive development. Two of these—Howard Gardner's theory of multiple intelligences and Robert Sternberg's triarchic model of intelligence—seem particularly significant.

Theory of Multiple Intelligences

Howard Gardner's (1993) **theory of multiple intelligences** helps to explain the diverse abilities of individuals who are capable of penetrating mathematical vision but who are baffled by the most obvious musical symbols. To explain this phenomenon, Gardner identified eight kinds of intelligence, any one of which may be outstanding in a particular individual (**Table 46-1**):

1. *Linguistic intelligence.* Gardner's first category is linguistic intelligence—that is, language. By studying damage to the language-related areas of the brain, researchers have identified the core operations of any language (phonology, syntax, semantics, and pragmatics).

2. *Musical intelligence.* The early appearance of musical ability (in individuals such as Yehudi Menuhin) suggests a biological basis for musical intelligence. The right hemisphere of the brain seems particularly important for music, and musical notation clearly indicates a basic symbol system.

3. *Logical–mathematical intelligence.* Logical–mathematical intelligence is probably what most people think of as intelligence. Gardner used Piaget's ideas to trace the evolution of scientific thinking.

4. *Spatial intelligence.* Gardner believed that the abilities to perceive the visual world accurately, to manipulate initial perceptions, and to recreate aspects of visual experiences identify spatial intelligence. Spatial intelligence becomes obvious during middle childhood, as children produce advanced drawings, explain the relationships on a map, and excel at putting puzzles together.

5. *Bodily–kinesthetic intelligence.* Control of bodily motions and an ability to handle objects competently are indications of bodily–kinesthetic intelligence. It is clear that intelligence is a critical component of expert physical performance. During middle childhood, children's

Table 46-1 Gardner's Types of Intelligence

Type of Intelligence	Meaning
Linguistic	Communication, a preeminent example of human intelligence
Musical	Linked to brain location and a basic symbol system
Logical–mathematical	What is usually meant by "intelligence"
Spatial	Linked to brain location and symbol systems
Bodily–kinesthetic	Smooth development of bodily movements and adaptation
Interpersonal and intrapersonal	Linked to frontal lobe of brain; recognize what is distinctive in others and self
Naturalist	Ability to discriminate among categories; classification skill; linked to brain's tendency to match patterns

Source: Adapted from Gardner, H. (1983). *Frames of mind.* New York: Basic Books; Gardner, H. (1995). *Leading minds.* New York: Basic Books; Gardner, H. (1997). Multiple intelligences as a partner in school improvement. *Educational Leadership, 55*(1), 20–21.

physical acts (e.g., throwing, catching) become highly coordinated. Some become so adept that even at this early age they are skilled athletes, dancers, and so on.

6, 7. *Interpersonal and intrapersonal intelligence.* These are the personal intelligences: Interpersonal intelligence builds on an ability to recognize what is distinctive in others, while intrapersonal intelligence enables people to understand their own feelings.

8. *Naturalist intelligence.* Gardner recently identified this eighth type of intelligence, which is the human ability to discriminate among living things as well as a sensitivity to the natural world.

Triarchic Model of Intelligence

Robert Sternberg (1988) designed a **triarchic model of intelligence**, which proposes that human intelligence has three primary aspects: analytical (analyzing, evaluating, comparing, contrasting, critiquing); creative (dealing with novel situations, discovering, inventing, imagining); and practical (using and applying information to day-to-day life.) He argues that a common set of processes underlies these aspects of intelligence: knowledge-acquisition components, metacomponents, and performance components (**Figure 46-1**).

> Robert Sternberg designed a **triarchic model of intelligence**, which proposes that human intelligence has three primary aspects: analytical (analyzing, evaluating, comparing, contrasting, critiquing); creative (dealing with novel situations, discovering, inventing, imagining); and practical (using and applying information to day-to-day life.) He argues that a common set of processes underlies these aspects of intelligence: knowledge-acquisition components, metacomponents, and performance components.

1. Knowledge-acquisition components help individuals acquire relevant knowledge in the first place so that they can solve problems via selective encoding (choosing what to take in), selective combination (putting it together), and selective comparison (selecting what is relevant).

2. Metacomponents help individuals to elect a strategy, construct a strategy, and coordinate strategies to solve problems.

3. Performance components help individuals to execute the strategy of the metacomponents: encoding, inference, mapping, and application.

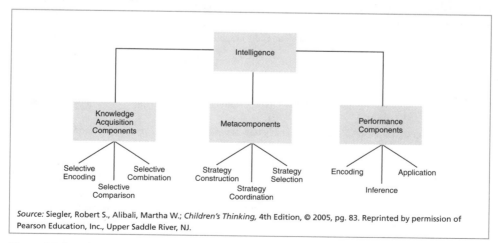

Source: Siegler, Robert S., Alibali, Martha W.; *Children's Thinking,* 4th Edition, © 2005, pg. 83. Reprinted by permission of Pearson Education, Inc., Upper Saddle River, NJ.

Figure 46-1 The Sternberg Model of Cognitive Development

These processes are highly interactive and generally act together. As an example, assume you need to develop a health teaching plan for a patient. The metacomponents help you decide which subjects to include, plan what to include, monitor the actual writing, and evaluate the final product. The performance components help you in the actual writing of the plan. You use the knowledge-acquisition components to do the research on the subjects for the plan.

> You use the knowledge-acquisition components to do the research on the subjects for the plan.

Sternberg's triarchic model also accounted for the role of individual experiences and context in intelligence. Experience improves the ability to deal with novel tasks and to use pertinent information to solve problems. On occasions when children must confront the unknown, their intelligence and problem-solving skills help them to face new challenges. The context of intelligence is the ability to adapt to the various environments individuals move through in their culture. The major thrust of contextual intelligence is adaptation: Either individuals adjust to current circumstances, change these conditions to meet their needs, or move on to new circumstances.

> Sternberg's triarchic model also accounted for the role of individual experiences and context in intelligence.

IMPLICATIONS FOR HEALTHCARE PROVIDERS

The work of Gardner and Sternberg should encourage you to view teaching patients in a new light. Not everyone learns by reading about a disease or by watching a demonstration of how to give an injection. Sternberg also reminds us that health teaching and learning are complex processes, not a rote exchange of information. It is important to understand how your clients learn so your teaching can become more effective. These theories go beyond IQ and stage models, such as that proposed by Piaget, to address different kinds of intelligence and the roles played by information processing, experience, and context in intelligence. When assessing patients' needs for health teaching, it is important to consider these elements as well as their stage of cognitive development.

> These theories go beyond IQ and stage models, such as that proposed by Piaget, to address different kinds of intelligence and the roles played by information processing, experience, and context in intelligence. When assessing patients' needs for health teaching, it is important to consider these elements as well as their stage of cognitive development.

SOURCES

Dacey, J., Travers, J., & Fiore, L. (2008). *Human development across the lifespan* (7th ed.). New York: McGraw-Hill.

Gardner, H. (1993). *Multiple intelligences: The theory in practice.* New York: Basic Books.

Gardner, H. (2004). *Frames of mind: The theory of multiple intelligences.* New York: Basic Books.

Sternberg, R. (1988). *The triarchic mind: A new theory of human intelligence.* New York: Viking.

Sternberg, R. (2005). *Cognition and intelligence: Identifying the mechanisms of the mind.* New York: Cambridge University Press.

QUICK LOOK AT THE CHAPTER AHEAD

- Central themes of problem solving include task analysis, encoding, mental models, domain-general and domain-specific knowledge, and processes of change.
- Problem-solving processes are planning, causal inference, analogy, and tool use.
- Common errors children make include failing to analyze the task and encode facts and failure to make a mental model or understand relationships in the problem.
- Good problem solvers have a positive attitude, are concerned with accuracy, can take a problem apart, and don't guess or jump at answers.

47

Problem Solving

TERMS
- ☐ **DUPE model**
- ☐ **Problem**

During middle childhood, youngsters use their emerging cognitive accomplishments to solve the problems they face in their daily lives. A great deal is known about problem-solving strategies, and this knowledge can be of great value to children. For example, simply reassuring childen that there is nothing to be afraid of when they face a problem and urging them to look carefully for the facts that are given in a problem may greatly improve their problem-solving abilities.

WHAT IS A PROBLEM?

Technically, a **problem** is a significant discrepancy between the actual circumstances or expected circumstances. Children know a problem exists when they cannot get where they want to go; a gap stretches before them. To solve the problem, they must construct some way of bridging the gap.

> Technically, a **problem** is a significant discrepancy between the actual circumstances or expected circumstances.

Central Themes

The following central themes are important in understanding how children solve problems:

- *Task analysis:* careful examination of the problem to identify what is needed to solve it.
- *Encoding:* identification of the critical information and use of it to build an internal representation of the problem.
- *Mental models:* construction of a model that accurately represents the structure of the problem (i.e., how its parts relate to one another). The child must reconcile personal experience with the contradictory information being provided.
- *Domain-general and domain-specific knowledge:* appropriate integration of these types of knowledge to solve problems.
- *Processes of change:* the evolution of newer and better problem-solving strategies is uneven, with older and new strategies existing side by side for some time. Both failure and interest in innovation for its own sake fuel change.

Problem-Solving Processes

Common problem-solving processes are described here:

- *Planning:* future-oriented problem-solving; requires inhibiting initial response; "think before you act"; compare the goal to the current situation and think ahead; keep several items in mind at one time, such as intervening steps.
- *Causal inference:* understanding contiguity (events occur together in time and space), precedence (cause comes before effect), and covariation (cause and effect occurred together in past).
- *Analogy:* identifying how two objects or events correspond in function or structure; brushing teeth is like brushing hair, a camera is like a video recorder.
- *Tool use:* Using objects and other people to solve problems.

THE KINDS OF ERRORS CHILDREN MAKE IN SOLVING PROBLEMS

Children can improve their problem-solving ability if they become aware of the kinds of errors they make in attempting to solve problems, such as not attending to details or being uncertain about how to begin. Some of the more common traps that children—and adults—fall into include the following:

- Failure to analyze the task and encode relevant facts of a problem. Children must learn to constantly search the problem for all the information they can get (**Figure 47-1**).
- Failure to plan ahead or use systematic, step-by-step procedures. Children often skip steps, ignore vital information, and leap to a faulty conclusion. They act without thinking.

Failure to plan ahead or use systematic, step-by-step procedures. Children often skip steps, ignore vital information, and leap to a faulty conclusion. They act without thinking.

- Failure to make a mental model or perceive vital relationships in the problem. Children ignore contradictory information rather than reconcile it, and they fail to search for patterns.

Failure to make a mental model or perceive vital relationships in the problem.

Two motorcyclists are 100 miles apart. At exactly the same moment, they begin to drive toward each other for a meeting. Just as they leave, a bird flies from the front of the first cyclist to the front of the second cyclist. When it reaches the second cyclist, it turns around and flies back to the first. The bird continues flying in this manner until the cyclists meet. The cyclists both travel at the rate of 50 miles per hour, while the bird maintains a constant speed of 75 miles per hour. How many miles will the bird have flown when the cyclists meet?

Figure 47-1 Example Problem 1

CHARACTERISTICS OF GOOD PROBLEM SOLVERS

Obviously, some people are better at problem solving than others, owing to their greater intelligence, experience, or education. Nevertheless, it is possible to improve anyone's ability to solve problems, even children's.

- Good problem solvers have a positive attitude toward problems, believing they can solve them by careful, persistent analysis.
- They are concerned with accuracy, which is a wonderful attitude to foster in children, and one that carries over to all aspects of their lives.
- They learn to take a problem apart, to break it down into its smallest, manageable parts, and then to integrate the parts into a manageable whole that leads to a solution.
- They learn not to guess and jump at answers, a valuable tool to remember whenever they are challenged by a problem, in or out of school (**Figure 47-2**).

These characteristics do not just appear. Rather, they require knowledge, work, and persistence to develop. One way of helping children improve their problem-solving skills is by teaching them simple rules to follow—that is, a model of problem-solving behavior.

THE DUPE MODEL

Many models have been proposed to help people solve a wide variety of problems. An easy acronym for children to remember is **DUPE**. Its intent is to convey the message, *don't let yourself be deceived*. The meaning of each letter is described here.

- *D is for determine.* Determine just exactly what the nature of the problem is. Too often, meaningless elements in the problem are deceptive; it is here that attention to detail is so important.
- *U is for understand.* Understand the nature of the problem. Realizing that a particular problem exists is not enough; you must also comprehend the essence of the problem if your plan for solution is to be accurate.

---

888 88 8 88 888 8

Group these numbers in such a way that when you
total the groups, they add up to the sum of 1000.

88888888

8 8 88 8 88

888 88 88 888

Figure 47-2 Example Problem 2

- *P is for plan.* Plan your solution. Now that you know that a problem exists and you understand its nature, you must select strategies that are appropriate for the problem. It is here that memory plays such an important role.

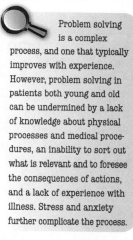

The DUPE model should remind you of the nursing process!

- *E is for evaluate.* Evaluate your plan, which usually entails two phases. First, you should examine the plan itself in an attempt to determine its suitability. Then, you must decide how successful your solution was.

IMPLICATIONS FOR HEALTHCARE PROVIDERS

Problem solving is a complex process, and one that typically improves with experience. However, problem solving in patients both young and old can be undermined by a lack of knowledge about physical processes and medical procedures, an inability to sort out what is relevant and to foresee the consequences of actions, and a lack of experience with illness. Stress and anxiety further complicate the process. A major step in helping patients toward recovery is to encourage patients to believe that they have the capability of aiding themselves. Encourage them to see their present difficulty as a problem, and then help them to understand and use the strategies discussed in this chapter. The DUPE model is a particularly effective means of identifying a problem and devising steps for its solution. The DUPE model should remind you of the nursing process!

Problem solving is a complex process, and one that typically improves with experience. However, problem solving in patients both young and old can be undermined by a lack of knowledge about physical processes and medical procedures, an inability to sort out what is relevant and to foresee the consequences of actions, and a lack of experience with illness. Stress and anxiety further complicate the process.

SOURCES

Bransford, J., & Stein, B. (1993). *The IDEAL problem solver.* New York: Freeman.

Siegler, R., & Alibali, M. (Eds.) (2005). *Children's thinking* (4th ed.). Upper Saddle River, NJ: Prentice Hall.

- Universal moral standards condemn actions such as lying, cheating, and murder.
- Conventional moral standards belong to a particular culture, religion, or other self-identified group, and condemn actions ranging from consumption of certain foods to sexual mores.
- Piaget identified changes in children's moral reasoning from learning right and wrong, to considering intent, and then understanding the principles behind rules.
- Kohlberg identified levels of moral reasoning in children and adults that increase in complexity.
- Gilligan distinguished between Kohlberg's morality of justice, which assumes the reasoner is an autonomous thinker, and an ethic of caring, which is based on relationships between the reasoner and the situation.

48

Moral Development

TERMS
- [ ] **Conventional moral standards**
- [ ] **Moral development**
- [ ] **Moral growth**
- [ ] **Moral philosophers**

Moral development refers to the emergence in children of universal moral standards that lead to the condemnation of such behaviors as lying, cheating, robbing, murdering, raping, and the like. **Conventional moral standards,** by contrast, refers to the ideas that a particular group, religion, or culture believe in but cannot demand that everybody else agree with them. For example, in India violations of food taboos are regarded as seriously as crimes against a person. Members of Western cultures may not accept this belief, but members of both cultures agree in condemning murder. Culture, with its powerful influence on conventional moral standards, is a recurrent theme in any analysis of moral development.

 Moral development refers to the emergence in children of universal moral standards that lead to the condemnation of such behaviors as lying, cheating, robbing, murdering, raping, and the like.

As we begin our analysis of children's moral progress, keep in mind that moral behavior is a complex mixture of cognition (thinking about what to do), emotion (feelings about what to do or what was done), and behavior (what is actually done).

THE PATTERN OF MORAL GROWTH

Piaget studied moral reasoning in children. Young children (from birth to about 2 or 3 years of age) begin to learn about right and wrong from their parents. During these early years, modeling is especially effective. Lacking cognitive sophistication, young children who have good relationships with their parents usually are impressed by what they see their parents doing.

The next phase of **moral growth** (about 2 to 6 years of age) reflects children's growing cognitive maturity and their developing ability to decide what is right or wrong. As they approach school age, they begin to understand intent as another factor in doing wrong—for example, dropping and breaking a dish "on purpose" versus "by accident."

As they approach school age, they begin to understand intent as another factor in doing wrong—for example, dropping and breaking a dish "on purpose" versus "by accident."

As children move into middle childhood (about 6 to 12 years of age), they interact with their siblings in their family lives, with their schoolmates in classroom experiences, and with their friends in games and other social activities. Here they again encounter the reality of rules—but rules not established by parental edict. Consequently, they learn about making and following regulations as well as deriving insights into the children who don't. School-aged children who are concrete thinkers tend to cling to absolute rules of right and wrong, whereas older school-aged children (10 to 13 years of age) begin to appreciate the principle behind the rules. For example, think about children of different ages playing a baseball game. A 9-year-old may declare that allowing the 5-year-old to stay at bat until he or she hits the ball is "unfair" and "breaking the rules," whereas the 13-year-old pitcher looks at the discrepancy in skill between the 5- and 9-year-olds, and handicaps the younger player in an effort to "level the playing field" among players.

School-aged children who are concrete thinkers tend to cling to absolute rules of right and wrong, whereas older school-aged children (10 to 13 years of age) begin to appreciate the principle behind the rules.

CAN CHILDREN BE MORAL PHILOSOPHERS?

Lawrence Kohlberg believed children can be moral. Fascinated with the study of children's moral development during his doctoral work at the University of Chicago, and especially by Piaget's work, Kohlberg (1966) developed his ideas by presenting children with a series of moral dilemmas and then asking them *what* they would do and *why* they would do it. The dilemmas were real or imaginary conflicts that forced children to make decisions based on their moral reasoning—that is, to become **moral philosophers**.

Kohlberg found that children begin to think about moral issues at about the age of 4 years as they pass through three levels of moral development. Each of these levels contains two stages; thus there are three levels and six stages of moral development. Take a few moments and study the levels and stages in **Table 48-1**. Remember, however, that even children who make it to the third level as adults may not always act in a moral manner. Knowing the right answer to a moral dilemma does not guarantee moral behavior, which is why we distinguish between knowing, feeling, and behaving. A person may be brilliant, but also morally destitute.

Table 48-1   Kohlberg's Stages of Moral Development

Level I. Preconventional (4–10 years)

During these years children respond mainly to cultural control to avoid punishment and attain satisfaction. There are two stages:

Stage 1.   Punishment and obedience. Children obey rules and orders to avoid punishment; there is no concern about moral rectitude.

Stage 2.   Naive instrumental behaviorism. Children obey rules but only for pure self-interest; they are vaguely aware of fairness to others but obey rules for their own satisfaction. Kohlberg introduces the notion of reciprocity here. "You scratch my back, I'll scratch yours."

Level II. Conventional (10–13 years)

During these years children desire approval, both from individuals and from society. They not only conform, but also actively support society's standards. There are two stages:

Stage 3.   Children seek the approval of others, the "good boy–good girl" mentality. They begin to judge behavior by intention: "She meant to do well."

Stage 4.   Law-and-order mentality. Children are concerned with authority and maintaining the social order. Correct behavior is "doing one's duty."

Level III. Postconventional (13 years and older)

If true morality (an internal moral code) is to develop, it appears during these years. The individual does not appeal to other people for moral decisions; these decisions are made by an "enlightened conscience." There are two stages:

Stage 5.   An individual makes moral decisions legalistically or contractually; that is, the best values are those supported by the law because they have been accepted by the whole society. If there is a conflict between human need and the law, individuals should work to change the law.

Stage 6.   An informed conscience decides what is right. People act not from fear, approval, or law, but from their own internalized standards of right and wrong.

Source: Based on Kohlberg, L. (1996). A cognitive-developmental analysis of children's sex-role concepts and attitudes. In E. Maccoby (Ed.), *The development of sex difference*. Stanford, CA: Stanford University Press.

GENDER AND MORAL DEVELOPMENT

Gilligan questioned the validity of Kohlberg's theory for women. She believed that Kohlberg's theory stressed the moral qualities of masculinity (autonomous thinking, clear decision making, and responsible action) and ignored those moral qualities associated with femininity. For example, the characteristics that define the traditional "good woman" (gentleness, tact, concern for others, display of feelings) all contribute to a different concept of morality.

Gilligan, Ward, & Taylor (1988, p. 7) argued strongly that different images of self lead to different interpretations of moral behavior. Girls, who are typically raised with the belief that attachment is desirable, fuse the experience of attachment (see Chapter 29) with the process of identity formation.

Consequently, women's moral decisions are based on an ethic of caring rather than a morality of justice. Gilligan, therefore, argued for a different interpretation of moral development for women. For males, separation from mothers is essential to the development of masculinity; for females, femininity is defined by attachment to mothers. Male gender identity is threatened by attachment, whereas female gender identity is threatened by separation. Women define themselves through a context of human relationships and judge themselves by their ability to care.

IMPLICATIONS FOR HEALTHCARE PROVIDERS

Many cultures consider children to be able to know right from wrong somewhere around age 7, when they can reason about cause and effect, and consider intent. Lying, stealing, and cheating are common temptations for all children and should not be tolerated. In some cases, however, they may indicate serious behavioral disturbances. Parents may express concerns during a routine visit, or you may hear children complain about a peer. Moral behavior is learned in a number of ways, but you do your part when you model honesty, fairness, and taking responsibility for your behavior.

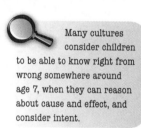

Many cultures consider children to be able to know right from wrong somewhere around age 7, when they can reason about cause and effect, and consider intent.

SOURCES

Gilligan, C. (1982). *In a different voice.* Cambridge, MA: Harvard University Press.

Gilligan, C., Ward, J., & Taylor, J. (1988). *Mapping the moral domain.* Cambridge, MA: Harvard University Press.

Kohlberg, L. (1966). A cognitive-developmental analysis of children's sex-role concepts and attitudes. In E. Maccoby (Ed.), *The development of sex differences.* Stanford, CA: Stanford University Press.

Piaget, J. (1965). *The moral judgment of the child.* New York: Free Press.

QUICK LOOK AT THE CHAPTER AHEAD

- Critical components of language include acquiring vocabulary and acquiring grammar, that is, the content and the structure of language.
- Vocabulary acquisition begins during the toddler years, increases dramatically beginning at age 2 so that by first grade a child understands 10,000 words, and by fifth grade understands 40,000 words.
- The sensitive period for grammar acquisition is between 18 months and puberty, although grammar acquisition for a second language begins to decline after age 7.
- Children who are truly bilingual—both vocabulary and grammar—learned both languages by the age of 3.
- Bilingual education involves teaching children subject matter in their native language and in English, whereas English as a Second Language (ESL) programs involve teaching English in a separate class.

49

Language Development

TERMS

- ☐ Bilingual education
- ☐ Bilingual Education Act of 1988
- ☐ Convergent semantic production
- ☐ Divergent semantic production
- ☐ English as a Second Language (ELS)
- ☐ Limited English proficiency (LEP)

By middle childhood, most children have acquired the critical components of their language and find themselves engulfed in a verbal world (**Figure 49-1**). During this period, both vocabulary and structural knowledge continue to expand. By first grade, a child understands about 10,000 words; by fifth grade, he or she understands 40,000 words. Between 18 months and puberty is considered by some to be a sensitive period for the mastery of grammar, the complex structure of communication using language. By the end of the middle childhood, children are similar to adults in their language usage. Children who experience language problems are at a serious disadvantage with their peers, at school, and in their overall relationships with others.

By first grade, a child understands about 10,000 words; by fifth grade, he or she understands 40,000 words.

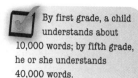
Between 18 months and puberty is considered by some to be a sensitive period for the mastery of grammar, the complex structure of communication using language.

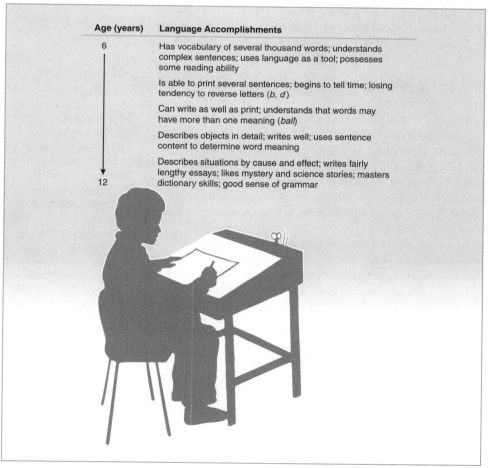

Age (years)	Language Accomplishments
6	Has vocabulary of several thousand words; understands complex sentences; uses language as a tool; possesses some reading ability
	Is able to print several sentences; begins to tell time; losing tendency to reverse letters (*b, d*)
	Can write as well as print; understands that words may have more than one meaning (*ball*)
	Describes objects in detail; writes well; uses sentence content to determine word meaning
12	Describes situations by cause and effect; writes fairly lengthy essays; likes mystery and science stories; masters dictionary skills; good sense of grammar

Figure 49-1 Typical Language Accomplishments: 6–10 Years

THE LANGUAGE EXPERT

During middle childhood, children communicate with others more effectively and realize that language is a powerful tool they can use to manipulate their world. Increasing visual discrimination is apparent in their accurate description of events and the elimination of letter reversals (e.g., "b" for "d"). Growth in cognitive ability is seen in the detection of cause and effect, and the appeal of science and mystery stories.

As their vocabulary continues to grow, children begin to demonstrate divergent and convergent language abilities. **Divergent semantic production** is seen in the wide variety of words, phrases, and sentences they use when discussing a topic, thereby bringing originality, flexibility, and creativity to their language. **Convergent semantic production** is seen when children use the right word in response to a specific, restricted question such as "What is the opposite of hot?" (Owens, 1996). Children also appreciate that a word can have different meanings (e.g., "watch" or "spring"), which allows them to expand their repertoire of jokes.

 Children also appreciate that a word can have different meanings (e.g., "watch" or "spring"), which allows them to expand their repertoire of jokes.

CHILDREN WHO SPEAK MORE THAN ONE LANGUAGE

Forty-seven million Americans (18% of the U.S. population), speak a language other than English at home. Twenty-one million Americans (8% of the population), have **limited English proficiency** (LEP). Twenty percent of children now live with at least one foreign-born parent. Forty percent of children with immigrant parents have origins in Mexico. Nearly half of all children in all immigrant families speak English fluently and another language at home; thus another half is not fluent in English.

Many children who do not speak the language of their school are taught by teachers who have no special proficiency or training in working with these children. Unfortunately, many of these children will not achieve up to their potential and drop out of school. In an effort to combat this problem, the **Bilingual Education Act of 1988** stipulated that students with LEP receive **bilingual education** until they can use English to succeed in school.

Forty-seven million Americans (18% of the U.S. population), speak a language other than English at home. Twenty-one million Americans (8% of the population), have **limited English proficiency** (LEP). Twenty percent of children now live with at least one foreign-born parent. Forty percent of children with immigrant parents have origins in Mexico. Nearly half of all children in all immigrant families speak English fluently and another language at home; thus another half is not fluent in English.

Bilingual Children

Children who are truly fluent in more than one language either learn two different languages simultaneously before the age of 3, or learn one language and then another in sequence, again usually before the age of 3. Studies indicate that the earlier they learn the second language, the better, in keeping with sensitive periods of language and grammar acquisition. Studies of Asian immigrants indicate that age of arrival in the United States is more closely related to language mastery, especially grammatical mastery, than is the length of time an immigrant child has been living in the United States. In these studies, immigrant children who arrived in the United States before the age of 7 eventually mastered English grammar as well as native-born adults. Among those arriving in the United States after age 7, there was a sharp decline in grammar acquisition, such that eventual mastery was poor for those arriving after age 15.

The better children speak both their native language and their second language, the better their level of cognitive attainment. The native language does not interfere with the second language, because the phonemic categories of the first language serve as a basis for learning the second language. Many adjustments are made in learning the second language. Given that the acquisition of languages is a natural part of the cognitive system, both first- and second-language acquisition seems to be guided by similar principles. In fact, the rate of acquisition of the second language seems to be related to the level of proficiency with the first language. With these ideas in mind, programs have been devised to help these children.

> Children who are truly fluent in more than one language either learn two different languages simultaneously before the age of 3, or learn one language and then another in sequence, again usually before the age of 3. Studies indicate that the earlier they learn the second language, the better, in keeping with sensitive periods of language and grammar acquisition.

Bilingual Education Programs

Two different techniques for aiding LEP students are apparent:

- The **English as a Second Language (ESL)** program usually removes students from the class and gives them special English instruction.
- With the bilingual technique, students are taught partly in English and partly in their native language. The objective is to help students learn English by subject matter instruction both in their own language and in English.

Bilingual education programs can be divided into two categories. The first type of programs (often called "transitional" programs) encourages the rapid development of English so that students switch as soon as possible to an all-English program. The second type of programs (sometimes referred to as "maintenance" programs) permits LEP students to remain in the program even after they have become proficient in English. The rationale for such programs is that students can use both languages to develop mature skills and to become fully bilingual.

Because the use of two languages in classroom instruction actually is bilingual education, several important questions arise:

- What acceptable level of English signals the end of a student's participation?
- Which subjects should be taught in each language?
- How can each language be used most effectively? (That is, how much of each language is to be used to help a student's progress with school subjects?)
- Should English be gradually phased in, or should students be totally immersed in the second language (which, for most of the students discussed here, would be English)?

IMPLICATIONS FOR HEALTHCARE PROVIDERS

Nurses should expect to work with children and families for whom English is not the primary language, and with native-English speakers who have language disabilities. Among native-English speakers, be alert for any articulation disorders, problems with the flow of speech, or speech usage that differs from that of typical children. Know how to connect families with the resources available for children with language disabilities.

Indications that a bilingual child is not progressing in his or her language development include lack of normal milestones in the first language, difficulty with word retrieval, long periods of time when the child does not speak or interact with others, and poor progress in school. If you work regularly with a non-English-speaking population, learn their language, become familiar with their cultural norms, use interpreter services, and identify other resources for newcomers in your area. Ask children about school, and/or develop a relationship with the local schools.

Language barriers often translate into poor health. Immigrant parents with limited English proficiency are three times more likely than English-proficient parents to have a child in fair or poor health, are more likely to be uninsured, and less likely to take their child to a doctor or clinic.

Language barriers often translate into poor health. Immigrant parents with limited English proficiency are three times more likely than English-proficient parents to have a child in fair or poor health, are more likely to be uninsured, and less likely to take their child to a doctor or clinic.

SOURCES

Center for Social and Demographic Analysis, University at Albany, State University of New York. (2007, April 12). *News release: Children in immigrant families firmly rooted in America.* Washington, DC: The Center.

Flores, G., Abreu, M., & Tomany-Korman, S. (2005). Limited English proficiency, primary language at home, and disparities in children's health care: How language barriers are measured matters. *Public Health Reports, 120*(4), 418–430.

Hakuta, K., & McLaughlin, B. (1996). Bilingualism and second language learning: Seven tensions that define the research. In D. Berliner & R. Calfee (Eds.), *Handbook of educational psychology.* New York: Macmillan.

Owens, R. (1996). *Language development: An introduction.* Needham, MA: Allyn & Bacon.

Siegler, R., & Alibali, M. (Eds.). (2005). *Children's thinking* (4th ed.). Upper Saddle River, NJ: Prentice Hall.

- Learning to negotiate peer relationships is central to social development in childhood and for later in life.
- Children's concept of friendship changes as they are able to take someone else's point of view, called a second-person perspective, and to understand how it is similar to and/or different from their own.
- Social cognition is the ability to read a social situation and to act accordingly. It is related to social skills such as conflict resolution.
- The term *playground politics* refers to how children negotiate the complex structure of the peer group, which involves competition, shifting alliances, and conflict, as well as cooperation and trust.

50

Peers and Social Development

TERMS
- ☐ Egocentric
- ☐ Second-person perspective
- ☐ Social cognition
- ☐ Unilateral

PEERS AND SOCIAL DEVELOPMENT

While the attitude of younger children is "The world is my oyster," school-age children believe that "The world is other kids." Peers are central to children's development. Whereas their relationships with adults and with children younger and older than themselves are vertical in nature and reflect a hierarchy of experience and authority, their relationships with peers are more horizontal. Peers may not be equal in ability or expertise or the same age. Nevertheless, they are of roughly equal status in the give-and-take of a relationship, the context for development of social and moral reasoning.

CONCEPT OF FRIENDSHIP AND PERSPECTIVE TAKING

How children think about themselves and friendships is related to cognitive development, and to the ability to take someone else's point of view (Selman & Schultz, 1991) (**Figure 50-1**).

Age 3–6	
A friend . . .	Is who I played with today; won't break my toys.
Perspective	Egocentric: "world is my oyster"; reads actions, not intentions.
Conflict	Is intrusive; impulse hitting; running away.
Feelings	Feelings are outside; smile means happy; feelings associated with events.
Age 5–9	
A friend . . .	Likes the same things as me; "Let's do this."
Perspective	Unilateral: "I win"; I know you have feelings, intents.
Conflict	You versus me; do this or else; "Do what I say or I'll tell the teacher."
Feelings	I can hide feelings inside, so can you; events cause feelings.
Age 7–12	
A friend . . .	Likes me and has the same experiences as me; won't leave me out; keeps secrets.
Perspective	Reciprocal, second-person perspective; I put myself in your shoes, you can put yourself in mine.
Conflict	Between me and you, I'll get you to see it my way; guilt tripping; persuasion.
Feelings	I have more than one feeling about an event; I can pretend to feel angry in order to fool you.
Age 8–15	
A friend . . .	Works to keep our friendship going; knows who I am.
Perspective	Mutual, third-person perspective: I see our friendship as part of a whole.
Conflict	Between us, work it out so the solution benefits both of us.
Feelings	Express multiple conflicting feelings; introspective; not sure how I feel.

Figure 50-1 Stages of Social–Emotional Development

Children ages 3 to 6 are aware that other people have feelings, but they focus on what other people do—not on their subjective experiences or intentions. Friendships are momentary physical interactions. Friends are people they played with this morning. Trust means their friend will not break their toys. Young children ascribe their own feelings to others. When shopping for a present for someone else, children will buy something they themselves want.

During the early school years, friendships become less **egocentric** and more **unilateral**. Children are aware of subjective experiences in others, but their own interests predominate. Friends like the things "I" like to do. "He didn't play fair" really means "He didn't do what I wanted." Teasing is an obnoxious type of verbal dominance behavior and, if left unchecked, turns into harassment.

By age 10, the development of a **second-person perspective** allows children to put themselves in other people's shoes and to experience things from another person's point of view. They expect, in turn, that friends will do the same for them. Children realize that if they can hide feelings and thoughts, so can others; social appearances can be deceiving. Friendships expand beyond sharing activities to sharing subjective experiences. Trust means they will not hurt their friend's feelings, that they understand the desire to be liked and accepted. Hurting people's feelings is understood to be intentional. Being excluded is painful.

Recognizing different perspectives means concrete thinkers can compare themselves with others. No longer is everybody the fastest runner—there can be only one fastest person. Older school-age children who reflect on their own abilities and feelings relative to others become very self-conscious. They are also very effective teachers for younger children and less-able peers because they are so attuned to the other's experience.

SOCIAL COGNITION

Social cognition is the ability to read a social situation and decide how to act accordingly. Whereas social cognition reflects underlying levels of cognitive development, social skills develop with experience, practice, and guidance. How well or how poorly children learn these skills determines their popularity and classroom performance, which in turn affects their self-concept.

Because preschool children focus on what is happening right now, they resolve conflicts by trying to alter circumstances: They impulsively act out, grab toys, withdraw, run away, or shut down emotionally. The consequences tell children that hitting is socially unacceptable and running away solves nothing.

In the early school years, conflict is experienced as unilateral dominance—that is, "Me against you" and "You started it!" The outcomes of unilateral social strategies are designed to favor only one party—me. These strategies include issuing verbal commands and threats, acting victimized, and appealing to powerful others (such as teachers) to intervene.

An appreciation for the second-person perspective during the later school years opens the door to new social skills. If I can see things from your point of view, I can persuade you to see them from mine. I might use my inadequacy as a tool to make you feel guilty. I could do it your way, and next time you'll do it my way. Or let's figure out a way to make it work for everybody. Influence, persuasion, and negotiation are sophisticated strategies that sustain friendships and activities among peers.

THE GAMES CHILDREN PLAY

The school-age years are the period of "playground politics" because children learn to negotiate the complex social structure of the peer group. Alliances shift. The rough-and-tumble play and physical aggression of early childhood give way to competitive games of mental and physical skill. School-age children are inflexible about the rules of competition because rules are a civilized way of resolving conflict and keeping aggressive tendencies in check. Competition can foster the development of social, mental, and physical skills through friendly rivalry. When the only goal is to win, however, competition fosters dominance behavior. Children need cooperative and competence-building activities. Hobbies, Girl and Boy Scout troops, and chores around the house promote cooperation, problem solving, and self-confidence.

 ## IMPLICATIONS FOR HEALTHCARE PROVIDERS

Children who do not have friends are at greater risk for behavioral and emotional difficulties. They may avoid going to school or do poorly in school. Peers also influence children's health behavior, such as eating habits, physical exercise, and risk taking. Always ask children about their friends when doing a health assessment. Ask children these questions as part of your assessment: "Who is your best friend? What kind of things do you like to do together? Is there someone you don't get along with?"

 Ask children these questions as part of your assessment: "Who is your best friend? What kind of things do you like to do together? Is there someone you don't get along with?"

 Children who do not have friends are at greater risk for behavioral and emotional difficulties. They may avoid going to school or do poorly in school.

SOURCES

Greenspan, S. (1993). *Playground politics: Understanding the emotional life of your school-age child.* Reading, MA: Addison-Wesley.

Selman, R., & Schultz, L. (1991). *Making a friend in youth.* Chicago: University of Chicago Press.

QUICK LOOK AT THE CHAPTER AHEAD

- School matters! Children learn not only the basics such as reading, writing, math, art, music, and science; they also learn how to learn, how to solve problems, and how to impose some order onto their thinking.
- Good schools have strong leaders who provide an orderly environment that is safe and supportive; are staffed by qualified teachers who teach a rigorous curriculum with high expectations; are equipped with the resources children need to succeed; and involve parents and the community.
- The No Child Left Behind Act holds schools accountable for students' academic achievement.

51

Schools and Learning

TERMS
- ☐ **Instructional leadership**
- ☐ **Orderly environment**

Schooling is important at any time in a child's life, but developmentally appropriate instruction and materials are especially crucial during middle childhood. Children's talents—abilities in science or mathematics, artistic talent, musical capability, and athletic skill—become apparent between ages 6 and 11. **Table 51-1** lists developmental tasks of middle childhood (note that several of these tasks cross domains).

Much is expected of U.S. schools today. The No Child Left Behind Act of 2001 (PL 107-110) holds schools accountable for students' academic achievement. States must test every child in grades 3 through 8 each year in reading and math, and publish yearly progress reports of their students' progress toward national benchmarks. The No Child Left Behind Act also requires that students be taught by a "highly qualified teacher" who holds at least a bachelor's degree, has obtained full state certification, and has demonstrated knowledge in the core academic subjects he or she teaches. Results of the act have been mixed to date; while progress has been made in some areas of the country, disparities continue to exist along socioeconomic lines. The National Center for Educational Statistics compiles data on all student performance through grade 12.

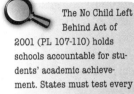

The No Child Left Behind Act of 2001 (PL 107-110) holds schools accountable for students' academic achievement. States must test every child in grades 3 through 8 each year in reading and math, and publish yearly progress reports of their students' progress toward national benchmarks.

SCHOOLS DO MAKE A DIFFERENCE

Schools make a profound difference in children's lives. During the past 25 to 30 years, a substantial body of literature has sharply defined the characteristics marking an effective school. Along with his colleagues, Michael Rutter (1979, 2002), an internationally respected researcher of children's issues, in a massive and meticulously conducted study of school effectiveness, found startling differences between schools. The data led to several conclusions, which have been upheld in follow-up studies (**Table 51-2**):

• Children are more likely to show good behavior and good scholastic achievement when they attend some schools but not others.

Table 51-1 Some Developmental Tasks of Middle Childhood

Physical	Learning the physical skills necessary for games
Cognitive	Building a healthy self-concept
	Learning an appropriate sex role
	Developing the fundamental skills–reading, writing, arithmetic
	Developing concepts for everyday living
Social	Learning to get along with others
	Learning an appropriate sex role
	Developing acceptable attitudes toward society
Personal–emotional	Buiidling a healthy self-concept
	Developing attitudes and values
	Achieving independence

Table 51-2 Characteristics of Good Schools

1. High expectations for every student
2. Parent and community support
3. A rigorous curriculum and fair assessments
4. Sufficient resources to help all students achieve
5. Safe, healthy, and supportive learning environments
6. Schools and classrooms equipped for teaching and learning
7. Qualified teachers in every classroom
8. Strong school leadership

- Differences between schools are not due to the size or age of the buildings, or to the space available.
- Differences between schools are due to a school's emphasis on academic success, teacher expectations of student success, time-on-task, skillful use of rewards and punishment, teachers who provide a comfortable and warm classroom environment, and teachers who insist on student responsibility for their behavior.

These criteria graphically demonstrate that good **instructional leadership** is critical, which means that principals, teachers, students, and parents agree on goals, methods, and content. Home–school cooperation supports good leadership, which in turn produces an **orderly environment** that fosters desirable discipline, academic success, and personal fulfillment. When teachers sense that they have the support of parents and administrators, they intuitively respond in a manner that promotes student achievement and adjustment, encourages collegiality among teachers, and produces a warm, yet exciting atmosphere.

WHAT WE KNOW ABOUT SCHOOLS

President John Kennedy once said that life is unfair. He was right—unfortunately, defective schools do exist. When visiting less-effective schools, an observer is immediately struck by the lack of communication among all the leading players. Everyone and everything seem compartmentalized. Students lack commitment to the school itself or its teachers, teachers lack any degree of collegiality, issues are not discussed, and decisions are rendered from above. Parental involvement is actively discouraged.

Conversely, the following features characterize high-achieving schools:

- A moderately authoritarian principal who works well with parents. The school's leader should have well-defined educational objectives and the motivation, inclination, and skill to achieve them.
- A principal who does not fear to be different if necessary to help students achieve to the best of their ability. A creative and realistic leader can help children to explore new and exciting topics, which merely heightens students' positive feelings toward school.

* A community that agrees with the school about high achievement as the top-priority objective. Principals and teachers should be sensitive to the need for jointly (parents, teachers, administrators) formulated school goals, because cooperation between home and school can further children's achievement and adjustment.
* An educational environment that has high expectations for student achievement. The critical role that expectations play in children's achievement has been a consistent finding of the research. When children know that much is expected of them, they respond to the challenge as well as their ability permits.
* Clearly stated rules and regulations that help students realize their goals. Well-run schools have a few basic rules that children know, understand, and follow. These serve as a guide to acceptable school behavior.
* Teachers, principals, and parents who are willing to fight for the policies and programs that lead to high achievement.

IMPLICATIONS FOR HEALTHCARE PROVIDERS

Schools and health care have long functioned in separate realms. The link between the two has typically been the school nurse, whose duties are often restricted to public health initiatives (immunization schedules, emergency needs of individual students), and who may not be in the school building on a regular basis. Because good health is key to school success, schools need to integrate student health issues with academic initiatives. Children who are malnourished, abused, depressed, or in poor health are at a disadvantage in school.

Children who are malnourished, abused, depressed, or in poor health are at a disadvantage in school.

SOURCES

Give Kids Good Schools. (n.d.). *Home.* Retrieved March 13, 2008, from www.givekidsgoodschools.org

National Center for Educational Statistics. (n.d.). *Welcome to NCES.* Retrieved March 13, 2008, from www.nces.ed.gov

Rutter, M., & Maughan, B. (2002). School effectiveness findings 1979–2002. *Journal of School Psychology, 40*(6), 451–475.

Rutter, M., Maughan, B., Mortimore, P., & Ouston, J. (1979). *Fifteen thousand hours.* Cambridge, MA: Harvard University Press.

U.S. Department of Education. (n.d.). *ED.gov.* Retrieved March 13, 2008, from www.ed.gov

- Creativity is not sudden inspiration; it involves a lot of hard work.
- Creative people have inquiring minds and supportive environments, are willing to look at problems from different perspectives, and have a lot of determination.
- The creative process includes knowledge not only about the subject at hand but about things that might be related to it, as well as the ability to recognize meaningful patterns and to visualize how parts of a pattern are related.
- Gifted children have an unusually high performance ability in a particular area, such as art, math, writing, or leadership, that is not directly related to schooling alone; and they also have a high level of commitment to performing well in this area.

52

Creativity in Children

TERMS
- ☐ Creative process
- ☐ Gifted
- ☐ Graphic imagery
- ☐ Knowledge
- ☐ Mental imagery
- ☐ Perceptual imagery
- ☐ Visualization

The essential ingredients of creativity include an inquiring mind, a supportive environment, a willingness to look at problems from a different perspective, determination that cannot be extinguished, and an acceptance of the risks accompanying novel ventures. It is not just academic or scientific fields that thirst for creative ideas; the way people relate to one another demands creativity, too. The strains of modern living frequently necessitate a new way of looking at relationships, which involves just as much creativity as the work Edison was engaged in. Can children growing up in a modern society retain that spark of creativity that adds a dynamic dimension to their lives?

CHARACTERISTICS OF CREATIVE CHILDREN

Most creative people exhibit several characteristics:

- Creative people learn the strategies needed to solve the problems they inevitably encounter.
- Creative people do not quit when the going gets tough; they persevere.
- Creative people are sensitive to problems.
- Creative people are more fluent than most other people. (They generate a large number of ideas, which is called ideational fluency.)
- Creative people propose novel ideas that are also useful.
- Creative people demonstrate considerable flexibility of mind.
- Creative people reorganize the elements.

Table 52-1 summarizes the more common characteristics of creativity.

THE CREATIVE PROCESS

Three elements are particularly important for understanding the **creative process**: knowledge, visualization, and the thinking process itself.

Knowledge

Knowledge (information) is one of the critical necessities of the creative process. Some children are usually more interested in one subject than in others. For example, some children are drawn almost immediately to physical activities in which they show early grace, skill, and coordination. Other children turn almost intuitively to artistry and demonstrate early talent. Still others are highly ver-

Table 52-1 Common Characteristics of Creativity

Tolerant of ambiguity	Insightful	Intuitive
Flexible	Visual ability	Self-critical
Original	Fluent	Risk taking
Intelligent	Sensitive	Knowledgeable
Independent	Imaginative	Analytical
Able to synthesize	Connected	Curious
Persistent	Resilient	Focused

bal almost from the time they begin to talk. Consequently, children need to acquire vital fundamental knowledge.

Visualization

Three kinds of visual thinking (**visualization**) cut to the heart of the creative process (McKim, 1972):

1. **Perceptual imagery.** Children do not respond to their surroundings on a one-to-one basis. For example, when someone asks you what time it is, do you carefully scrutinize all of the minute markings and the second hand on your watch? No, your familiarity with telling time leads you immediately to the important section where the hands and numbers are. Children do exactly the same thing: They try to form meaningful patterns to help them understand everything going on around them.

2. **Mental imagery.** The information children obtain from their perceptual imagery is stored in the form of a representation. The word "car" is a representation; it *represents* a certain idea (something with wheels, that moves, and so on). Given the tremendous flexibility children have with language, the representation of this object could be stored in many other forms: "auto," "automobile," or "wheels." For each form, however, the information represented remains the same.

3. **Graphic imagery.** Sometimes merely seeing the pieces of a puzzle, or visualizing how words or symbols connect to each other, or even sketching the physical location of people and seeing how they relate to each other will change a pattern and put individuals on track to solve the problem at hand.

BEING GIFTED

The term "gifted and talented" when used in respect to students, children, or youth means students, children, or youth who give evidence of high performance capability in areas such as intellectual, creative, artistic, or leadership capacity, or in specific academic fields, and who require services or activities not ordinarily provided by the school to fully develop such capabilities (P.L. 103–382, Title XIV, p. 388). The definition of **gifted** has three intersecting parts (**Figure 52-1**): above-average IQ, high levels of creativity, and high levels of commitment to a task. Giftedness is manifested in academics, creative thinking, leadership, visual/performing arts, and psychomotor abilities. Approximately 5% of children can be considered gifted, which should not be confused with precociousness. Being gifted does not guarantee later success. Motivation, opportunity, and diligence play a role.

The definition of **gifted** has three intersecting parts (**Figure 52-1**): above-average IQ, high levels of creativity, and high levels of commitment to a task. Giftedness is manifested in academics, creative thinking, leadership, visual/performing arts, and psychomotor abilities.

IMPLICATIONS FOR HEALTHCARE PROVIDERS

AIDS research? Causes of cancer? Urban renewal? Diplomatic breakthroughs? Just think of what is needed to solve these problems: enormous knowledge stored in the researcher's memory; the

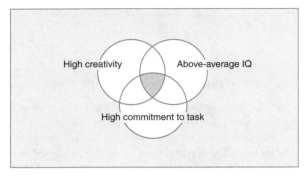

Figure 52-1 Three-Ring Concept of Giftedness

ability to identify crucial relationships in the information; the availability of strategies to attack the problem; a talent for visualizing patterns in a vast array of data; and the skill to recombine elements—that is, move A to M, M to Z, and Z to A. If children's creativity is encouraged early in their lives, they will learn to apply creative thinking to the problems they face, helping them to enjoy richer, more meaningful lives.

SOURCES

Josephson, M. (1959). *Edison.* New York: Wiley.

McKim, R. (1972). *Experiences in visual thinking.* Monterey, CA: Brooks/Cole.

Sternberg, R. J. (Ed.). (1988). *The nature of creativity: Contemporary psychological perspectives.* Cambridge, UK: Cambridge University Press.

- Classic studies of deprivation include the stories of Genie, the Koluchova twins, and Lebanese orphans.
- Recent studies of deprivation have focused on orphans adopted from Romania.
- Resilience has been studied among children on the Isle of Wight in England and on the island of Kauai in Hawaii, and among underprivileged urban youth in American cities, especially Chicago.
- Characteristics of resilience fall into three major categories: characteristics of the child, such as social skills; characteristics of the family, such as a competent, organized parent; and characteristics of the community, such as a supportive school or religious institution where the child finds competent adults interested in his or her ability to do well.
- Resilience is not hardiness of individual character; it is the relationship among the child, family, and community over time.

53

Resilience in Childhood

TERMS
- ☐ **Chronic stress**
- ☐ **Resilience**

Resilience is of interest to nurses for two reasons. First, developmentalists believe there are sensitive periods for attaining certain milestones—for example, attachment. When circumstances interfere with development, how far off the normal developmental path can children stray before the likelihood of recovery is lost? Second, it is important to learn which factors contribute to resilience among children who are subject to **chronic stress** from poverty, abuse, or illness.

DEPRIVATION AND TRAUMA: HOW FAR OFF THE PATH?

Researchers have learned about the effects of deprivation on development by studying children who have been subject to it and then rescued. Three classic examples from the 1970s follow.

The story of Genie, a girl in California, is well known. Genie was tied up alone in a locked room by her father between ages 2 and 13. Food was left but no one spoke to her. When rescued, she could not walk, was not toilet trained, made no sounds, and displayed no emotion. With care, her health recovered, and Genie became responsive to selected people. She never developed normal language, however, and has lasting cognitive deficits.

In Czechoslovakia, twin boys were locked away together as toddlers. Rescued at age 6—and referred to as the Koluchova twins after the researcher who studied them—they could barely talk and lagged cognitively. Unlike Genie, they displayed fear and wariness. After being placed in a home with younger children with whom they could more easily interact, they were adopted and recovered developmentally by age 14.

In Lebanon, babies were abandoned in orphanages and were left to languish in cribs. Those adopted before age 2 recovered. Those adopted at age 4 fared slightly less well. Those subjected to deprivation throughout childhood were functionally retarded by adolescence.

More recently, the adoption of Romanian orphans into stable families in the United Kingdom has allowed researchers to more carefully study patterns of adaptation. Orphans who experienced profound institutional deprivation lasting longer than the first 6 months of life exhibited the same patterns of impairment and normal functioning at ages 6 and 11, albeit to different degrees. Problems with attachment behaviors, attention, and social/peer relationships were the most commonly observed. Orphans who experienced deprivation for less than 6 months had more normal patterns of development. The 6-month cut-off surprised researchers.

These cases indicate that the sensitive period for attachment may possibly be extended to age 4 and language development to age 6 if it is followed by high-quality nurturing. They also illustrate the importance of a biopsychosocial model for understanding development. The deprived Lebanese orphans strayed farther from the normal developmental path than did the Koluchova twins. The twins were developing normally prior to their ordeal, they were confined together and not socially isolated, and they received optimal care afterward. The Romanian orphans were subject to particularly severe deprivation.

> More recently, the adoption of Romanian orphans into stable families in the United Kingdom has allowed researchers to more carefully study patterns of adaptation. Orphans who experienced profound institutional deprivation lasting longer than the first 6 months of life exhibited the same patterns of impairment and normal functioning at ages 6 and 11, albeit to different degrees. Problems with attachment behaviors, attention, and social/peer relationships were the most commonly observed. Orphans who experienced deprivation for less than 6 months had more normal patterns of development. The 6-month cut-off surprised researchers.

CHRONIC STRESS: RISK AND PROTECTIVE FACTORS

Studies of children subjected to chronic adversity have identified which factors increase the risk of poor developmental outcome and which factors protect against the same risk (**Table 53-1**). For example, the children at greatest risk for abuse are those with health problems, especially premature infants; those younger than age 3; those with irritable, defiant, or hyperactive personalities; and those who come from homes chronically stressed by poverty. Girls suffer more sexual abuse than boys. Estimates are that 2 million children are seriously abused in the United States each year.

The Isle of Wight studies in England (Rutter, Yule, Morton, & Bagley, 1975) identified four risk factors that contribute to delinquency, school failure, and mental health problems: (1) serious family discord; (2) parental deviance (criminal activity, mental illness); (3) low socioeconomic status and overcrowded living conditions; and (4) poor school environment. Negative effects are not additive but multiplicative; that is, having two factors increases the risk by 400%, not 200%. Boys are at greater risk than girls.

In a longitudinal study of disadvantaged children on the island of Kauai in Hawaii, 30% prospered better than expected. Children who proved to be resilient had good cognitive and social skills, as well as easy-going personalities that attracted adults and peers, who in turn provided guidance and friendship. Despite the low socioeconomic status, their families were cohesive, with a multigenerational network of family members and friends who helped care for children. The network provided structure, rules, and expectations (e.g., household chores, caring for siblings, doing homework). Although poorly educated, mothers of resilient children often worked outside the home, providing children with competent role models. Resilient children came from communities in which there were adult-run church and school programs, as well as health clinics.

Table 53-1 Risk and Protective Factors in Disadvantaged Children

Risk Factors	Protective Factors
Child	**Child**
Male	Female
Irritable, hyperactive	Easy-going personality
Poor self-control	Good self-control
Learning impairment	Good cognitive skills
Poor social skills	Good social skills
Difficulty making friends	Has friends
Family	**Family**
Family discord/divorce	Cohesive family
Criminal activity in father	Network of friends
Mental illness in mother	Competent mother
Overcrowded living space	Religious affiliation
More than four children, spaced less than 2 years apart	Less than four children, spaced more than 2 years apart
Community	**Community**
Poor school environment	School/community programs
No positive adult role models	Adult guidance

THEORIES OF RESILIENCE

Resilience should not be confused with being "hardy" or "invulnerable." It is not a character trait, but rather a dynamic process arising from interactions between children and the events and people in their lives. The key characteristic of resilience in children is connectedness—to family, friends, and other adults who can provide guidance, hope, and stability. Serendipity also plays a role. In some family circumstances, being the oldest child is a protective factor; in others, it carries risk.

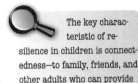

The key characteristic of resilience in children is connectedness—to family, friends, and other adults who can provide guidance, hope, and stability.

Resilience does not imply that there are no harmful effects from adversity. In the face of adversity, resilient children and families are better able to reorganize and to stay on the developmental path.

IMPLICATIONS FOR HEALTHCARE PROVIDERS

For a long time, health care has focused on what goes wrong in human development. Studies on risk and resilience tell us what works—that is, what goes right. Policies and programs that promote and support good health, good schools, nurturing families, and safe neighborhoods that are invested in children's welfare will produce normal, healthy children.

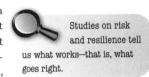

Studies on risk and resilience tell us what works—that is, what goes right.

SOURCES

Dennis, W. (1973). *Children of the creche*. New York: Appleton-Century-Crofts.

Jana, M., Kreppner, J., Rutter, M., Beckett, C., Castle, J., Colvert, E., et al. (2007). Normality and impairment following profound early institutional deprivation: A longitudinal follow-up into early adolescence. *Developmental Psychology, 43*(4), 931–946.

Koluchova, J. (1976). A report on the further development of twins after severe and prolonged deprivation. In A. M. Clarke & A. D. Clarke (Eds.), *Early experience: Myth and evidence*. London: Open Books.

Rutter, M., Yule, B., Morton, J. & Bagley, C. (1975). Attainment and adjustment in two geographical areas. III: Some factors accounting for area differences. *British Journal of Psychiatry, 126*, 520–533.

Werner, E., & Smith, R. (1992). *Overcoming the odds: High risk children from birth to adulthood*. Ithaca, NY: Cornell University Press.

QUICK LOOK AT THE CHAPTER AHEAD

- Developmental disabilities represent an alteration in either the sequence of and/or the resulting integration among three areas: motor, cognitive (which includes language), and neurobehavioral development.
- Mental retardation is characterized by below average intellect *and* limitations in two or more adaptive skills, such as inability to live alone or to manage personal finances.
- Children with learning disabilities have normal intelligence but below average achievement in a particular area, such as reading.
- The Individuals with Disabilities Education Act (IDEA) calls for children with disabilities to be educated in local schools along with same-age peers.
- Children with chronic medical conditions, such as diabetes, represent a growing population facing unique challenges during childhood.

54

Children with Challenges

TERMS
- ☐ Developmental delay
- ☐ Developmental disabilities
- ☐ Dissociation
- ☐ Learning disabilities
- ☐ Mental retardation
- ☐ Other health impaired (IDEA)

As human development unfolds, development in one area is tied to development in other areas. Play behavior shows an integration of language, visuomotor, and problem-solving skills. Of course, not all children follow the typical developmental path. Three groups are exceptions. According to the Social Securities Act of 1985, "children with special health care needs" account for three overlapping groups: those with developmental disabilities, mental retardation, and learning disabilities; those with chronic illness, such as diabetes and asthma; and those with emotional/behavioral difficulties, including attention-deficit disorder (ADD).

DEVELOPMENTAL DISABILITIES, MENTAL RETARDATION, AND LEARNING DISABILITIES

Developmental disabilities represent alterations in the typical developmental sequence in one or more of three areas: motor, cognitive, and neurobehavior (**Figure 54-1**). "Motor" includes gross motor, fine motor, and visuomotor coordination. "Cognitive" includes central processing, problem solving, and language. "Neurobehavior" refers to self-help, self-regulatory, and social skills. These developmental disabilities are characterized by delay, dissociation, and/or deviation from the norm (Capute & Accardo, 1996).

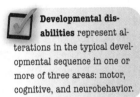

Developmental disabilities represent alterations in the typical developmental sequence in one or more of three areas: motor, cognitive, and neurobehavior.

A **developmental delay** is a significant lag in meeting milestones; for example, motor delays may indicate cerebral palsy. **Dissociation** is a difference between the rate of development in two aspects of one area—for example, between expressive and receptive language in children who are deaf. When the sequence of development in one or more areas deviates sufficiently from the norm, the overall pattern that emerges over time represents a different developmental path. In children with autism, the development of language, social, and problem-solving skills is so skewed that the pattern of play behavior and peer interactions that emerges is very different from the norm.

Mental retardation is characterized by "subaverage intellectual functioning" along with limitations in two or more adaptive skills (e.g., academics, communication, ability to live on one's own, social skills, leisure, and work.) Mental retardation is a distinctive feature of fragile X syndrome, Down syndrome, and fetal alcohol syndrome. The current definition of mental retardation reflects

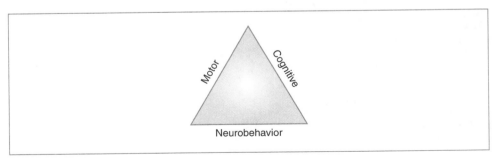

Figure 54-1 Triangle of Developmental Disabilities

a new approach that broadens the previous emphasis on IQ scores to include abilities and adaptive skills.

Learning disabilities are characterized by a discrepancy between ability as measured on intelligence tests and actual achievement. The most common learning disabilities involve language function and metacognitive abilities, such as memory and problem solving. It is estimated that 3% to 15% of all U.S. school children have a learning disability.

 Learning disabilities are characterized by a discrepancy between ability as measured on intelligence tests and actual achievement.

CHRONIC MEDICAL ILLNESS AND CHRONIC HEALTH CONDITIONS

Chronic health conditions are biologically based, involve organ systems, and last for at least 3 to 12 months. They compromise day-to-day functioning; and/or require special diets, medications, or assistive devices; and/or require more health care than is routine. In the United States, as many as 30% of people younger than age 21 have one of a wide range of chronic health conditions, which include disabilities and chronic illness (**Table 54-1**); the prevalence is highest among the rural poor. Approximately 6% to 15% of youth have a chronic illness, which includes diabetes, cancer, and hemophilia. Asthma affects 4% of U.S. children.

Families of children with chronic illness and disability have similar risk and protective factors (**Table 54-2**). Poor developmental outcome is linked to unresolved family discord, lack of structure and organization, lower socioeconomic class, and functional dependence on parents by the child for routine care, such as feeding. Contrary to popular belief, severity of illness or disability alone is not a factor.

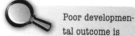 Poor developmental outcome is linked to unresolved family discord, lack of structure and organization, lower socioeconomic class, and functional dependence on parents by the child for routine care, such as feeding. Contrary to popular belief, severity of illness or disability alone is not a factor.

Factors that protect children with health problems include families that are cohesive and organized, and that promote autonomy. Such families are typically connected to the community through work. The better educated the mother, the better off the child. Educated mothers are adept at finding the resources medically ill children need, and their families tend to be of a higher socioeconomic class.

Table 54-1 Common Disabilities and Illnesses Affecting U.S. Children

Common Disabilities	Common Illnesses	Laws to Know
Autism	Asthma (4.3%)	1973: Section 504 of the Rehabilitation Act
Blind, vision disorders	Cancer	
Deaf, hearing impairments	Cystic fibrosis	1975: PL 142-92 IDEA
Cerebral palsy	Diabetes	1990: ADA
Down syndrome	Hemophilia	1997: Reauthorization of IDEA
Mental retardation	Juvenile rheumatoid arthritis	Medicaid laws (by state)
Spina bifida	Sickle-cell anemia	Social Security (by state)

Table 54-2 Risk and Protective Factors in Adaptation to Chronic Illness

Risk Factors: Disease/Disability	Resistance Factors
Functional dependence	Child: social competence, problem-solving skills, stress
Involvement of brain	appraisal and coping
Impaired cognitive fuctioning	Social: cohesive family, support for mother, social network,
Poor bowel/bladder control	practical resources (money, insurance) child has friends,
Visible, especially the face	activities
Chronicity, daily hassles	

BEHAVIORAL/EMOTIONAL DIFFICULTIES

Self-regulation in response to demands from people, settings, and events is key to adaptive behavior. While many children occasionally have difficulties, approximately 9% of U.S. children have serious conduct disorders, and 4% to 6% have attention-deficit/hyperactivity disorder (ADHD). Post-traumatic stress disorder (PTSD) is often found in children who have been abused. The prevalence of behavior and attention disorders is higher in boys and in lower socioeconomic groups.

Post-traumatic stress disorder (PTSD) is often found in children who have been abused. The prevalence of behavior and attention disorders is higher in boys and in lower socioeconomic groups.

Treatment of ADHD is controversial. It is easier to medicate a child with Ritalin (methylphenidate) than to change the classroom environment.

Approximately 2% of children and 5% of adolescents in the United States are clinically depressed. Depression in youth is underdiagnosed by health professionals, who minimize the symptoms as a passing phase or a natural response to a stressful event. Left untreated, it may lead to social withdrawal, school failure, self-destructive behavior, and suicide.

Approximately 2% of children and 5% of adolescents in the United States are clinically depressed.

SOCIAL POLICY ISSUES

The emphasis must be on the child first and the condition second. The accepted reference is to "children with mental retardation"—not "retarded children." Children are not "cancer victims" nor do they "suffer" from spina bifida. Advocates are also responsible for a wide range of reform efforts.

The Individuals with Disabilities Education Act of 1975 (IDEA; reauthorized by Congress in 1997) allows children with disabilities to be educated in local schools rather than forcing them to be warehoused in institutions. The IDEA includes a category of disability called "**other health impaired**," which addresses children with chronic illness. The Americans with Disabilities Act of 1990 (ADA) makes it illegal to discriminate against people with disabilities, especially in the workplace and in school.

SOURCES

Capute, A., & Accardo, P. (Eds.). (1996). *Developmental disabilities in infancy and childhood* (2nd ed.). *Volume I. Neurodevelopmental diagnosis and treatment.* Baltimore: Paul Brookes.

Ireys, H. (1994). *Children with special health care needs: Evaluating their needs and relevant service structures.* Unpublished paper. Institute of Medicine, Johns Hopkins University, Baltimore, MD.

Kronenberger, W., & Thompson, R. (1990). Dimensions of family functioning in families with chronically ill children: A higher order factor analysis of the Family Environment Scale. *Journal of Clinical Child Psychology, 19*(4), 380–388.

Parker, S., & Zuckerman, B. (Eds.). (1995). *Behavioral and developmental pediatrics: A handbook for primary care.* Boston: Little, Brown.

PART V • QUESTIONS

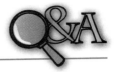

For each of the following questions, choose the **one best** answer.

1. By what age can children typically ride a two-wheel bicycle?
   a. 5 years
   b. 7 years
   c. 9 years
   d. 11 years
2. Malnourished children in the United States tend to be obese, not thin, because
   a. they consume a lot of junk food.
   b. they watch too much television.
   c. they eat too many packaged foods.
   d. All of the above.
3. What did Piaget mean by "concrete operations"?
   a. Children's thinking is perceptually bound.
   b. Causal reasoning is based on association.
   c. Children's thinking is very matter-of-fact.
   d. Children can do mentally what had to be done physically before.
4. Boys of about ages 9 to 10 love to collect and sort baseball cards. Which characteristic of concrete thought contributes to this activity?
   a. Hierarchical classification skills
   b. Matrix classification skills
   c. Abstract thinking
   d. Set identity
5. Sternberg's theory is based on
   a. context.
   b. gender.
   c. age.
   d. biology.
6. Gardner's theory of intelligence includes _____ types of equal intelligence.
   a. two
   b. four
   c. six
   d. eight
7. A well-known model of problem solving is
   a. HOME.
   b. DUPE.
   c. NATO.
   d. SAC.

8. Everyone should attempt to internally represent solutions to problems.
   a. True
   b. False
   c. Uncertain
9. Kohlberg used a method called
   a. cognitive structuring.
   b. contextual determinism.
   c. moral dilemmas.
   d. contingencies of reinforcement.
10. Gilligan believed that Kohlberg's work was too _____ oriented.
    a. age
    b. culture
    c. neutral
    d. male
11. LEP refers to those students whose primary language is not
    a. English.
    b. Spanish.
    c. French.
    d. Vietnamese.
12. To work with LEP students, many school systems are trying to decide between ESL programs and
    a. separate systems.
    b. bilingual education.
    c. native-born instructors.
    d. curricular insertion.
13. By about what age do children develop reciprocity in their friendships?
    a. 6 years
    b. 8 years
    c. 10 years
    d. 12 years
14. Which of the following statements best describes children's games during middle childhood?
    a. Children are inflexible about the rules of competition.
    b. Rules help to keep aggression in check.
    c. Competition can foster social, mental, and physical development.
    d. All of the above are correct.
15. Good schools are characterized by their emphasis on
    a. building conditions.
    b. recreational facilities.
    c. amount of materials.
    d. academic success.

16. The author of an influential study of school effectiveness was
    a. Rutter.
    b. Piaget.
    c. Bruner.
    d. Skinner.
17. Creativity is also known as
    a. critical thinking.
    b. convergent thinking.
    c. divergent thinking.
    d. vertical thinking.
18. Among the characteristics of creativity are visualization, thinking processes, and
    a. knowledge.
    b. contingency.
    c. laterality.
    d. symmetry.
19. What is the sensitive period for the development of language?
    a. Up to 2 years old
    b. Up to 4 years old
    c. Up to 6 years old
    d. Up to 8 years old
20. Which triad of factors contributes to resilience in children at risk?
    a. Family discord, low socioeconomic status, poor school environment
    b. Cohesive family, easy-going personality, competent adults in community
    c. Mothers who work, absent fathers, good social skills
    d. Being in foster care, concerned case worker, visits with mother
21. Developmental disabilities represent alterations in the typical developmental sequence of which three areas?
    a. Fine motor, gross motor, intelligence
    b. Problem solving, language, motor coordination
    c. Motor, cognitive, neurobehavior
    d. Neurobehavior, intelligence, gross motor
22. Which of the following characteristics describes children who are gifted?
    a. Above-average IQ
    b. High levels of creativity
    c. High levels of commitment to a task
    d. All of the above

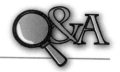

PART V · ANSWERS

1. **The answer is b.** The organization of the central nervous system in school-age children is like that in adults, contributing to better physical coordination. There is an increase in muscle mass relative to body weight. Body proportions change during the school years. Children have a lower center of gravity. There is an increase in leg length, a decrease in head size, and a decrease in waist size relative to height. All of these changes contribute to physical agility, so that riding a bike, kicking a soccer ball, or hiking a mountain trail is easier and more coordinated.

2. **The answer is d.** Malnourished children in the United States tend to be obese, not thin, because they consume too much fat and sugar, mostly in junk foods. Their families use more high-fat, low-cost packaged foods, such as macaroni and cheese, and eat fewer fresh fruits and vegetables. Also, the average child who watches 4 hours of television per day is not playing outside, expending energy, strengthening muscles and bones, and increasing aerobic capacity.

3. **The answer is d.** In school-age children, concrete operational thinking consists of mental operations that allow children to do mentally what had to be experienced physically before. Actions can be played out in their minds, giving them more flexibility for solving problems than during the preschool years. Concrete thought is characterized by decreasing centration, reversibility of a mental sequence, set identity, conservation of physical properties, classification skills, and inability to think abstractly.

4. **The answer is b.** "Hierarchical classification" refers to the ability to understand the relationship between subordinate and superordinate classes. Matrix classification skills are more complex. Children can categorize things along two dimensions simultaneously—for example, baseball teams by player positions. A 2-by-2 matrix might consist of two rows of teams (Red Sox and Yankees) and 2 columns of positions (pitchers and catchers). This matrix can expand or be rearranged to include multiple teams, positions, years, and players.

5. **The answer is a.** Sternberg recognized that intelligence reflects the context in which it is embedded. That is, different cultures value different skills and place a greater premium on them.

6. **The answer is d.** Gardner believed that we can no longer view intelligence as a unitary concept. Rather, different tasks require different intelligences.

7. **The answer is b.** The DUPE model offers several clear guidelines for solving problems in a logical manner.

8. **The answer is b.** No one should be forced to use a technique with which he or she is uncomfortable. Both children and adults, depending on their personality and experience, will determine what is best for them.

9. **The answer is c.** Kohlberg relied on moral dilemmas to discover the level of a person's moral development. This method forced subjects to indicate why they thought as they did.

10. **The answer is d.** Gilligan believed that Kohlberg's dependence on male subjects neglected women's viewpoints. She argued that women traveled a different path of moral development.

11. **The answer is a.** LEP stands for limited English proficiency. With the great wave of immigration that has swept across the United States, many children in U.S. classrooms now have difficulty with English.

12. **The answer is b.** Controversy rages concerning the most effective means of teaching LEP students. Bilingual education seems to be gaining favor as the preferred method.

13. **The answer is c.** By age 10, the development of a second-person perspective allows children to put themselves in the other person's shoes and experience things from their point of view. They expect that friends will do the same for them. Children realize that if they can hide feelings and thoughts, so can others; social appearances can be deceiving. Friendships expand beyond sharing activities to include sharing subjective experiences. Trust means that the child does not hurt his or her friend's feelings, and that the child understands the desire to be liked and accepted. Consequently, hurting people's feelings is understood to be intentional. Being excluded is painful.

14. **The answer is d.** The school-age years are the period of "playground politics," during which children learn to negotiate the complex social structure of the peer group. There are different kinds of friends for different occasions, alliances shift, and secrets are kept. The rough-and-tumble play and physical aggression of early childhood give way to competitive games of mental and physical skill. School-age children are inflexible about the rules of competition because such rules offer a civilized way of resolving conflict and keeping aggressive tendencies in check. Competition can foster the development of social, mental, and physical skills through friendly rivalry. When the only goal is to win, however, competition fosters dominance behavior.

15. **The answer is d.** A school's emphasis on academic success sets it apart from other similar schools that lack this emphasis. Other qualities are secondary to academic success.

16. **The answer is a.** Rutter's work is a widely quoted study of school success that has had far-reaching implications. Its major conclusion stressed the significance of instructional excellence and emphasis on academic success.

17. **The answer is c.** Creative or divergent thinking is marked by a search for novel ideas and products. Creative individuals are not afraid to diverge from customary paths.

18. **The answer is a.** Unless a person has knowledge of a subject, it is difficult—if not impossible—for him or her to engage in divergent thinking.

19. **The answer is c.** Case histories of children who were subject to early deprivation reveal that the sensitive period for language development can be extended to age 6 if it is followed by high-quality nurturing.

20. **The answer is b.** Children who are resilient have good cognitive and social skills, as well as easy-going personalities. Their families are cohesive, with a multigenerational network of family members and friends that provides structure, rules, and expectations. Resilient children come from communities in which there are adult-run church and school programs, as well as health clinics.

21. **The answer is c.** Developmental disabilities represent alterations in the typical developmental sequence in one or more of three areas: motor, cognitive, and neurobehavior. The motor area includes gross motor, fine motor, and visuomotor coordination. The cognitive area includes central processing, problem solving, and language. Neurobehavior refers to self-help,

self-regulatory, and social skills. This triangle of developmental disabilities is characterized by delay, and/or dissociation, and/or deviation from the norm.

22. **The answer is d.** The definition of "gifted" has three intersecting parts: above-average IQ, high levels of creativity, and high levels of commitment to a task. Giftedness is manifested in academics, creative thinking, leadership, visual/performing arts, and psychomotor abilities. Approximately 5% of U.S. children can be considered gifted, which should not be confused with precociousness.

VI

Adolescence

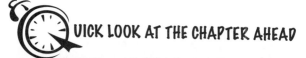

- Puberty is characterized by the release of female and male hormones, which bring reproductive organs to full maturity and are responsible for sexual characteristics, such as pubic hair.
- Tanner's description of the stages of puberty is still used by healthcare providers.
- The average age of the onset of menarche among girls in the United States is age 12, compared to age 17 about 100 years ago.
- The timing of the onset of puberty has social implications for boys and girls, with early maturing girls and late maturing boys experiencing the most difficulty.
- Precocious puberty occurs when the signs of puberty appear before the age of 8 years, and may be due to tumors or to fat intake and environmental contaminants.

55

Puberty

TERMS

☐ Estrogen
☐ Follicle-stimulating hormone (FSH)
☐ Gonadotropin-releasing hormone (GnRH)
☐ Luteinizing hormone (LH)
☐ Postpubescence
☐ Prepubescence
☐ Progesterone
☐ Puberty
☐ Testosterone

287

Physically, adolescence is bounded by the beginning and end of puberty, the period of physical maturation of the reproductive organs. These borders are imprecise, because puberty occurs in stages over time, beginning at ages 10 to 12 (in girls) and ending at ages 18 to 20 (in boys). The physical changes of puberty underlie the cognitive, social, and emotional changes that have earned adolescence the reputation for being a tumultuous and bittersweet time of life.

The term **puberty** refers to sexual maturity, which in girls means the onset of menstruation and in boys is harder to define. **Prepubescence** is the 2-year period of preliminary changes that occur prior to the onset of puberty. **Postpubescence** extends another 2 years or so beyond puberty, during which time bone growth is completed and the reproductive organs become fully mature. The sequence of sexual maturation has been described by Tanner (1990), whose Sexual Maturity Rating Scale is used by healthcare providers to track the development of breasts in girls and of the penis and scrotum in boys (**Table 55-1**).

> The term **puberty** refers to sexual maturity, which in girls means the onset of menstruation and in boys is harder to define.

SEX CHARACTERISTICS AND HORMONES

Puberty begins when the hypothalamus starts to produce **gonadotropin-releasing hormone (GnRH)**, which is transported via the bloodstream to the pituitary gland. The pituitary gland releases **luteinizing hormone (LH)**, which stimulates the production of sex hormones by the gonads (ovaries and testes) and other endocrine glands in both males and females. Primary sexual characteristics (i.e., maturation of the ovaries, breasts, uterus, penis, and testes) develop in the reproductive organs as a result of sex hormone production. Secondary sexual characteristics (i.e., development of facial, body, and pubic hair; deepening voice; and distribution of fat and muscle), accompany hormonal changes but are not directly involved in reproduction.

> Puberty begins when the hypothalamus starts to produce **gonadotropin-releasing hormone (GnRH)**, which is transported via the bloodstream to the pituitary gland.

Male sex hormones, called androgens, are produced by the cells of Leydig in the testes. The principal androgen is **testosterone**. In the male fetus, testosterone is responsible for development of the male reproductive organs. At puberty, testosterone stimulates overall growth, including muscles, vocal cords, and body hair, in addition to promoting maturation of the reproductive system. During this time, semen production begins, and the male is able to experience erection and ejaculation. Boys experience "wet dreams" when they ejaculate semen during sleep.

In females, GnRH also stimulates the release of **follicle-stimulating hormone (FSH)** from the pituitary. Together, FSH and LH are responsible for the production of female sex hormones, **estrogen** and **progesterone**, from the ovaries. Recall that a girl's ovaries attain their full complement of egg cells—approximately 2 million—during prenatal development. Puberty marks the beginning of the menstrual cycle, during which an egg cell matures and is released into the uterus, making it available for fertilization from male sperm.

The menstrual cycle, which averages about 28 days, is complex and highly regulated by hormones. The cycle begins on day 1 with the onset of the menstrual flow. The first 13 days are called the follicular phase, during which FSH stimulates the follicles in the ovary to develop. As one follicle becomes more dominant and begins to secrete estrogen, the egg cell it contains matures. The

Table 55-1 Composite of the Sexual Maturity Rating Scale

Stage	Genital Development in Males	Pubic Hair Development in Males and Females	Breast Development in Females
1	Testes, scrotum, and penis are about the same size and shape as in early childhood.	The vellus over the pubes is not further developed than over the abdominal wall; in other words, there is no pubic hair.	There is elevation of the papilla only.
2	Scrotum and testes are slightly enlarged. The skin of the scrotum is reddened and changed in texture. There is little or no enlargement of the penis at this stage.	There is sparse growth of long, slightly pigmented, tawny hair, straight or slightly curled, chiefly at the base of the penis or along the labia.	Breast bud stage. There is elevation of the breast and the papilla as a small mound. Areolar diameter is enlarged over that of stage 1.
3	Penis is slightly enlarged, at first mainly in length. Testes and scrotum are further enlarged than in stage 2.	The hair is considerably darker, coarser, and more curled. It spreads sparsely over the function of the pubes.	Breast and areola are both enlarged and elevated more than in stage 2 but with no separation of their contours.
4	Penis is further enlarged, with growth in breadth and development of glans. Testes and scrotum are further enlarged than in stage 3; scrotum skirt is darker than in earlier stages.	Hair is now adult in type, but the area covered is still considerably smaller than in the adult. There is no spread to the medial surface of the thighs.	The areola and papilla form a secondary mound projecting above the contour of the breast.
5	Genitalia are adult in size and shape.	The hair is adult in quantity and type with distribution of the horizontal (or classically "feminine") pattern. Spread is to the medial surface of the thighs but not up the linea alba or elsewhere above the base of the inverse triangle.	Mature stage. The papilla projects but the areola is recessed to the general contour of the breast.

increase in estrogen causes the lining of the uterus to thicken; it also triggers a surge of LH at about day 14. The follicle ruptures and the egg cell, called the oocyte, is released into the fallopian tubes—an event called ovulation.

The second half of the menstrual cycle, about days 14 to 28, is the luteal phase. The ruptured follicle collapses, forming the corpus luteum, which secretes progesterone and small amounts of estrogen. Progesterone causes the uterine lining to mature in preparation for implantation of a fertilized embryo; it also inhibits the production of FSH, which would trigger the beginning of a new cycle. If fertilization does not occur, the increase in progesterone from the corpus luteum also shuts down production of LH, which sustains the corpus luteum itself. As the corpus luteum begins to disintegrate and progesterone levels fall, FSH production is no longer inhibited and begins anew. Without progesterone, the lining of the uterus cannot be sustained, and it is shed in the form of the menstrual flow. The menstrual cycle then begins again.

CAUSES AND EFFECTS OF THE TIMING OF PUBERTY

The production of sex hormones and of GnRH in the hypothalamus is influenced by genetics, nutritional and health status, chronic stress, and environmental factors. Today, the average age at the onset of menstruation among North American girls is 12 years, compared to age 17 about 100 years ago. For boys, the average age of puberty is 14 years, down from almost age 16 a century ago.

The trend toward earlier onset of puberty has been attributed to better nutrition, especially fat intake, and to increased exposure to natural and artificial light. The brain may interpret the increase in light as evidence of environmental changes that support the growth of the food supply. Conversely, the female body responds to a drastic drop in body weight and fat by shutting down menstruation, regardless of whether the cause is famine, illness, excessive exercise, or anorexia nervosa. Males may also experience a drop in sperm production in response to undue stress or illness.

The timing of puberty has important social implications. Early-maturing girls and late-maturing boys have the most difficulty adjusting. Girls who begin puberty at age 10 or 11 are a year or more ahead of their female peers, and 3 to 4 years ahead of their average male peers. The difference in physical maturity highlights the greater discrepancy in social, emotional, and cognitive maturity.

The late-maturing male still looks like a boy at age 15 or 16. Such males have difficulty competing with their physically mature male peers both in sports and in the social arena, undermining their self-confidence. Ironically, the late-maturing male may eventually grow to be larger than his early-maturing male peers.

IMPLICATIONS FOR HEALTHCARE PROVIDERS

Is puberty coming too early? Some studies have found that the mean age for onset of breast development is 8.87 years for African American girls and 9.96 years for white girls; for onset of pubic hair development, mean ages were 8.78 years and 10.51 years, respectively—that is, Tanner Stage 2. Precocious puberty means having the signs of puberty (development of breasts, testes, and pubic and underarm hair; body odor; menstrual bleeding; and increased growth rate) appear before age 8 in a girl or 9½ in a boy. Other than evidence of pathology (e.g., tumor), most causes of precocious

Is puberty coming too early? Some studies have found that the mean age for onset of breast development is 8.87 years for African American girls and 9.96 years for white girls; for onset of pubic hair development, mean ages were 8.78 years and 10.51 years, respectively—that is, Tanner Stage 2. Precocious puberty means having the signs of puberty (development of breasts, testes, and pubic and underarm hair; body odor; menstrual bleeding; and increased growth rate) appear before age 8 in a girl or 9 ½ in a boy. Other than evidence of pathology (e.g., tumor), most causes of precocious puberty are not identified; researchers are studying obesity, high fat intake, and environmental contaminants.

puberty are not identified; researchers are studying obesity, high fat intake, and environmental contaminants.

SOURCES

Herman-Giddens, M. E., Slora, E., Wasserman, R. C., Bourdony, C. J., Bhapkar, M. V., Koch, G. G., et al. (1997). Secondary sexual characteristics and menses in young girls seen in office practice: A study from the pediatric research in office settings network. *Pediatrics 99*(4), 505–512.

Tanner, J. M. (1990). *Foetus into man*. Cambridge, MA: Harvard University Press.

University of Michigan Medical School and Health System. (2008). *Home*. Retrieved March 13, 2008, from www.med.umich.edu

- The National Youth Risk Behavior Surveillance Survey is conducted by the Centers for Disease Control (CDC) each year.
- The survey collects data on several behaviors, including nutrition and exercise; use of tobacco products, alcohol, and illicit drugs; and sexual behavior.
- Compared to 10 years ago, consumption of fresh fruits and vegetables, exercise, binge drinking, and smoking are down among adolescents, whereas riding in a car with a friend who had been drinking is up.

56

Healthy and Risky Behaviors

TERMS
☐ Alcohol
☐ Drugs
☐ Healthy People 2010
☐ Nutrition

The U.S. Department of Health and Human Services has a national health promotion and disease prevention campaign called **Healthy People 2010**. Objectives are set for 10-year periods; those relevant to school-age children and adolescents are shown in **Table 56-1**. The Centers for Disease Control and Prevention (CDC) regularly conduct a nationwide Youth Risk Behavior Surveillance Survey among more than 10,000 students in grades 9 to 12. The data cited in this chapter compare the 1995 and 2005 reports (updated as of April 2007). Data are from 2005 unless noted otherwise.

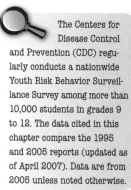

The Centers for Disease Control and Prevention (CDC) regularly conducts a nationwide Youth Risk Behavior Surveillance Survey among more than 10,000 students in grades 9 to 12. The data cited in this chapter compare the 1995 and 2005 reports (updated as of April 2007). Data are from 2005 unless noted otherwise.

NUTRITION AND EXERCISE

Boys have higher caloric needs than girls because boys have a greater proportion of lean body mass to adipose tissue. A rapidly growing athletic 15-year-old boy may need as many as 4000 calories per day just to maintain his weight. By contrast, an inactive 15-year-old girl, whose growth is almost completed, may need fewer than 2000 calories a day to avoid gaining weight. Half of adult bone structure is deposited during adolescence, requiring 1200 mg of calcium per day.

In 1995, 27% of adolescents ate the five or more recommended servings of fresh fruits and vegetables (foods rich in calcium, iron, and vitamins) in a 24-hour period; in 2005, only 20% did so. In 1995,

In 2005, 16% of boys and 10% of girls were considered overweight (based on BMI ≥ 95th percentile by age and gender), with the greatest prevalence among Hispanic males (21.3%) and black females (16%).

Table 56-1 Healthy People 2010 Baselines and Targets, Grades 9–12

	Baseline (year)	Target 2010
Tobacco Products		
Adolescents who used any tobacco products in past month	40% (1999)	21%
Adolescents who used cigarettes in past month	35% (1999)	16%
Alcohol and Drugs		
High school seniors who have *never* used alcohol	19% (1998)	24%
High school seniors who have *never* used illicit substances	46% (1998)	56%
Adolescents who rode in a car with a driver who had been drinking alcohol	33% (1999)	30%
Adolescents who used marijuana in past 30 days	8.2% (2002)	0.7%
Adolescents who engaged in binge drinking in past 2 weeks	32% (1998)	11%
Adolescents who *have not* used alcohol or illicit substances in past 30 days	78% (2002)	91%
Exercise and Nutrition		
Adolescents who engage in regular activity, either moderate or vigorous	32% (1997)	50%
Adolescents who are overweight/obese	16% (2002)	5%

boys (32%) ate more fruits and vegetables than girls (22.7%) did; in 2005, that was still true, but the total percentages had decreased for both genders, to 21.4% and 18.3% respectively. Boys simply eat more food, although they are less likely to consider themselves overweight (25%) than girls (38%). In 2005, 16% of boys and 10% of girls were considered overweight (based on BMI ≥ 95th percentile by age and gender), with the greatest prevalence among Hispanic males (21.3%) and black females (16%).

In 1995, 63% of teens exercised vigorously at least three times per week, with boys (74%) doing so more than girls (52%), and whites (67%) doing so more than blacks (53%). In 2005, only 35.8% met the new standard of 60 minutes or more exercise for 5 days a week, again with males (43.8%) reporting more activity than females (27.8%), and whites (38.7%) reporting more exercise than blacks (29.5%) and Hispanics (32.9%). Black females were least likely to exercise (21.3%). At the same time, the 2005 survey found that black females are also most likely to watch more than 3 hours of TV each day (64.5%), compared to white females (28.1%), who are the least likely TV watchers among all youth. Participation in exercise of any kind, and in team sports in particular, tends to decline from 9th to 12th grade, as work and other activities begin to take precedence.

Teens who eat diets high in starches and fats and who are overweight and sedentary are at greater risk for dying before the age of 70 from heart disease, stroke, and colon cancer, compared to their leaner and more active peers. Efforts to reduce the risk for disease range from healthier school lunches and **nutrition** education to early screening for high blood pressure and cholesterol.

> In 1995, 63% of teens exercised vigorously at least three times per week, with boys (74%) doing so more than girls (52%), and whites (67%) doing so more than blacks (53%). In 2005, only 35.8% met the new standard of 60 minutes or more exercise for 5 days a week, again with males (43.8%) reporting more activity than females (27.8%), and whites (38.7%) reporting more exercise than blacks (29.5%) and Hispanics (32.9%).

SMOKING

While both incidence and frequency of smoking cigarettes increase as students get older, smoking has declined among youth between 1995 and 2005. In 1995, 63.4% of 9th graders had tried cigarettes, whereas 75.8% of 12th graders had done so; in 2005, those numbers were 48.7% and 60.3%, respectively. In 1995, 9.6% of 9th graders smoked frequently, rising to 20.9% by 12th grade; in 2005, prevalence had decreased to 6.9% and 13.2%, respectively. While there is no difference between males and females in total (9.3% for both), white girls are most likely to smoke (11.7%), and black girls are least likely (2.4%) to do so.

The best predictors of smoking behavior are having parents and friends who smoke, with the influence of friends being greater earlier in adolescence rather than later. Advertisements—especially those that implicate smoking with thinness in women—also play a role. The decrease in smoking over the 10-year period could be at-

> In 1995, 63.4% of 9th graders had tried cigarettes, whereas 75.8% of 12th graders had done so; in 2005, those numbers were 48.7% and 60.3%, respectively. In 1995, 9.6% of 9th graders smoked frequently, rising to 20.9% by 12th grade; in 2005, prevalence had decreased to 6.9% and 13.2%, respectively.

tributed to a number of factors, from education programs that warn students about the long-term risks of smoking to fewer displays of smoking behavior on television and in movies. Adolescents are not inclined to change their current behavior based on information alone, however. Instead, successful smoking prevention programs have combined information about the dangers of tobacco with efforts to improve social skills and change attitudes about the social merits of smoking.

The decrease in smoking over the 10-year period could be attributed to a number of factors, from education programs that warn students about the long-term risks of smoking to fewer displays of smoking behavior on television and in movies.

ALCOHOL AND DRUGS

As is the case with cigarette smoking, **alcohol** use increases with age. By 12th grade, the majority of students (81.7%) have had at least one alcoholic drink, and half of all high school seniors (50.8%) report using alcohol within the past month. In 2005, 43.3% of all students in grades 9 through 12 reported having used alcohol at some time during the previous 30 days, a decline from 51.6% in 1995. Statistics indicate that white (46.4%) and Hispanic (46.8%) students are still more likely to drink than are black students (31.2%). Binge drinking has decreased among 12th graders, from 39% reporting this behavior in 1995 to 32.8% in 2005. However, in 2005, drinking was an equal-opportunity behavior among boys (43.8%) and girls (42.8%), although boys were somewhat more likely to engage in binge drinking than were girls (27.5% and 23.5%, respectively). Of serious concern is the finding that 28.5% of all students in 2005 reported riding in a car driven by someone who had been drinking, with Hispanic youths (36.1%) most likely to take this risk.

Use of marijuana and other **drugs** is still more prevalent among boys than among girls, and more prevalent among Hispanic students than among white students and black students. While 38.4% of students in grades 9 through 12 in 2005 had tried marijuana, 22% of males had used it within the past month, compared to 18% of girls, with the highest prevalence among Hispanic males (28%). Twelve percent of Hispanic students have tried cocaine, compared to 7.6% of white students and 2.3% of black students.

By 12th grade, the majority of students (81.7%) have had at least one alcoholic drink, and half of high school seniors (50.8%) report using alcohol within the past month.

Twelve percent of Hispanic students have tried cocaine, compared to 7.6% of white students and 2.3% of black students.

IMPLICATIONS FOR HEALTHCARE PROVIDERS

Alcohol use is strongly associated with other unhealthy behaviors, such as using drugs and tobacco and engaging in unprotected sex. Youth who indulge in one risky behavior are more likely to indulge in others, compounding their risk. For example, teens who use alcohol and drugs tend to become sexually active at an earlier age and have more partners than teens who do not use these substances regularly. Sex while under the influence of drugs and alcohol is usually unprotected, placing adolescents at risk for sexually transmitted diseases (STDs) and unwanted pregnancy. Questions about substance use and abuse should be part of every adolescent health assessment.

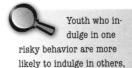

Youth who indulge in one risky behavior are more likely to indulge in others, compounding their risk.

Adolescent drug and alcohol problems are commonly associated with erosions in social values, economic viability, and family structure. Risk factors include family history of alcoholism, low academic aspirations, and antisocial behavior or social isolation during childhood. Nevertheless, studies dispute the all-too-easy association between risky behavior and lower socioeconomic status. Affluent youth who see themselves as popular, feel the pressure to perform academically and socially, or feel protected from the consequences of risky behavior by virtue of greater resources may, in some cases, take greater risks.

QUESTION TO ASK

Questions about substance use and abuse should be part of every adolescent health assessment.

The National Youth Risk Behavior Surveillance survey contains far more data than are cited here. In addition, it is only one survey; many other studies have addressed youth behaviors and accounted for socioeconomic status, family demographics, personality factors, and more specific race/ethnic profiles. For example, Healthy People 2010 collects data differently. Many theories exist regarding risk taking and health-related behaviors among youth, and many prevention programs targeting family, community, and peers have been implemented and evaluated. Healthcare providers should become familiar with data in their own patient populations.

SOURCES

Centers for Disease Control and Prevention. (2007). *YRBSS: Youth risk behavior surveillance system.* Retrieved March 13, 2008, from www.cdc.gov/HealthyYouth/yrbs/index.htm

Centers for Disease Control and Prevention. (2008). *WONDER online databases.* Retrieved March 13, 2008, from http://wonder.cdc.gov/

Stein, K. F., Roeser, R., & Markus, H. R. (1998). Self-schemas and possible selves as predictors and outcomes of risky behaviors in adolescents. *Nursing Research, 47*(2), 96–106.

Suniya, L., & Latendresse, S. (2002). Pathways to positive development among diverse youth. In R. Lerner, C. Taylor, & A. von Eye (Eds.). *New directions for youth development: Theory practice research* (pp. 101–121). San Francisco: Jossey-Bass.

QUICK LOOK AT THE CHAPTER AHEAD

- The development of a healthy adolescent sexuality involves body image, managing sexual arousal, and making wise choices about sexual behavior.
- The National Youth Risk Behavior Surveillance Survey on sexual behavior indicates that while the prevalence of sexual intercourse increases with age, the use of condoms *decreases*. That is, younger teens are less likely to be sexually active, but when they are, they are more careful.
- Teen birthrates and pregnancy rates has decreased, but the United States still has the highest rates in the industrialized world.
- Sexually transmitted diseases remain a significant problem among sexually active youth.

57

Sexuality

TERMS
- ☐ Body image
- ☐ Safe sex
- ☐ Sexual arousal
- ☐ Sexual behavior
- ☐ Teenage pregnancy

During adolescence, physical and social factors influence the development of a sexual identity that incorporates body image, feelings of sexual arousal, and choices regarding sexual behavior. Religion, marriage customs, and attitudes about the sexual roles of men and women set the cultural context in which adolescents come to terms with their sexual identities.

DEVELOPMENTAL CHALLENGES OF ADOLESCENT SEXUALITY

Although it is normal to forge a sexual identity during the teen years, adolescent sexuality has often been viewed as a "problem waiting to happen." Parents, healthcare providers, and educators warn teens about pregnancy, date rape, and sexually transmitted diseases (STDs). Less attention has been paid to how a healthy sexual identity develops. Brooks-Gunn and Paikoff (1993) proposed that adolescent sexual well-being is an integration of physical, social, cognitive, and emotional factors. They identify four developmental challenges.

Puberty and Body Image

The first challenge occurs with the onset of puberty. Girls who develop early and boys who develop late are most unhappy with their bodies, and they tend to feel less attractive to the opposite sex. Satisfaction with **body image** is also influenced by cultural norms. American girls are particularly self-conscious about their weight. Boys want to be athletic and muscular.

Managing Sexual Arousal

The second challenge is the management of **sexual arousal**. It is normal to be flooded with desire, yet teens receive mixed messages about how to deal with their feelings. Boys are most readily aroused by visual stimuli—hence their interest in sexually explicit magazines. Sexual arousal in girls, however, is not as openly acknowledged—and may also be more complex. While girls are attracted to handsome boys, being the object of male desire also makes girls feel sexy. Overt displays of sexuality in girls, and discussion of their desires, remain taboo.

Sexual Behavior

The third developmental challenge involves **sexual behavior**. Heterosexual behavior refers to sexual interactions with the opposite sex, which range from hand holding to intercourse. Homosexuality refers to a sexual preference for members of one's own sex. Adolescents need to learn how to negotiate sexual situations so that they do not engage in risky sexual behaviors.

Safe Sex

The fourth challenge is to avoid the unnecessary risks of pregnancy and STDs by practicing **safe sex** or by abstaining from intercourse (**Table 57-1** and **Table 57-2**) (Centers for Disease Control and Prevention, 2005).

Table 57-1 Contraceptive Use

Method	Who	Use
Condoms	All adolescent couples	62.8%
	Grade 9	62.9%
	Grade 12	49.5%
	Black students	66.1%
	White students	52.5%
	Hispanic students	44.4%
Birth control pills	All adolescent couples	17.6%
	Grade 9	7.5%
	Grade 12	25.6%
	Black students	10%
	White students	22.3%
	Hispanic students	9.8%

Source: Centers for Disease Control and Prevention, 2005.

SEXUAL BEHAVIOR

Expectations regarding adolescent "romantic" relationships have changed over the past 100 years. In many cultures, the onset of puberty was traditionally accompanied by mating rituals, and girls were expected to be virgins when they married, often in their teens. Today, especially in industrialized countries, a decade or more separates the onset of puberty and marriage. There increasingly is a mismatch between adolescents' sexual desires, their opportunities for sexual behavior,

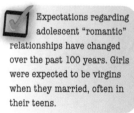

Expectations regarding adolescent "romantic" relationships have changed over the past 100 years. Girls were expected to be virgins when they married, often in their teens.

Table 57-2 Sexually Transmitted Diseases

Disease	Causes/Symptoms/Risk	Prevalence
Chlamydia		498/100,000 all females aged 10–65
		2796.6/100,000 females aged 15–19
		2691/100,000 females aged 20–24
Gonorrhea		115.6/100,000 all persons
		624.7/100,000 females aged 15–19
		581.2/100,000 females aged 20–24
		261.2/100,000 males aged 15–19
		436.8/100,000 males aged 20–24
Genital herpes		20% of adolescents have been infected
HIV/AIDS		1255 reported cases in 33 states, age 13–19
		3876 reported cases in 33 states, age 20–24
		32,031 reported cases in 33 states, age ≥ 25

Source: Centers for Disease Control and Prevention, 2005.

and their psychological and economic ability to deal with these desires and possible consequences. American culture has not helped them. On the one hand, teenagers are bombarded by messages in movies, music, and advertisements that promote casual sex without restraint; on the other hand, there is open discussion about HIV/AIDS and condoms.

There increasingly is a mismatch between adolescents' sexual desires, their opportunities for sexual behavior, and their psychological and economic ability to deal with these desires and possible consequences.

Data from the 2005 Youth Risk Behavior Surveillance Survey indicate that 46.8% of students in grades 9 through 12 have had sexual intercourse at some time, with the prevalence increasing with age; however, the use of condoms *decreases* with age (Table 57-1; Centers for Disease Control and Prevention, 2007). In general, the prevalence of intercourse is higher among black students (74.6% males/61.2% females) than among Hispanic (57.6%/44.4%) and white students (43.2%/43.7%). However, black students also are *more likely* to use condoms than their white and Hispanic peers (Table 57-1). Although more boys than girls in 9th grade have had intercourse (39.3% and 29.3%, respectively), by 12th grade the numbers are almost even (63.8% and 62.4%, respectively). Interestingly, high school senior girls are more likely to have had more than one partner than are boys (51.7% and 47% respectively), and black students (47.4%) are more likely to have had multiple partners than are white (32%) and Hispanic students (35%). There is an important caveat when considering these data: Adolescents are not always reliable reporters of their sexual behavior. Bravado may prompt exaggeration, especially among younger boys, whereas older teens may revise their sexual history to appear more moderate.

Data from the 2005 Youth Risk Behavior Surveillance Survey indicate that 46.8% of students in grades 9 through 12 have had sexual intercourse at some time, with the prevalence increasing with age; however, the use of condoms *decreases* with age

Perhaps because of fears about HIV/AIDS and pregnancy, and as a result of the emphasis on casual sex in the media, a new sexual phenomenon has appeared among adolescents: "friends with benefits." Heterosexual adolescents who are not in or are not looking for steady relationships "hook up" with one another for casual sex, which may be intercourse or the girl performing oral sex on one or more boys (Kan & Cares, 2006). National surveys have not collected data on this behavior, but it has certainly captured the attention of newspapers, magazines, and popular music.

Many studies indicate that teens who come from stable families in which parents demonstrate responsible behavior and are open to discussing sex with their children, and who strongly identify with a religious belief, are less likely to engage in premarital sex. Those who do are older at first coitus. Risk factors for earlier sexual activity include families that are disorganized and/or in which communication between parents and children is not optimal; lack of future planning on behalf of the adolescent; and norms among one's peers and community. Similar factors influence the use of contraceptives (Table 57-1) and incidence of teen pregnancy.

Many studies indicate that teens who come from stable families in which parents demonstrate responsible behavior and are open to discussing sex with their children, and who strongly identify with a religious belief, are less likely to engage in premarital sex.

TEENAGE PREGNANCY

The United States has the highest rates of **teenage pregnancy** and births in the Western industrialized world. After reaching a high of 117 pregnancies per 1000 females aged 15–19 in 1990, the pregnancy rate *decreased* to 75 pregnancies per 1000 females in 2000. (Pregnancy data include births, abortions, and miscarriages.) Thirty-one percent of young women become pregnant at least once before they reach the age of 20—about 750,000 per year; 80% percent of these pregnancies occur in unmarried teens. Teen birth rates have also decreased from a high of 96.3 per 1000 females in 1957 to a new low of 40 per 1000 females in 2005. Of the 4.1 million infants born in 2004, approximately 342,000 were born to unmarried teenage girls aged 15–19. Only one third of unmarried teen mothers completes high school, and 80% end up on welfare.

Thirty-one percent of young women become pregnant at least once before they reach the age of 20—about 750,000 per year; 80% percent of these pregnancies occur in unmarried teens.

The United States has the highest rates of **teenage pregnancy** and births in the Western industrialized world. After reaching a high of 117 pregnancies per 1000 females aged 15–19 in 1990, the pregnancy rate *decreased* to 75 pregnancies per 1000 females in 2000. (Pregnancy data include births, abortions, and miscarriages.)

IMPLICATIONS FOR HEALTH CARE PROVIDERS

Youths who engage in early and casual sexual behavior are at increased risk for STDs and pregnancy, which can have lifelong consequences for themselves, their partners, their families, and any children they bear. Prevention efforts do work; nevertheless, most youth will engage in potentially risky sexual behavior before marriage. Healthcare providers should include sexual history as part of every adolescent health assessment rather than ask these questions only when the visit focuses on reproductive health. Table 57-1 suggests that youth are *less likely* to protect themselves as they get older.

Healthcare providers should include sexual history as part of every adolescent health assessment rather than ask these questions only when the visit focuses on reproductive health.

SOURCES

Brooks-Gunn, J., & Paikoff, R. L. (1993). "Sex is a gamble, kissing is a game": Adolescent sexuality and health promotion. In S. Millstein, A. Petersen, & E. Nightingale (Eds.), *Promoting the health of adolescents: New directions for the twenty-first century* (pp. 180–208). New York: Oxford University Press.

Centers for Disease Control and Prevention. (2005). *Chlamydia prevalence monitoring project annual report 2005.* Retrieved February 5, 2008, from http://www.cdc.gov/STD/Chlamydia2005/CTSurvSupp2005Short.pdf

Centers for Disease Control and Prevention. (2007). *YRBSS: Youth risk behavior surveillance system.* Retrieved March 13, 2008, from www.cdc.gov/HealthyYouth/yrbs/index.htm

Denizet-Lewis, B. (2004, May 30). Friends, friends with benefits and the benefits of the local mall. *New York Times.*

Kan, M. L., & Cares, A. C. (2006). From "friends with benefits" to "going steady": New directions in understanding romance and sex in adolescence and emerging adulthood. In A. C. Crouter & A. Booth (Eds.), *Romance and sex in adolescence and emerging adulthood: Risks and opportunities* (pp. 241–258). Mahwah, NJ: Lawrence Erlbaum Associates.

National Center for Health Statistics. (2008). *Home.* Retrieved March 19, 2007, from www.cdc.gov/nchs

Upchurch, D. M., Lillard, L. A., Aneshensel, C. S., & Li, N. (2002). Inconsistencies in reporting the occurrence and timing of first intercourse among adolescents. *Journal of Sex Research, 39*(3), 197–206.

QUICK LOOK AT THE CHAPTER AHEAD

- Piaget's stage of formal operations reflects an ability to think abstractly and to consider possibilities, especially regarding future events.
- Some features of formal operational thinking include the ability to separate the real from the possible, to state propositions and back them up with data arranged in all possible combinations (i.e., they argue because they can), and to think about thinking.
- Adolescents have more domain-specific knowledge than when they were in mid-childhood.
- Adolescents have a greater information processing capacity than when they were in mid-childhood.
- The adolescent brain changes dramatically between ages 13 and 18.

58

Cognitive
Development

TERMS
☐ Formal operational period
☐ Piaget's stage of formal operations

Piaget's stage of formal operations is a fruitful beginning for any analysis of adolescent thought. According to Piaget, the **formal operational period**, during which the beginnings of logical, abstract thinking appear, commences at about the age of 11 or 12 years.

PIAGET'S STAGE OF FORMAL OPERATIONS

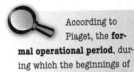

During adolescence and the appearance of formal operations, youngsters demonstrate an ability to reason realistically about the future and to consider possibilities that they actually doubt. Teenagers look for relations, they separate the real from the possible, they test their mental solutions to problems, and they feel comfortable with verbal statements. In short, the period's great achievement is a release from the restrictions of the tangible and the concrete (Elkind, 1994) (**Table 58-1**).

According to Piaget, the **formal operational period**, during which the beginnings of logical, abstract thinking appear, commences at about the age of 11 or 12 years.

Some adolescents, however, may still be in the concrete operational stage or just beginning the initial stages of formal operations. They have just consolidated their concrete operational thinking and continue to use it consistently. Unless they find themselves in situations that demand formal operational thinking (such as science and math classes), they continue to be concrete operational thinkers. As Elkind (1994, p. 221) noted, learning how to use formal operations takes time and practice with a blend of concrete and abstract materials.

FEATURES OF THE FORMAL OPERATIONAL PERIOD

There are several essential features of **formal operational thinking**:

- The ability to separate the real from the possible distinguishes the formal operational thinker from the concrete operational thinker. Adolescents try to discern all possible rela-

Table 58-1 Cognitive Development in Adolescence

Thinking
- Thinking applies to possibilities as well as the realistic.
- Thinking relates to the future as well as the present.
- Thinking is evident in hypothetical-deductive statements.
- Thinking demonstrates logical reasoning.
- Thinking illustrates the use of abstract concepts.

Ability
- Ability to consider possibilities.
- Ability to consider alternatives.
- Ability to engage in propositional thinking.
- Ability to combine pertinent facts.
- Ability to apply concrete data.
- Ability to acquire needed data.
- Ability to improve existing competencies.

tions in any situation or problem and then, by mental experimentation and logical analysis, attempt to discover which are true.

- Adolescent thinking is propositional, which means that adolescents use not only concrete data, but also statements or propositions that contain the concrete data. Dealing with abstract concepts no longer frustrates them. Also, their increasing ability to deal with "If this . . . then that" statements may cause them to argue more vigorously about any controversial matter such as drug use, school programs on sexual conduct, or political issues.
- Adolescents attack a problem by gathering as much information as possible and then making all possible combinations of the variables that they can. They proceed as follows:

1. They organize data by concrete operational techniques (classification, seriation).
2. They use the results of concrete operational techniques to form statements or propositions.
3. They combine as many of these propositions as possible.
4. They test these combinations to determine which are true.

OTHER CHARACTERISTICS OF ADOLESCENT THOUGHT

Flavell, Miller, and Miller (1993) identified several other features of adolescent thought:

- *An increase in domain-specific knowledge.* Adolescents simply have accumulated more knowledge in many subjects than have younger children.
- *Greater information-processing capacity.* Development seems to be the key explanation here. The speed of information processing increases, which leads to an expansion of functional capacity.
- *Advances in metacognition.* "Thinking about thinking" becomes an important part of adolescent thought. Children gradually acquire knowledge about cognitive functioning—that is, how people process information.
- *Improvement of existing competencies.* Adolescent thought is distinguished not only by the acquisition of new abilities (e.g., propositional thinking), but also by an improvement in the competencies already possessed (Table 58-1).

THE ADOLESCENT BRAIN

The adolescent brain undergoes dramatic changes during adolescence. Considerable asynchrony among the different lobes is apparent in early adolescence, around age 13 to 14, with greater synchrony appearing at about age 17 to 18. The brain as a whole undergoes pruning of brain cells and a thinning of the cortex; at this time, myelination is completed. The result is a reorganized brain. The frontal lobes, which are responsible for executive processing such as planning ahead, increase in their information-processing capacity. Waves of hormones also wash over the amygdala, the site of emotion and anxiety. Hence the mood swings and unclear thinking often associated with adolescence likely have some neurological foundation.

 Neurological changes may be necessary for developing higher-order executive processes and abstract thinking, but they are not enough. Clear thinking, advanced problem solving, and making good decisions take practice.

Neurological changes may be necessary for developing higher-order executive processes and abstract thinking, but they are not enough. Clear thinking, advanced problem solving, and making good decisions take practice.

IMPLICATIONS FOR HEALTHCARE PROVIDERS

The adolescent years are a time of rapid change. If you find yourself dealing with teenagers, learn as much as possible about all aspects of adolescent development. In most cases, adolescents retain the fears of a child when faced with the consequences of an accident or disease. Simultaneously, they try to muster up the bravado that these years demand. Be honest, and answer questions as fully as possible. Do not hesitate to ask direct questions: Are you using birth control pills? Listen carefully to your patients' answers and do not dismiss any warning signs as "typical teenage talk." All too often, throw-away statements such as "I'd like to kill myself" have turned out to be tragically prophetic.

When working with adolescents, be careful not to exaggerate their abilities. Keep in mind that while adolescents are capable of abstract thought, not all of them will exercise this ability, especially when faced with a stressful situation or when new information is being presented. Do not be afraid to explain things in concrete terms, including the consequences of the condition that brought the adolescent to you. Observe your patients' reactions as they answer your questions or describe symptoms, and use these questions to guide your observations.

- Can they separate the real from the possible? Some adolescents will still have a difficult time.
- Are they comfortable with propositional thinking?
- Can they help you gather as much data as needed and combine clues, helping you to make vital decisions?

SOURCES

Elkind, D. (1994). *Understanding your child*. Boston: Allyn & Bacon.

Flavell, F., Miller, P., & Miller, S. (1993). *Cognitive development*. Englewood Cliffs, NJ: Prentice Hall.

Nagel, B. J., Medina, K. L., Yoshii, J., Schweinsburg, A. D., Moadab, I., & Tapert, S. F. (2006). Age-related changes in prefrontal white matter volume across adolescence. *Developmental Neuroscience, 17*(13), 1427–1431.

Piaget, J., & Inhelder, B. (1969). *The psychology of the child*. New York: Basic Books.

Selekman, J. (2005). The teen brain as a work in progress: Implications for nurses. *Pediatric Nursing, 31*(2), 144–148.

- Elkind has described the ability to think abstractly as "thinking in a new key."
- When adolescents feel that everyone is scrutinizing them, they are responding to an imaginary audience.
- The personal fable enables adolescents to think of themselves as unique.
- The third person perspective enables adolescents to watch themselves as they play many roles.
- Adolescents argue for the sake of arguing; it sharpens their thinking.

59

Adolescent Thought

TERMS
- ☐ Imaginary audience
- ☐ Personal fable
- ☐ Perspective taking
- ☐ Social schemas

Adolescents can think abstractly. Younger adolescents appreciate that symbols can represent reality, such as the use of metaphor in poetry. Older adolescents manipulate systems of symbols: They appreciate themes in literature and discuss complex ideas, such as justice. Over time, adolescents' ability to reason becomes more systematic. They use hypothetical reasoning to ask, "What if?" This approach to problem solving is akin to the scientific method.

The emergence of abstract thinking has several important implications for social and psychological development (**Table 59-1**). Elkind (1984) referred to the increased complexity of cognitive processing during adolescence as "thinking in a new key."

EGOCENTRIC THINKING: IMAGINARY AUDIENCE AND PERSONAL FABLE

Adolescents spend a lot of time thinking, and thinking about their thinking. They tend to see themselves not as others see them, but rather as they think others must see them. Being absorbed in their own experience, adolescents think that others think they are unique and fascinating, or awful and stupid.

Table 59-1 Characteristics of Adolescent Thought

Characteristic	Explanation and Implication
Egocentric thinking	Thinking more about oneself than about others. Adolescents become self-absorbed.
Imaginary audience	Thinking everyone is looking at oneself. Adolescents are painfully self-conscious.
Personal fable	Seeing oneself as unique and powerful. Adolescents' belief in their abilities is inflated.
Social cognition	The ability to think about interpersonal relationships, to make sense of other people's behavior. Adolescents learn to manipulate the rules of social engagement.
Second-person perspective	The ability to see an event from someone else's point of view. Adolescents understand exclusion from the group is deliberate and intended to be hurtful.
Third-person perspective	The ability to observe oneself playing out a role in a social situation in relationship to others. Adolescents scrutinize themselves.
Betrayal	When an understanding between two parties is violated. Adolescents feel betrayed when they act in accordance with what they think are the rules of a relationship, and find that the other party did not.
Disillusionment	When an established social schema is proved false. Adolescents learn their idols have flaws.

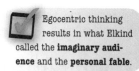

Egocentric thinking results in what Elkind (1984) called the **imaginary audience** and the **personal fable**. Younger adolescents in particular are extremely self-conscious (Selman & Schultz, 1991)—they are sure that everybody is looking at them. They perform for an audience that exists in their imaginations, and use it to anticipate the reactions of other people to their behavior.

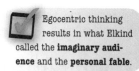

Egocentric thinking results in what Elkind called the **imaginary audience** and the **personal fable**.

Adolescents also feel different from everyone else. Believing that they are unique means that others—especially anyone older—cannot understand their thoughts and feelings. If adolescents are alone in their experience, they also need to perceive themselves as all-powerful and indestructible. The personal fable enables adolescents to create stories in which they are capable of great and important things. Adolescents also appreciate and deny their own mortality. Personal fables afford adolescents the opportunity to play with alternative social scenarios mentally and can sharpen their social cognitive abilities.

SOCIAL COGNITION AND PERSPECTIVE TAKING

Social cognition has two aspects (Fiske & Taylor, 1984): **social schemas** and how they change. Social schemas are mental representations of the roles that people play in different situations and relationships. Schemas are based on personal experiences and how people organize them, and they change with experience and maturity.

Social cognition has two aspects (Fiske & Taylor, 1984): **social schemas** and how they change. Social schemas are mental representations of the roles that people play in different situations and relationships. Schemas are based on personal experiences and how people organize them, and they change with experience and maturity.

Perspective taking influences social cognition and the development of schemas (Selman & Schultz, 1991). When older children and young adolescents take a second-person perspective, they see an event from someone else's point of view; this viewpoint gives them some insight into others' intentions and feelings. The third-person perspective refers to the ability of older adolescents to step outside of themselves and watch how they play out their roles in different situations. It is related to later abstract thinking, when adolescents can think in terms of interactions within and between systems.

Both types of perspective taking challenge existing social schemas. Adolescents understand that exclusion from the group is intended to be deliberate and hurtful. They see that some groups are more open to new membership than are others. Members of a group learn to jockey for position. Adolescents also discover that girls and boys approach relationships with different expectations. Teens learn the strategic manipulations of social survival. Those who misunderstand the rules, and those who follow the rules when others do not, feel betrayed and disillusioned.

Adolescents become disillusioned when they realize their idols have flaws. The "big man on campus" is shallow; the admired teacher has a drinking problem. In time and with greater maturity, adolescents use the third-person perspective to scrutinize themselves. They relinquish the personal fable and replace it with more realistic, yet still idealized expectations. The importance of the imaginary audience fades, and adolescents begin to develop their own set of standards to guide their behavior. Changing social schemas can lead to greater self-understanding in those adolescents who can negotiate the emotional discomfort that such psychological and social adjustments entail.

ARGUMENT AND DEBATE

Adolescents appreciate the art and science of debate. They approach problems systematically, collect the relevant facts, find the logic in them, and make their case with passion and an unshakable belief that they are right. They love to exercise their new cognitive abilities and to outmaneuver opponents with carefully crafted strategies. In other words, adolescents argue for the sake of arguing.

As painful as adolescent argumentativeness is for adults, it can help teenagers sharpen their cognitive and social skills. Once adults recognize argument as a form of mental exercise, they can help adolescents to argue constructively, to focus on the principles under discussion, and to defuse the emotion.

IMPLICATIONS FOR HEALTHCARE PROVIDERS

Adolescence is probably the most difficult time at which to have serious health problems. The excessive attention to adolescent patients' physical health feeds into their self-centeredness and self-consciousness. Adolescents may correctly perceive themselves as different from peers. A very real threat to mortality challenges their personal fables about invulnerability. The ability to live in one's mind means that "just thinking" about illness is stressful. The frustration and anger associated with the illness experience, added to their natural tendency to argue, can make life difficult for adolescents and the people who care for them (Thies & Walsh, 1999).

SOURCES

Elkind, D. (1984). *All dressed up and no place to go*. Reading, MA: Addison-Wesley.

Fiske, S., & Taylor, S. (1984). *Social cognition*. New York: Random House.

Selman, R., & Schultz, L. (1991). *Making a friend in youth: Developmental theory and pair therapy*. Chicago: University of Chicago Press.

Thies, K., & Walsh, M. F. (1999). A developmental analysis of cognitive appraisal of stress in children and adolescents with chronic illness. *Child Health Care, 28*(1), 15–32.

 QUICK LOOK AT THE CHAPTER AHEAD

- Peers are either similar in age, or similar in physical, cognitive, or social abilities.
- The ability to assume a second and third person perspective shapes a child's relationships with peers.
- Children and teens often gravitate toward peer groups in which the members are much like themselves because it feels familiar.
- Adolescents may have several different peer groups based on their activities and affililations.
- "Peer pressure" can be positive or negative.

60

Peer Relationships

The importance and the influence of **peers** in development cannot be exaggerated. In the 1940s, Anna Freud (Sigmund Freud's daughter) and Sophie Dann worked with six German Jewish orphans whose parents had died in the Nazi gas chambers. The six children spent several years together in a concentration camp, enduring horrible conditions, with few adult contacts. When the war ended, the children were taken to England to recover. Although they showed some effects of their ordeal— thumb sucking, fearfulness, restlessness—they were strongly attached to each other, to the point where they comforted each other when disturbed and became upset when separated. With the loving care that the children received over the subsequent years, coupled with their continued relationships with their peers, they gradually showed normal patterns of development (Freud & Dann, 1951).

THE MEANING OF PEER

We typically use the word "peer" to refer to those who are similar in age, usually having been born within 12 months of each other. But equal in age does not mean equal in everything—for example, intelligence, physical ability, or social skills. Also, research shows that many peer interactions involve individuals who are more than 12 months older.

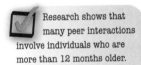

Research shows that many peer interactions involve individuals who are more than 12 months older.

Most adolescents still want to remain close to parents, but the forces of separation and independence are powerful, leading to strains in the home. The attraction of peer relationships grows intense and assumes a sensitivity and sense of belongingness that challenges adults to remain "sensitively responsive." Adolescents whose parents are warm, responsive, and consistent disciplinarians are more competent with peers than those whose parents are harsh and rejecting or overly permissive.

Teenagers are acutely aware that they must get along with their peers, which forces them to think about their relationships—a major step in social development. For example, they begin to make definite judgments about the behavior of their peers and become more astute at detecting meaning in facial expressions and in the way something is said. Their increasing social skills and cognitive maturity enable them to recognize that other points of view exist.

SOCIAL PERSPECTIVE TAKING

Selman (1980) believed that people's views on relationships cannot be separated from their personal theories about the psychological characteristics of others. Selman identified several levels of **social perspective taking** and noted that youngsters gradually comprehend that other people are different and have ideas of their own. As they move into adolescence, their views of a relationship include self, someone else, and the kind of relationship between them. At this point in their development, the desire to conform becomes achingly important. Selman's five-level analysis of interpersonal understanding is illustrated in **Table 60-1.**

THE FORMATION OF PEER GROUPS

The view of adolescence has changed in recent years. Although the adolescent period brings challenges, anxiety, excitement, and even upsets, for most adolescents it is not a time of great stress, tur-

Table 60-1 Do Parents Know What Their Teens Are Doing?

Do you think that your child . . .	Parental Myth	Teen Reality
Has contemplated suicide?	9%	26%
Has cheated on a test?	37%	76%
Has had sex?	9%	19%
Has friends with drug problems?	12%	36%
Has driven a car while drunk?	22%	46%

moil, and trouble (Lerner & Galambos, 1998). More frequently than not, the **peer group** becomes a positive force during these years and exercises many positive functions.

Tracing the changes in the nature of peer groups from childhood to adolescence, Brown (1990) noted the following:

- Adolescents spend much more time with their peers than do children, and during high school they spend twice as much time with their peers as with their parents and other adults.
- Adolescent peer groups are subject to much less adult supervision than groups of children are. This is especially the case with groups that are accessed through the Internet.

 Adolescent peer groups are subject to much less adult supervision than groups of children are. This is especially the case with groups that are accessed through the Internet.

- More-frequent interactions with peers of the opposite sex occur as time with parents decreases.
- Adolescents tend to identify with a particular interest group (sports, drama, music, adventure seekers), and make friends with peers much like themselves in terms of interests, values, and goals. Even so, adolescents often have different groups of friends at the same time—for example, from history class, from the drama club, from the team, from the church youth group.

Biological, psychological, and social changes in adolescence occur simultaneously and can cause considerable anxiety and insecurity (Lerner & Galambos, 1998). As a consequence, turning to others who share the same experiences is a natural inclination for most teenagers. Their dependence on parents lessens, and their dependence on their peers increases.

 Adolescents tend to identify with a particular interest group (sports, drama, music, adventure seekers), and make friends with peers much like themselves in terms of interests, values, and goals. Even so, adolescents often have different groups of friends at the same time—for example, from history class, from the drama club, from the team, from the church youth group.

PEER PRESSURE: MYTHS AND REALITIES

Peers are not necessarily a negative influence on adolescents; in fact, parents want their children to spend time with peers they regard as good influences. Even so, the myth that peer pressure means peers persuade one another to engage in risky behavior persists. Research suggests matters are not that simple. Adolescents may consciously adopt certain behaviors and attitudes to enhance their social and personal power within a group. Groups often take greater risks together than any of the members would individually or in pairs.

Table 60-2 addresses some of the myths and realities about peer pressure.

IMPLICATIONS FOR HEALTHCARE PROVIDERS

Working with teenagers can be both frustrating and fulfilling—frustrating in that adolescents feel they must maintain the appearance of independence, and fulfilling because if you gain their confidence, you can accomplish so much. Remembering the adolescent characteristics discussed in this chapter will help you to develop and maintain good relationships with them. To paraphrase Erikson (1968), adolescents need enough freedom to make their own rules and learn from their mistakes, but enough structure that they know which rules they are choosing and the mistakes do not jeopardize their futures. A routine health history should include questions about friends and group activities. If friends drink alcohol, are sexually active, or use drugs, your patient likely does as well.

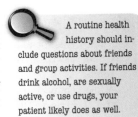

A routine health history should include questions about friends and group activities. If friends drink alcohol, are sexually active, or use drugs, your patient likely does as well.

Many adolescents with health conditions worry what their peers may think of them, and they may be tempted to take shortcuts in a therapeutic regimen in an attempt to "fit in." Try to capitalize on adolescents' relationships with their peers by urging them to discuss their condition with friends they trust, and connect them to others who may have experienced a similar health problem, especially others in their twenties.

Here are some tips for helping teens negotiate peer groups:

- Foster positive relationships not just with parents, but also with other responsible adults who value the teens and can serve as role models and sources of support.
- Encourage teens to have several types of relationships, crossing gender, socioeconomic status, ethnicity, religion, and interest groups. Exposure to multiple identities and styles pro-

Table 60-2 Peers, Parents, and Pressure

Myth	Reality
Parent–child relationships are undermined by peer relationships.	Parents remain the chief positive source of support and influence for most teens.
When parents and teens argue, they grow apart as teens turn to their peers.	Parents who continue to communicate with their teens, especially in conflict, maintain closer relationships.
Teens who fall in with the "wrong crowd" succumb to pressure from those of higher status in the group to engage in risky behaviors.	Teens often choose a group based either on shared values and interests, or because group membership increases their social and personal power. In fact, friendships are often a healthy path to positive development. It is "groupthink" to which teens succumb, and not individual incidents of manifest persuasion.

vides models to emulate or reject, helps them develop different aspects of their own identity, and teaches them how to get along with a variety of people—a good life skill.

• Help teens to develop the social and cognitive skills they need to negotiate risky situations *before* those situations arise so they have an exit strategy already planned—for example, what to say or do if they are at a party where alcohol is present, how to turn down cigarettes or drugs, or how to resist sexual advances.

• Help them to see that some peer behaviors may be rooted in the same insecurities that they themselves may feel.

SOURCES

Brown, B. (1990). Peer groups and peer cultures. In S. Feldman & G. Elliot (Eds.), *At the threshold: The developing adolescent* (pp. 171–196). Cambridge, MA: Harvard University Press.

Brown, B. B., & Klute, C. (2006). Friendships, cliques and crowds. In G. R. Adams and M. D. Berzonsky (Eds.), *Blackwell handbook of adolescence* (pp. 330–348). Malden, MA: Blackwell.

Erikson, E. (1968). *Identity: Youth and crisis*. New York: W.W. Norton.

Freud, A., & Dann, S. (1951). An experiment in group upbringing. *Psychoanalytic Study of Child, 6,* 127–168.

Lerner, R., & Galambos, N. (1998). Adolescent development: Challenges and opportunities for research, programs, and policies. In J. Spence, J. Darley, & D. Foss (Eds.), *Annual review of psychology*. Palo Alto, CA: Annual Reviews.

Selman, R. (1980). *The growth of interpersonal understanding: Developmental and clinical analysis*. New York: Academic Press.

Ungar, M. T. (2000). The myth of peer pressure. *Adolescence, 35*(137), 167–180.

- Erikson was the originator of the terms *identity* and *identity crisis*.
- Erikson referred to adolescence as the period of "identity vs. identity confusion."
- Self-schemas are complex ways of constructing the self through a variety of experiences.
- Self-esteem develops when real success is found through hard work.
- The formation of identity occurs by building on strengths and recognizing weaknesses, communicating with supportive adults, and becoming a competent person.

61

The Search for Identity

TERMS
- ☐ **Identity achievement**
- ☐ **Identity confusion**
- ☐ **Identity diffusion**
- ☐ **Identity foreclosure**
- ☐ **Identity moratorium**
- ☐ **Self-esteem**
- ☐ **Self-schemas**

For many years, adolescence had been thought of as a time of tremendous turmoil. Recently, however, theorists and researchers have concluded that upset and turmoil are *not* the defining characteristics of adolescence. Rather, most adolescents adjust well to the socialization demands of family, school, and society. They have also acquired friends who, for the most part, share these values. Nevertheless, the process of passing through these years introduces a certain tension for all adolescents, particularly with regard to their identity.

IDENTITY OR DOUBT

The adolescent years, from about ages 12 to 18, have come to be identified with Erikson's (1968) colorful description of them as the time of "identity versus identity confusion." Recall from Chapter 2 that Erikson believed personality development occurred through a series of conflicts, both inner and outer, and that individuals emerge from each crisis with a greater sense of inner unity, an increase in good judgment, and a growing tendency to live by personally significant standards.

Erikson (1968) viewed the adolescent years as the end of childhood and the beginning of adulthood. Teenagers display an acute sensitivity about what others think of them, and peer opinion plays a large part in how they think of themselves. If uncertainty at this time results in identity confusion, a bewildered youth may withdraw, run away, or turn to drugs. Youngsters who are faced with the question "Who am I?" may be unable to answer it. The challenges are new; the tasks are difficult; the alternatives are bewildering. Needless to say, adults must have patience and understanding with youths of this age. Erikson noted that the primary developmental task of adolescence is construction of an adult identity (**Table 61-1**).

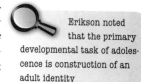

Erikson noted that the primary developmental task of adolescence is construction of an adult identity

IDENTITY VERSUS IDENTITY CONFUSION

Faced with a combination of physical, sexual, and cognitive changes, joined with heightened adult expectations and peer pressure, adolescents understandably feel insecure about themselves—who they are and where they are going. By the end of adolescence, those who have resolved their personal crises have achieved a sense of identity: They know who they are. Those who remain locked in doubt and insecurity experience what Erikson calls **identity confusion**. Erikson's views on identity have generated considerable speculation, theorizing, and research.

Table 61-1 Development of an Adult Identity Requires . . .

- Inhibiting or modifying behaviors to avoid negative future consequences
- Initiating, persisting, and sequencing steps toward goals
- Navigating complex social situations despite strong affect
- Self-regulating affect and complex behavior to serve long-term goals

For example, Marcia (1966, 1980) concluded from a series of studies that adolescents respond to the need to make choices about their identity (particularly regarding career, religion, or politics) in one of four ways:

1. **Identity diffusion,** or the inability to commit oneself; the lack of a sense of direction. Adolescents experiencing identity diffusion lack a cohesive, consistent whole; they simply do not have a genuine identity of their own.

2. **Identity foreclosure,** or making a commitment only because someone else has prescribed a particular choice; being "outer-directed." That is, adolescents have not identified and re-solved a crisis, but have accepted the dictates—usually of parents—about the direction of their lives.

3. **Identity moratorium,** or the desire to make a choice at some time in the future but being unable to do so. These adolescents are actively grappling with an identity crisis, but as yet have not resolved it.

4. **Identity achievement,** or the ability to commit oneself to choices about identity and main-taining that commitment under all conditions.

Table 61-2 summarizes Marcia's views on identity status.

SELF-SCHEMAS AND SELF-ESTEEM

A concept related to identity is that of self-schemas. **Self-schemas** are complex ways of constructing the self as a result of experience across domains that incorporate evaluation of the self by self and others. For example, a self-schema may involve body concepts, such as fat, thin, athletic, or clumsy. Other self-schemas may in-clude popularity, academics, work ethic, and so on. While self-schemas refer to the current self, possible selves are future wishes or expectations for the self. A great deal of research has addressed the extent to which self-schemas come before or after certain be-haviors. Young teens who consider themselves to be popular may take more risks, which when successfully executed may foster more risk taking, leading in turn to a deviant self-schema by mid-adolescence.

Self-esteem refers broadly to one's evaluation of self. While "poor self-esteem" is an often-used sweeping statement, it is not a global all-

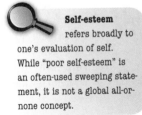

Self-schemas are complex ways of constructing the self as a result of experience across domains that incorporate evaluation of the self by self and others.

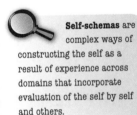

Self-esteem refers broadly to one's evaluation of self. While "poor self-esteem" is an often-used sweeping state-ment, it is not a global all-or-none concept.

Table 61-2 Identity Status

	Diffusion	Foreclosure	Moratorium	Achievement
Crisis	Absent	Absent	Present	Present
Commitment	Absent	Present	Absent	Present
Period of adolescence	Early	Middle	Middle	Late

or-none concept. Rather, it has many facets and can be both an antecedent to and a consequence of behavior. Perhaps the best definition of self-esteem comes from William James (1890), the 19th-century U.S. philosopher and psychologist. His formula is

$$\text{Self-esteem} = \text{Success} \div \text{Pretense}$$

That is, self-esteem is success divided by pretense. Success refers to authenticity and competence that is earned, and not conferred.

HELPING ADOLESCENTS FIND THEIR IDENTITY

Adults can help adolescents acquire psychosocial maturity by adopting the following strategies:

- Treat them as almost adult: Provide them with independence, freedom, and respect, but don't overestimate their maturity.
- Challenge and affirm their choices: Are their current choices and activities compatible with future goals?
- Help them to develop competence In a variety of life skills and activities, such as cognitive and social skills, as well as in a hobby, talent, or sport.
- Address the issues related to identity versus identity diffusion: Help them discover their strengths and weaknesses.
- Parents and teachers and healthcare providers should work together: Open communication among responsible adults helps keep teens on track.
- Support communication between teens and their parents, and between teens and their friends: If they are able to express how they feel and what they think, and by learning how to listen, teenagers will realize that they are not alone.

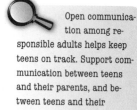

Open communication among responsible adults helps keep teens on track. Support communication between teens and their parents, and between teens and their friends.

IMPLICATIONS FOR HEALTHCARE PROVIDERS

Today's adolescents are maturing in a time of social turbulence in their life spans. Sex, drugs, alcohol, personal relationships, career choices, and interactions with parents pose daily challenges to adolescents.

Probably the most important strategy to remember in working with teenagers is to treat them as "almost adults." That is, adolescents are increasingly faced with adult situations that call for adult decisions, but they may not have the experience needed to negotiate these situations on their own—and may not realize it. Listen—really listen—to them. Do not talk down to them. Rather, explain in clear, nonemotional terms the nature and dimensions of the problem brought to you. This may be the crisis that crystallizes the adolescent's sense of identity.

SOURCES

Erikson, E. (1968). *Identity: Youth and crisis*. New York: W. W. Norton.

James, W. (1890). *The principles of psychology*. New York: Holt, Rinehart and Winston.

Marcia, J. E. (1966). Development and validation of ego identity status. *Journal of Personality and Social Psychology, 3*, 551–558.

Marcia, J. E. (1980). Identity in adolescence. In J. Adelson (Ed.), *Handbook of adolescent psychology*. New York: John Wiley.

- Motivation enables individuals to organize, direct, and sustain their own effortful behavior.
- Cognitive theories posit that individuals are motivated by excitement of discovery.
- Attribution theories identify four reasons to which individuals attribute their performance: ability, effort, task difficulty, and luck.
- Behavior theories focus on external reinforcement as the source of individuals' motivation.
- Intrinsic motivation theories posit that motivation arises from an internal need for competence and autonomy.
- Social cognitive theories emphasize the importance of role models and self-efficacy for motivation.

62

Motivating Adolescents

TERMS
- ☐ Attribution theory
- ☐ Motivation
- ☐ Social learning theory

People who set their sights on realistic goals and believe they have the ability to reach them have taken a major step on the path to success. This is as true for adolescents as for members of any other age group. Determination, positive attitude, and feelings of competence contribute powerfully to academic achievement, good relations with others, and positive interactions with parents, teachers, and other adults. One of the most significant psychological contributors to successful passage through adolescence is motivation.

THE MEANING OF MOTIVATION

When people ask about motivation, their intent is usually to discover what causes people to act in a particular way, what their inner feelings about their situation are, and what they want—what their goal is. It is difficult to specify just what motivation is, but a good, working definition is as follows: **Motivation** arouses, sustains, directs, and integrates behavior.

Another way of coming to grips with the meaning of motivation is to examine several motivational theories (**Table 62-1**). Review Chapter 6 for more on this topic.

COGNITIVE PSYCHOLOGY AND MOTIVATION

Cognitive theorists believe that internal processes, such as thinking, control human behavior. Jerome Bruner (1966), one of the leading cognitive theorists of the twentieth century, believed that there is an ideal level of arousal between apathy and wild excitement.

Bruner turned to the notion of discovery as a means of furthering intrinsic motivation. Arguing that discovery leads to new insights, Bruner believed that people learn to manipulate their environment more actively and achieve considerable gratification from personally coping with problems.

ATTRIBUTION THEORY AND MOTIVATION

All people attribute their behavior to a specific cause, and these attributions then serve as a guide to their expectations for future success or failure. **Attribution theory** rests on three basic assumptions (Weiner, 1980):

Table 62-1 Motivation: Theories and Themes

Theorist	Theory	Theme	Key Idea
Maslow	Humanistic	Needs hierarchy	Need satisfaction
Bruner	Cognitive	Intrinsic processes	Mixed motives
Weiner	Attribution	Causes of behavior	Perceived causes of behavior
Skinner	Behaviorism	Reinforcement	Schedules of reinforcement
Bandura	Social cognitive	Observation	Modeling
Deci and Ryan	Intrinsic motivation	Self-determination	Competence and autonomy

1. People want to know the causes of their own behavior and that of others.
2. People do not randomly assign causes to their behavior; rather, they assume there is a logical explanation for the causes to which they attribute their behavior.
3. The causes that people assign to their behavior influence subsequent behavior.

Individuals tend to attribute their performance to one of four elements (**Figure 62-1**):

- *Ability.* Adolescents' assumptions about their abilities are usually based on past experience. When they have a history of failure, they often make the devastating assumption that they lack ability.
- *Effort.* Adolescents (like all humans) judge their efforts by how well they did on a particular task.
- *Task difficulty.* Task difficulty usually is judged by the performance of others on the task. If many succeed, the task is perceived as easy, and vice versa. If individuals consistently succeed on a task at which others fail, they will attribute their success to ability. But if their success is matched by the success of others, then the source of the success is seen as the task (it was easy).
- *Luck.* If there is no tangible link between behavior and goal attainment, the tendency is to attribute success to luck.

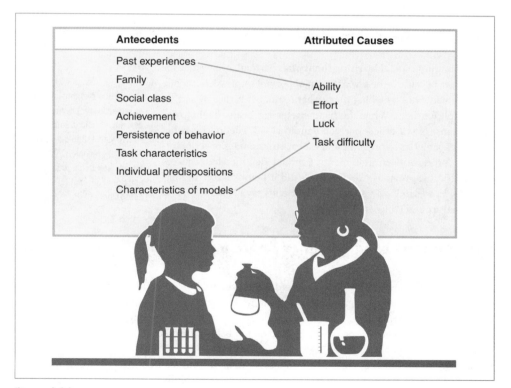

Figure 62-1 Attribution of Performance

BEHAVIORAL PSYCHOLOGY AND MOTIVATION

One of the great behaviorists of our time, B. F. Skinner (1971), stated that if you ask people why they go to the theater and they reply that they feel like going, you are usually satisfied. It would be more revealing, however, if you knew what happened when they previously attended the theater, what they had read about the play, and what else induced them to go.

According to Skinner, if adolescents obtain reinforcement for certain behavior, they tend to repeat it with vigor. If they do not obtain reinforcement, they tend to lose interest and their performance suffers.

INTRINSIC MOTIVATION AND SELF-DETERMINATION

Deci and Ryan (1985) posit that when a behavior arises from the need to feel effective (i.e., competent) and the need to master the environment independently (i.e., autonomy), that behavior is intrinsically motivated. The competent person knows what behavior is successful, feels able to execute or at least try this behavior, and wants to do so, continually learning from new experience. Intrinsic motivation is related to internal control, internalized values, and the inherent pleasure of success.

BANDURA AND SOCIAL COGNITIVE LEARNING

Albert Bandura's **social learning theory** has particular relevance for motivation, because he believed that an important impression is made on adolescents not by telling them what to do, but rather by setting an example for them. When this happens, teenagers also begin to develop a sense of self-efficacy, which Bandura (1997) defined as belief in one's capabilities to organize and execute the courses of action required to produce given attainments. Bandura identified four sources of self-efficacy: previous experience ("I did it before"), role models ("She did it; so can I"), persuasion ("My friends say I can do it"), and emotional arousal ("I like doing this").

Bandura identified four sources of self-efficacy: previous experience ("I did it before"), role models ("She did it; so can I"), persuasion ("My friends say I can do it"), and emotional arousal ("I like doing this").

IMPLICATIONS FOR HEALTHCARE PROVIDERS

Understanding what motivates adolescents can help you to develop more effective health teaching strategies. Tap into their inherent motivation to understand the world and themselves, and to be competent and independent. Role models, persuasion, and emotion play major roles in adolescents' motivation. Reinforce positive steps and do not belittle mistakes, because learning from mistakes is key to self-determination.

An eclectic approach to teenagers would seem to be the best solution. For example, whenever possible, reinforce any positive efforts they make, such as faithfully doing prescribed exercises or taking medication as scheduled. Encourage them to think about the reasons why they came to see you so that they see themselves as personally involved in planning what is needed to treat their condition or prevent poor outcomes. Most importantly, help them to develop a sense of personal efficacy. Once they feel confident in their ability to succeed in whatever program you design for them, they will have a much greater chance of improving their health.

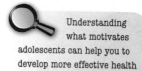

Understanding what motivates adolescents can help you to develop more effective health teaching strategies.

SOURCES

Bandura, A. (1997). *Self-efficacy: The exercise of control.* New York: Freeman.

Bruner, J. (1966). *Studies in cognitive growth.* New York: Wiley.

Deci, E. L., & Ryan, R. M. (1985). *Intrinsic motivation and self-determination in human behavior.* New York: Plenum.

Skinner, B. F. (1971). *Beyond freedom and dignity.* New York: Knopf.

Weiner, B. (1980). *Human motivation.* New York: Holt, Rinehart and Winston.

QUICK LOOK AT THE CHAPTER AHEAD

- Delinquency, aggression, and violence have many roots: physical, temperamental, attitudinal, psychological, and sociocultural.
- Contrary to popular belief, increased testosterone does not by itself cause aggression.
- Bullies need to dominate their victims, for whom they feel no empathy even at close range.
- A lack of self-control in young children may foreshadow troubled behavior in adolescence.
- Positive youth development refers to the opportunities for adolescents to become engaged in their communities and to interact with competent peers and adults.

63

Delinquency and Violence

TERMS
- ☐ Delinquency
- ☐ Impulsive behavior

The increasing violence in U.S. society has focused attention on the issues of juvenile delinquency, youth gangs, random aggression, and drug use in this country. Although most youths never become involved with law enforcement agencies, the extent of youth crime and violence cannot be ignored. The 2005 Youth Risk Behavior Surveillance Survey indicated that 18.5% of U.S. youth carried a weapon, 5.4% carried a gun, 6% avoided school out of fear, and 36% had been in a physical fight (Centers for Disease Control and Prevention, 2007). Bullying has become a public health problem. Youths who are African American or non-white Hispanic are disproportionately represented among troubled adolescents and their victims.

Delinquency may be defined as behavior that the public at any specific time thinks is in conflict with its best interests. (This definition includes behavior that is personally nonadaptive, albeit legally sanctioned.) The causes of delinquency defy easy categorization. Usually it is difficult to identify just what propelled a boy or girl along the troubled path to delinquency. One of the most disturbing characteristics of juvenile crime is its increasing tendency toward violence.

> The 2005 National Youth Risk Behavior Surveillance Survey indicated that 18.5% of U.S. youth carried a weapon, 5.4% carried a gun, 6% avoided school out of fear, and 36% had been in a physical fight. Bullying has become a public health problem. Youths who are African American or non-white Hispanic are disproportionately represented among troubled adolescents and their victims.

THE ROOTS OF DELINQUENCY, AGGRESSION, AND VIOLENCE

Not all aggression is meant to be violent, but all violence is aggressive and meant to cause harm. Theories that address the roots of aggressive and violent behavior include ethology, biology, social learning theory, self-control, and developmental contextualism (**Table 63-1**).

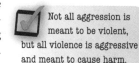

> Not all aggression is meant to be violent, but all violence is aggressive and meant to cause harm.

In their massive and now-classic study of crime and human nature, Wilson and Herrnstein (1985) found clear evidence of a positive association between past and future antisocial behavior; that is, the best predictor of violence is past antisocial behavior. Although the causes of violent and criminal behavior are multiple and complex, most modern scientists believe that a tendency to commit crime is established early in life, *perhaps as soon as the preschool years*, and that the behaviors of these children provide ample clues to their possible future antisocial behavior.

A critical age for early signs of emerging delinquency is 7 to 12 years, when children begin to develop self-schemas that are aligned with risky behavior and to search for friends who may affirm this behavior. They may be drawn to a particular group because a friend is a member; it may be a sign of rebellion ("My mother doesn't like those kids, but I think they're neat"); or it may just seem a daring thing to do.

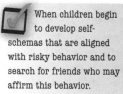

> When children begin to develop self-schemas that are aligned with risky behavior and to search for friends who may affirm this behavior.

THE CHARACTERISTICS OF DELINQUENTS

In their lifelong studies, the Gluecks (1950) found that delinquents were distinguishable from non-delinquents in several ways:

Table 63-1 Theories About Youth Violence

Theory	Theme	Key Ideas
Ethology	Adaptive for competition for limited resources	Close physical proximity plays a role in initiating (threat) and stopping (empathy for victim) physical aggression short of death.
Biology	Role of testosterone and limbic system	Testosterone may be necessary for aggression but does not cause aggression. Fear and anxiety live in the amygdala: impulsive reaction to stimuli. Impulse control lives in the frontal lobes: mediated behavior.
Social learning theory	Behavior is learned from role models	Influence of parents, friends, and culture is key in setting acceptable norms for behavior.
Self-control	Self-regulation of impulses and desires	Self-control is cognitively mediated and is learned through practice and guidance.
Developmental contextualism	Role of multiple systems in development	It takes a village to raise a healthy productive person and to intervene when one goes astray.

- *Physically.* They were more muscular and vigorous.
- *Temperamentally.* They were restless, energetic, impulsive, extroverted, aggressive, and destructive.
- *Attitudinally.* They were hostile, defiant, resentful, and stubborn, and resented authority.
- *Psychologically.* They were more interested in the concrete than the abstract and were generally poor problem solvers.
- *Socioculturally.* They were more often reared in homes that offered little understanding, affection, stability, or moral standards.

Many recent studies have reached similar conclusions.

BULLYING

Bullying is aggressive behavior in which the bully, who is usually physically stronger than the peers, needs to dominate his or her victims, for whom the bully feels no empathy even at close range. Bullies' victims are more anxious, passive, and insecure than their peers, and often lonely. Interestingly, bullies are often leaders, and either are not adept at picking up the social cues that would stop their aggression or are particularly good at doing so to enhance their power in the group.

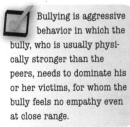

Bullying is aggressive behavior in which the bully, who is usually physically stronger than the peers, needs to dominate his or her victims, for whom the bully feels no empathy even at close range.

SELF-CONTROL AND IMPULSIVE BEHAVIOR

Impulsivity (**impulsive behavior**) seems to be a continuous thread running through delinquent behavior. When studying impulsivity, researchers have placed children in a position in which they were presented with something they enjoy—candies, toys—and told that if they did not eat the candy or play with the toy until the researcher returned, they could have two pieces of candy or an even bigger toy. The researchers then left the room, and observers watched the children through one-way mirrors. The results were as one would expect: Some children ate the candy immediately or played with the toy; others resisted by trying to distract themselves.

The amazing part of this work, however, was the follow-up research. The same children who displayed impulsivity at age 4 years were more troubled adolescents: They had fewer friends; they experienced more psychological difficulties; and they were more irritable and aggressive, more prone to delinquent behavior, and less able to cope with frustration. The 4-year-olds who delayed their gratification could better handle frustration, were more focused and calm when challenged by any obstacle, and were more self-reliant and popular as adolescents.

THE ROLE OF THE COMMUNITY

While parents and peers are important influences on adolescents, recent research indicates that the larger environment of neighborhood and community is equally important in fostering productive young adults and preventing deviant behavior. Lerner, Almerigi, Theokas, and Lerner's (2005) work on "positive youth development" has addressed the community assets that help to produce competent, confident, and caring youth who are of good character and who feel connected to other people. Opportunities to engage youth in civic-minded activities in which they give of themselves and interact with competent peers and adults are among those assets.

IMPLICATIONS FOR HEALTHCARE PROVIDERS

Begin screening for poor self-control in young children. They often are impulsive, difficult to manage in the classroom and at home, and do not have many friends. Intervening at this point is critical. Be alert to the signs of the major risky behaviors in adolescence: drug and alcohol abuse, unsafe sex and teenage pregnancy, school underachievement, and delinquency, crime, and violence. Also be alert for signs of victimization. Recognize that the causes of and treatment for troubling behavior are multifaceted. Become familiar with community programs that are designed to foster healthy and productive adolescents, and that help troubled adolescents before they become troubled adults.

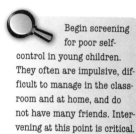

Begin screening for poor self-control in young children. They often are impulsive, difficult to manage in the classroom and at home, and do not have many friends. Intervening at this point is critical.

SOURCES

Bandura, A. (1997). *Self-efficacy: The exercise of control.* New York: Freeman.

Barrett, J., & Walsh, M. E. (2005). The roots of violence and aggression. In K. Thies, & J. Travers (Eds.), *The handbook of human development for health professionals* (pp. 355–377). Sudbury, MA: Jones and Bartlett.

Centers for Disease Control and Prevention. (2007). *YRBSS: Youth risk behavior surveillance system.* Retrieved March 13, 2008, from www.cdc.gov/HealthyYouth/yrbs/index.htm

Glueck, S., & Glueck, E. (1950). *Unraveling juvenile delinquency.* Cambridge, MA: Harvard University Press.

Lerner, R., Almerigi, J. B., Theokas, C., & Lerner, J. V. (2005). Positive youth development: A view on the issues. *Journal of Early Adolescence, 25*(1), 10–16.

Stein, K. F., Roeser, R., & Markus, H. R. (1998). Self-schemas and possible selves as predictors of risky behaviors in adolescents. *Nursing Research, 47*(2), 96–106.

Wilson, J., & Herrnstein, R. (1985). *Crime and human nature.* New York: Simon and Schuster.

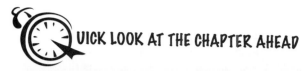

- One in 10 children and adolescents in the United States suffers from mental illness.
- Risk factors for depression in adolescence include significant loss, health problems, family history, abuse, and alcohol use.
- Depression in adolescents is not normal.
- Girls attempt suicide more often than boys, but boys are five times as likely to die from suicide.
- The comorbidities of alcohol use, emotional disorder, and sexual acting out are predictors of adolescent suicidal behavior.
- Do not hesitate to ask adolescents if they are suicidal; it may be a relief to them that someone notices how desperate they feel.

64

Mental Health Problems

TERMS
☐ Depression
☐ Suicide

According to the National Institute for Mental Health (2006), in the United States today, one in 10 children and adolescents suffers from mental illness severe enough to result in significant functional impairment. By 2020, childhood neuropsychiatric disorders are expected to rise by more than 50% internationally to become one of the five most common causes of morbidity, mortality, and disability among youth.

Teens are an age group that many consider at risk for **depression** simply by virtue of their developmental period. Normative changes may be accompanied by dissatisfaction with body type, disappointment in love, uncertainty about the future, anxiety about sexuality, and conflict with family. For some, however, their feelings of despair and hopelessness are out of proportion to developmental events. When that happens, the risk for **suicide** increases.

CHARACTERISTICS AND INCIDENCE OF DEPRESSION IN ADOLESCENCE

Figure 64-1 lists the criteria for a diagnosis of major depression according to the fourth edition of the *Diagnostic and Statistical Manual of Mental Disorders (DSM-IV*; 1994; *DSM-V* is due to be published in 2011). Social/emotional symptoms include dejected mood, loss of pleasure, social withdrawal, and crying spells. Physical symptoms include fatigue, sleep disturbance, and loss of appetite. Cognitive symptoms include difficulty concentrating, indecisiveness, and distorted perceptions about events and relationships. Cognitive difficulties may result in poor academic performance. Teens may withdraw into sleep, television, or video games.

Although the incidence of depression increases with age, a meta-analysis by the National Institutes of Mental Health (2001) indicates that the overall prevalence of depression has remained

---

A. Five or more of the following symptoms have been present during the same 2-week period and represent a change from previous functioning. At least one symptom is either (1) depressed mood or (2) loss of interest or pleasure.

   1. Depressed mood; in adolescents can be irritable mood

   2. Diminished interest or pleasure in all or almost all activities

   3. Significant weight loss without dieting or weight gain (e.g., 5% in a month)

   4. Insomnia or hypersomnia every day

   5. Psychomotor agitation or retardation nearly every day

   6. Fatigue or loss of energy nearly every day

   7. Feelings of worthlessness or excessive or inappropriate guilt nearly every day

   8. Diminished ability to think or concentrate, or indecisiveness, nearly every day

   9. Recurrent thoughts of death, recurrent suicidal ideation without specific plan, or a suicide attempt or specific plan for committing suicide

B. Symptoms do not meet criteria for mixed episode (i.e., depressive and manic symptoms).

C. Symptoms cause significant distress or impairment in social, occupational, or other areas of functioning.

D. Symptoms are not due to the physiological effects of a substance or medical condition.

E. Symptoms are not accounted for by bereavement.

Figure 64-1 Criteria for Major Depressive Disorder, Single Episode

steady for almost 30 years. Among youths aged 13 to 18, 5.6% of teens have been *diagnosed* with depression, with girls (5.9%) being diagnosed more frequently than boys (4.6%). However, about 28% of teens report feeling sad or hopeless, with girls (36.7%) feeling that way more than boys (20.4%). Hispanic girls (46.7%) are at greatest risk, followed by girls from Asian, Native American and Pacific Islander backgrounds (41.5%).

Although the incidence of depression increases with age, a meta-analysis by the National Institutes of Health indicates that the overall prevalence of depression has remained steady for almost 30 years. Among youths aged 13 to 18, 5.6% of teens have been *diagnosed* with depression, with girls (5.9%) being diagnosed more frequently than boys (4.6%). However, about 28% of teens report feeling sad or hopeless, with girls (36.7%) feeling that way more than boys (20.4%). Hispanic girls (46.7%) are at greatest risk, followed by girls from Asian, Native American and Pacific Islander backgrounds (41.5%).

Moderate and severe depression are not simply "more depression" than mild symptoms. Major depression represents a significant and negative alteration in how individuals think about themselves, their future, and life experiences. That is, major depression can become self-sustaining, shaping future experiences.

RISK FACTORS FOR DEPRESSION

Risk factors for depression in adolescence include significant loss, health problems, family history, abuse, and alcohol use. Loss can take the form of the death of a loved one, rejection in love, or dashed hopes and dream. Teens with serious health problems are 2.5 times more likely than healthy peers to experience significant depression and anxiety (Wallander & Varni, 1992). A history of abuse (especially sexual abuse) and a family history of depression (especially in a parent) increase this risk. Adolescents who use drugs or alcohol are also more likely to suffer from depression. Likewise, a lack of perceived emotional and social support magnifies risk factors.

Girls are at greater risk for depression than boys, although the suicide rate among boys is higher. Girls are more likely to be dissatisfied with their body type and to blame themselves for their failures. They feel responsible for maintaining relationships, and they may experience a greater sense of loss and failure when things do not work out as expected. Girls internalize their feelings and ruminate over negative experiences and feelings. Boys blame others or bad luck for their failures. They externalize their feelings, expressing them with action and often with aggression.

SUICIDE AND ADOLESCENTS

According to the Centers for Disease Control and Prevention (2007), in 2004 suicide was the third leading cause of death among youths and young adults aged 10 to 24 years in the United States, accounting for 4599 deaths. From 1990 to 2003, the combined suicide rate for persons aged 10 to

24 years declined from 9.48 to 6.78 per 100,000 persons. From 2003 to 2004, the rate increased from 6.78 to 7.32 per 100,000 persons—the largest single-year increase during the 1990–2004 period. Females ages 10 to 14 and 15 to 19 and males 15 to 19 accounted for this upward trend. Girls attempt suicide more often than boys, but boys are five times more likely to die from suicide. During their suicide attempts, girls are more likely to use hanging or poison (e.g., an overdose of pills or alcohol, or both), whereas boys resort to more violent and lethal methods, such as firearms. Boys who commit suicide may be more emotionally disturbed than girls, and more determined to die.

According to the National Youth Behavior Surveillance Survey (2005), 21.8% of female adolescents and 12% of male adolescents seriously considered suicide in the previous 12 months, with 10.8% and 6%, respectively, making a real attempt. Hispanic youths and those from other backgrounds, such as Native American, Asian, and Pacific Islanders, are at highest risk, especially females.

According to the Centers for Disease Control and Prevention (2007), in 2004 suicide was the third leading cause of death among youths and young adults aged 10 to 24 years in the United States, accounting for 4599 deaths. From 1990 to 2003, the combined suicide rate for persons aged 10 to 24 years declined from 9.48 to 6.78 per 100,000 persons. From 2003 to 2004, the rate increased from 6.78 to 7.32 per 100,000 persons—the largest single-year increase during the 1990–2004 period.

RISK FACTORS FOR SUICIDE

Risk factors for suicide include a history of emotional or psychiatric disturbance, especially affective disorders, such as depression and bipolar disorder. Adolescent girls who commit suicide are also more likely to suffer from borderline personality disorder, whereas boys manifest antisocial and conduct disorders. Adolescents who die from suicide have histories that include early and frequent use of alcohol and other substances, especially cocaine, and early and frequent sexual activity. Among males in particular, concerns about homosexuality are a risk factor for suicide.

Risk factors for suicide include a history of emotional or psychiatric disturbance, especially affective disorders, such as depression and bipolar disorder.

The comorbidity of alcohol use and emotional disorder, especially coupled with sexual acting out, are powerful predictors of suicidal behavior. The best predictor, however, is a previous attempt. Almost 50% of adolescents who die by suicide made a previous attempt. **Figure 64-2** lists the warning signs for possible suicide in adolescents.

IMPLICATIONS FOR HEALTHCARE PROVIDERS

Screen for depression and other mental health disorders as part of every health assessment. Somatic symptoms can mask depression, or they may be an excuse to talk to a healthcare provider, especially the school nurse.

Do not hesitate to ask adolescents if they are suicidal. Asking the question does not give them the idea, but rather may provide a sense of relief to the teen. Ask if there is a plan; the more detailed and possible the plan, the greater the immediate risk. If you believe that an

Screen for depression and other mental health disorders as part of every health assessment. Somatic symptoms can mask depression, or they may be an excuse to talk to a healthcare provider, especially the school nurse.

1. Talking about killing oneself: "I wish I were dead." "My family would be better off without me."
2. Preoccupation with death, in music, art, poetry, personal writings; talking about "not being" or not having a future: "I have nothing to live for." "It won't get any better, so what's the use."
3. Disturbances in eating or sleeping habits.
4. Declining grades in school, lack of interest in school or hobbies.
5. Giving away prized possessions.
6. Withdrawal from family and friends, feeling alienated from others.
7. Significant changes in usual behavior or demeanor (e.g., the shy person becomes an extrovert).
8. Series of "accidents" or impulsive risk-taking activities.
9. Pervasive sense of gloom, hoplessness, helplessness.

Figure 64-2 Warning Signs for Possible Suicide in Adolescents

adolescent is suicidal, do not leave him or her alone, even if he or she claims to be okay: Get immediate help. Your actions will indicate that you take the adolescent seriously, and at the very least will open a line of communication.

SOURCES

Centers for Disease Control and Prevention. (2007). *YRBSS: Youth risk behavior surveillance system.* Retrieved March 13, 2008, from www.cdc.gov/HealthyYouth/yrbs/index.htm

Centers for Disease Control and Prevention. (2007, September 7). Suicide trends among youths and young adults aged 10–24 years—United States, 1990–2004. *Morbidity and Mortality Weekly Review, 56*(35), 905–908.

Costello, J., Erkanli, E., & Angold, A. (2006). Is there an epidemic of child or adolescent depression? *Journal of Child Psychology & Psychiatry & Allied Disciplines, 47*(12), 1263–1271.

Diagnostic and statistical manual of mental disorders (4th ed.). (1994). Washington, DC: American Psychiatric Association.

National Institute of Mental Health. (2001). *Blueprint for change: Research on child and adolescent mental health.* Bethesda, MD: Author.

Wallander, J., & Varni, J. (1992). Adjustment in children with chronic physical disorders. In A. LaGreca, L. Siegel, J. Wallander, & C. Walker (Eds.), *Stress and coping in child health* (pp. 279–298). New York: Guildford Press.

PART VI • QUESTIONS

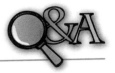

For each of the following questions, choose the **one best** answer.

1. Which of the following is an example of secondary sexual characteristics?
   a. Onset of menstruation in girls
   b. Growth of breasts in girls
   c. "Wet dreams" in boys
   d. Growth of facial hair in boys

2. Which hormone is responsible for the onset of menstrual flow?
   a. Estrogen
   b. Progesterone
   c. Follicle-stimulating hormone (FSH)
   d. Luteinizing hormone (LH)

3. What are the caloric needs of a rapidly growing adolescent boy?
   a. 1500 calories per day
   b. 2000 calories per day
   c. 3000 calories per day
   d. 4000 calories per day

4. Which of the following has the greatest influence on adolescents' decision to smoke cigarettes?
   a. Advertisements showing celebrities smoking
   b. Having parents who smoke
   c. Having friends who smoke
   d. Having good social skills

5. Who among the following is apt to be least happy with their bodies?
   a. Early-maturing boys and early-maturing girls
   b. Early-maturing girls and late-maturing boys
   c. Late-maturing boys and late-maturing girls
   d. Late-maturing girls and early-maturing boys

6. Which of the following factors is most influential in adolescents' decision to become sexually active?
   a. Family environment
   b. Difficulty managing sexual arousal
   c. Values depicted in the media
   d. Peer pressure

7. An ability to think about the future and consider negative possibilities is a feature of Piaget's
   a. sensorimotor period.
   b. preoperational period.
   c. concrete operational period.
   d. formal operational period.

8. Adolescents demonstrate an increase in
   a. searching ability.
   b. information-processing capacity.
   c. classroom sophistication.
   d. unilateral methodology.

9. A young adolescent refuses to walk through the mall with his mother, saying he is old enough to take care of himself in a public place. According to Elkind, this is an example of
   a. the imaginary audience.
   b. the personal fable.
   c. the second-person perspective.
   d. social cognition.

10. Why do adolescents argue so much?
    a. They like to argue.
    b. They are capable of propositional reasoning.
    c. They enjoy outmaneuvering their opponents.
    d. All of the above are correct.

11. When adolescents want to do something themselves, this is an example of
    a. persistence.
    b. logical processing.
    c. internal motivation.
    d. search and discovery.

12. Adolescents tend to attribute their performance to ability, effort, task difficulty, or
    a. luck.
    b. influence.
    c. diligence.
    d. peers.

13. "Peer" usually refers to those who are within _____ months of each other in terms of age.
    a. 10
    b. 12
    c. 18
    d. 24

14. The work of _____ is associated with social perspective taking.
    a. Selman
    b. Skinner
    c. Vygotsky
    d. Freud

15. Erikson's famous term for what adolescents may experience is
    a. discovery crisis.
    b. assimilated identity.
    c. structured ego.
    d. identity crisis.

16. The expression "adolescent egocentric thinking" is associated with
    a. Piaget.
    b. Marcia.
    c. Bruner.
    d. Elkind.
17. One of the most disturbing features of today's delinquency is its increasing
    a. spread.
    b. violence.
    c. hidden nature.
    d. family directedness.
18. Delay-of-gratification studies attempt to identify _____ children.
    a. impulsive
    b. delayed
    c. emotionally disturbed
    d. aggressive
19. Depression affects three major areas of functioning in adolescents. Which of the following are examples of symptoms in those areas?
    a. Crying, loss of pleasure, social withdrawal
    b. Fatigue, weight loss, trouble sleeping
    c. Drop in grades, cannot think straight, cannot make decisions
    d. Loss of pleasure, sleep disturbance, difficulty concentrating
20. What is the best predictor of suicide among adolescents?
    a. Psychiatric disorder
    b. Abuse of alcohol and drugs
    c. Early sexual activity
    d. A previous suicide attempt

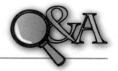

PART VI · ANSWERS

1. **The answer is d.** Primary sexual characteristics involve the reproductive organs as a result of sex hormone production (i.e., maturation of the ovaries, breasts, uterus, penis, and testes). Secondary sexual characteristics accompany hormonal changes but are not directly involved in reproduction. They include development of facial, body, and pubic hair; deepening voice; and distribution of fat and muscle.

2. **The answer is b.** Progesterone causes the uterine lining to mature in preparation for implantation of a fertilized embryo, and it inhibits the production of FSH, which would trigger the beginning of a new cycle. If fertilization does not occur, the increase in progesterone from the corpus luteum also shuts down the production of LH, which sustains the corpus luteum itself. As the corpus luteum begins to disintegrate and progesterone levels fall, FSH production is no longer inhibited and begins anew. Without progesterone, the lining of the uterus cannot be sustained, and it is shed in the form of the menstrual flow. The menstrual cycle then begins again.

3. **The answer is d.** Boys have higher caloric needs than girls because boys have a greater proportion of lean body mass relative to adipose tissue. A rapidly growing, athletic, 15-year-old boy may need as many as 4000 calories per day just to maintain his weight. By contrast, an inactive 15-year-old girl whose growth is almost completed may need fewer than 2000 calories per day to avoid gaining weight.

4. **The answer is b.** The best predictor of smoking behavior is having parents who smoke. The influence of friends is greater earlier in adolescence than later during this period. Advertisements—especially those that link smoking with thinness in women—also play a role. Adolescents who are socially skilled are more self-confident and less likely to succumb to the influence of peers to engage in risky behaviors.

5. **The answer is b.** The timing of puberty can significantly influence how adolescents feel about their new bodies. Girls who develop early and boys who develop late are most unhappy with their bodies, and tend to feel less attractive to the opposite sex. Early-maturing girls are self-conscious about their bodies and subject to teasing from boys, who typically develop later than the average girl. Late-maturing boys appear to be boys among the women and young men in their class, and have more difficulty competing in athletics and socially.

6. **The answer is a.** Of the many factors that influence adolescents' choice to become sexually active, the family environment is the most significant. Teens who come from stable families in which parents demonstrate responsible behavior and are open to discussing sex with their children are less likely to engage in premarital sex. Those who do are older at first coitus. Teens whose families are poor, are disorganized, and endorse the view that women are subservient to male dominance tend to become sexually active at an earlier age. Adolescent girls who have goals for their future involving education and career also delay first coitus.

7. **The answer is d.** Reversibility and ability to speculate about things that seem impossible help to identify formal operational thinking.

8. **The answer is b.** Most adolescents acquire a greater ability to process data during this stage of development than they had as children. For example, they usually can store greater amounts of information in memory.

9. **The answer is a.** Egocentric thinking results in what Elkind calls the "imaginary audience." Younger adolescents in particular are extremely self-conscious, sure that everybody is looking at them. Hence, they may act as if on stage, performing for an audience that exists only in their imaginations. They may use the audience to anticipate the reactions of other people to their own behavior.

10. **The answer is d.** Adolescents argue for the sake of arguing. Propositional reasoning—that is, analyzing the logic of propositions—means adolescents appreciate the art and science of debate. They approach problems systematically, collect the relevant facts, find the logic in them, and make their case. They invest the presentation of their case with passion and an unshakable belief that they are in the right. They love to exercise their new cognitive abilities, to see different perspectives, to discuss abstract principles, to analyze the intentions that underlie behavior, and to outmaneuver opponents with carefully crafted strategies.

11. **The answer is c.** Individuals who want to do something themselves do not need external rewards such as praise, recognition, or anything tangible. They are driven by a desire to accomplish a particular task, to excel, to discover.

12. **The answer is a.** Individuals who believe luck is the basis of any success they achieve typically lack self-esteem. They believe that control is out of their hands.

13. **The answer is b.** Interestingly, although 12 months is thought of as the age criterion for a peer, many relationships are formed on the basis of mutual interests and likes or dislikes.

14. **The answer is a.** The significance of Selman's work lies in its insights into psychosocial development. When children and adolescents begin to realize that others have their own opinions and ideas, it affects how they relate to those around them.

15. **The answer is d.** Teenagers who are uncertain as to their own self (i.e., identity crisis) have difficulty in resolving the personal crises that arise during these years.

16. **The answer is d.** Elkind's expression aptly captures the egocentrism of adolescence. Besieged by physical and emotional changes, adolescents tend to think that everything revolves around them.

17. **The answer is b.** Those concerned with the delinquency problem are alarmed at the growing violence. Whether due to changed societal conditions, a breakdown in authority, or televised aggression, new kinds of intervention are needed to counteract this trend.

18. **The answer is a.** Research showing how impulsivity is linked to achievement demonstrates its importance in all phases of development.

19. **The answer is d.** The criteria for depression address three major areas of functioning. Social/emotional symptoms include dejected mood, loss of pleasure, social withdrawal, and crying spells; depressed individuals lose interest in the routines of daily living. Physical symptoms include fatigue, sleep disturbance, and loss of appetite. Cognitive symptoms include difficulty concentrating, indecisiveness, and distorted perceptions about events and relationships.

20. **The answer is d.** The comorbidity of alcohol use and emotional disorder, especially when coupled with sexual acting out, are powerful predictors of suicidal behavior. The best predictor, however, is a previous attempt. Almost 50% of adolescents who die by suicide made a previous attempt.

VII
Adulthood

QUICK LOOK AT THE CHAPTER AHEAD

- Most young adults in the United States are in good physical condition.
- The health habits developed during these years are reliable indicators of future health conditions.
- Pregnancy and childbirth are significant physical events during these years.
- The condition of the cardiovascular and pulmonary systems depends on activity level, high versus low fat concentrations, and the decision whether to smoke.
- Prevention measures to safeguard healthy young people are becoming more widely adopted.
- The goal of health promotion is to improve one's well-being through healthy lifestyle choices.

65

Early Adulthood: Physical Health

TERMS
- ☐ **Cardiovascular system**
- ☐ **Musculoskeletal system**
- ☐ **Primary prevention**
- ☐ **Pulmonary system**

Humans are at the peak of physical development and performance between ages 20 and 30. The built-in reserve of vital capacity in major organs and biological systems remains robust until about age 30, after which it experiences varying rates of decline (**Figure 65-1**). The health habits that individuals develop during this period are excellent predictors of how humans will weather the physical changes and diseases that typically emerge in the middle and later years. **Figure 65-2** lists the seven health habits most closely associated with good health.

> The health habits that individuals develop during their 20s are excellent predictors of how humans will weather the physical changes and diseases that typically emerge in the middle and later years.

CHARACTERISTICS OF BIOLOGICAL SYSTEMS

Body Mass, Height, and Weight

The average woman in the United States is 5 feet, 4 inches, tall, and reaches that height by age 18. Men reach the average height of 5 feet, 9 inches, at age 20. The typical weight gain of 10 to 15 pounds between ages 18 and 30 is largely due to the maturing of muscles, bones, and internal organs and an increase in fatty tissue. Overindulgence in food and alcohol is the major reason for obesity during this period.

Skin, Hair, and Teeth

As total body water begins to decrease, and time spent in the sun accumulates, skin becomes drier. Male pattern balding, which begins with hair loss at the crown and is genetically determined, begins in men's twenties and thirties. Wisdom teeth often cause problems that lead to their removal.

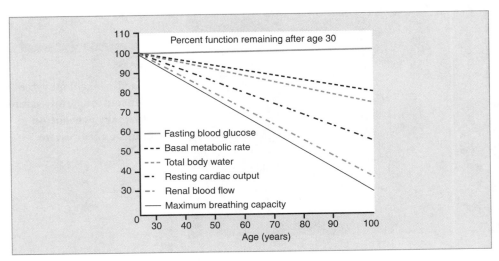

Figure 65-1 Rate of Decline in Organ Reserve

Eat breakfast almost every day

Rarely or never eat between meals

Sleep 7–8 hours daily

Maintain normal weight adjusted
for height, age, and sex

Never smoke cigarettes

Avoid alcohol or use it moderately

Engage in regular physical activity

Figure 65-2 Health Practices Associated with Good Health

Musculoskeletal System

Fusion of the epiphyses of the long bones occurs between ages 18 and 25, which is also the peak of muscle performance. After age 26, muscle strength begins to decline and reaction time levels off. Declines in muscle mass and body water content may be masked by an increase in fatty tissue, giving a false impression of vigor. Decline in water content in the joints results in small skeletal changes after age 30, increasing a person's vulnerability to knee, ankle, and shoulder injuries.

The average woman in the United States is 5 feet, 4 inches, tall, and reaches that height by age 18. Men reach the average height of 5 feet, 9 inches, at age 20.

Cardiovascular and Pulmonary Systems

The heart and lungs can achieve 100% capacity when required to do so during a person's twenties. After age 30, the rate of decline depends on activity level and smoking status. The risk for developing heart and lung diseases in middle age depends largely on the choices made in youth. The long-term effects of smoking, lack of exercise, a diet high in fat, and overuse of alcohol are the major contributors to heart disease and stroke (see Chapter 68).

Fusion of the epiphyses of the long bones occurs between ages 18 and 25, which is also the peak of muscle performance.

The heart and lungs can achieve 100% capacity when required to do so during a person's twenties.

Reproduction

Pregnancy and childbirth are major physical events for many women in their twenties and thirties. After age 30, women's fertility rates decline and the incidence of birth defects and complications during labor rise.

The risk for developing heart and lung diseases in middle age depends largely on the choices made in youth. The long-term effects of smoking, lack of exercise, a diet high in fat, and overuse of alcohol are the major contributors to heart disease and stroke (see Chapter 68).

Pregnancy results in multiple changes in all body systems. Blood volume and cardiac output increase by 25% to 50%, and oxygen consumption increases by 20%. The residual volume of the lungs decreases by 20%, however, so fatigue and shortness of breath are not uncommon. As the uterus increases in size, it displaces the stomach and intestines, leading to heartburn and constipation. Toward the end of pregnancy, the pelvic ligaments and joints soften to facilitate birth, which may cause difficulty walking. Most women benefit from engaging in moderate exercise throughout pregnancy.

 # HEALTH PROMOTION

During the past half-century, the death rate for young adults has been nearly cut in half. Unfortunately, accidents account for the most deaths for young Americans up to the age of 44. These are the years in which behavioral habits—eating, smoking, exercising—combined with a person's genetic influence, begin to shape health conditions for the coming years.

Unfortunately, accidents account for the most deaths for young Americans up to the age of 44.

Primary prevention refers to efforts to prevent disease and injury in healthy people. Examples include immunizations, use of seat belts, and breast self-examination. Health promotion is directed at increasing one's well-being, in part through healthy lifestyle choices. The U.S. Department of Health and Human Services has identified its top four priority areas for health promotion and disease prevention as physical activity and fitness, nutrition, tobacco use, and alcohol use. Other areas of high interest include mental health, family planning, and violence.

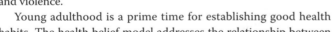

Primary prevention refers to efforts to prevent disease and injury in healthy people. Examples include immunizations, use of seat belts, and breast self-examination. Health promotion is directed at increasing one's well-being, in part through healthy lifestyle choices.

Young adulthood is a prime time for establishing good health habits. The health belief model addresses the relationship between health and behavior (Rosenstoch, 1974). The first and second components of this model are perception of susceptibility to a particular illness and perception of the seriousness of the illness; the third component is weighing the costs and benefits of taking preventive action.

For example, if your father died of heart disease at age 55 and you are 45 years old, a smoker, and overweight, you would perceive yourself to be susceptible to a serious disease in the near future. The perceived benefits of losing weight and quitting smoking might outweigh your costs in time, money, and aggravation. If you have no personal experience with heart disease and are younger than age 30, you would not perceive yourself as being susceptible. The hassle of watching your diet and giving up cigarettes would, in this case, outweigh the perceived benefits.

For example, if your father died of heart disease at age 55 and you are 45 years old, a smoker, and overweight, you would perceive yourself to be susceptible to a serious disease in the near future.

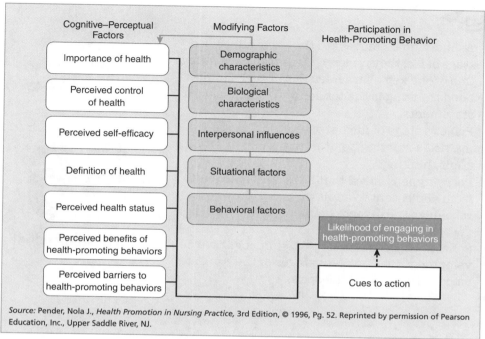

Source: Pender, Nola J., *Health Promotion in Nursing Practice*, 3rd Edition, © 1996, Pg. 52. Reprinted by permission of Pearson Education, Inc., Upper Saddle River, NJ.

Figure 65-3 Health Promotion Model

The health promotion model (Pender, 1996) (**Figure 65-3**) addresses the likelihood of choosing to adopt health-enhancing behaviors. Cognitive perceptual factors include perception of how healthy one is, how much control one has over health, whether one thinks one is capable of changing habits, and the benefits of healthy behaviors. These are modified by factors such as age, interpersonal influences, social group, and education. For example, if you want to lose weight but believe you have inherited your weight problem, you would not perceive yourself as being in control of your health and, therefore, are less likely to change your eating habits.

Cognitive perceptual factors include perception of how healthy one is, how much control one has over health, whether one thinks one is capable of changing habits, and the benefits of healthy behaviors. These are modified by factors such as age, interpersonal influences, social group, and education.

SOURCES

Belloe, N., & Breslow, L. (1972). Relationship of physical health status and health practices. *Preventive Medicine, 1*, 409–421.

Pender, N. (1996). *Health promotion and nursing practice* (3rd ed.). Norwalk, CT: Appleton-Century-Crofts.

Rosenstoch, I. (1974). Historical origin of the health belief model. *Health Education Monograph, 2*, 334.

- As individuals move into the early adulthood stage of life, they undergo three transformations.
- One of the key characteristics of early adulthood thinking is the tendency to analyze verbal statements.
- Piaget's stage of formal operations has remained a starting point in any analysis of adult thinking.
- Perry hypothesized that as adolescents shift from adolescent to adult thinking, they begin to recognize the diverse opinions and multiple perspectives of others.
- Schaie proposed a theory of adult cognitive development that involves stages of thinking at various times in the lifespan.

66

Early Adulthood: Cognitive Development

TERMS
- ☐ Achieving stage
- ☐ Formal operational stage
- ☐ Postformal thought
- ☐ Reflective thinking

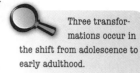

Three transformations occur in the shift from adolescence to early adulthood:

1. The structure of thought changes as young adults, using the foundation of earlier cognitive development, turn to distinct ways of thinking.

2. Young adults concentrate on acquiring advanced knowledge in a particular field as they begin their careers.

3. The path of intellectual development may remain relatively stable or decline sharply during the adult years.

Three transformations occur in the shift from adolescence to early adulthood.

THE TRANSITION TO ADULT THINKING

One major feature of adult thinking, beginning in adolescence and becoming more firmly rooted in early adulthood, is the tendency to analyze verbal statements and to evaluate their validity as formal propositions. When faced with a problem, adults immediately search for possibilities. They examine the situation carefully, look for all possible solutions, and then analyze those options to determine which is the best possible answer. They follow the steps of scientific reasoning. (See Chapter 47 for a discussion of problem solving.)

Another notable component of adult thought is the acquisition of specific knowledge combined with a greater capacity for information processing. Both of these features, plus greater speed and accuracy, contribute to the reasoning abilities needed in problem solving. With improvement in memory, for example, adults solve problems more readily by remembering similar problems and the ways in which they were solved.

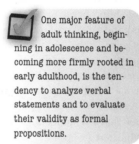

One major feature of adult thinking, beginning in adolescence and becoming more firmly rooted in early adulthood, is the tendency to analyze verbal statements and to evaluate their validity as formal propositions.

Another notable component of adult thought is the acquisition of specific knowledge combined with a greater capacity for information processing.

EXPLANATIONS OF ADULT THOUGHT

Several theories have been proposed to explain changes in adult thinking that move beyond Piaget's work. These theoretical endeavors have examined a person's improved ability to engage in **reflective thinking**. New research has also probed the dimensions of **postformal thought**, which includes emotion and practical experience.

Nevertheless, Piaget's (1950, 1971; Inhelder & Piaget, 1958; Piaget & Inhelder, 1969) interpretation of adult thought demands initial consideration. Piaget's final stage—the **formal operational stage**—represents his interpretation of adolescent and adult thought. Piaget believed that formal operational thinking has several essential features:

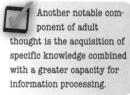

These theoretical endeavors have examined a person's improved ability to engage in **reflective thinking**. New research has also probed the dimensions of **postformal thought**, which includes emotion and practical experience.

• Individuals at this stage of cognitive development can separate the real from the possible. They try to identify all possible relations in any problem and then, by mental experimentation and logical analysis, discover which are true.

- Formal operational thinking is propositional; that is, individuals can use statements and propositions to reach conclusions.
- Formal operational thinkers attack a problem by gathering all available information and then combining as many variables as possible.

Piaget believed that formal operational thinking has several essential features.

Among the theorists who concentrated on adult cognitive development was William Perry (1970, 1981), who interviewed 67 Harvard and Radcliffe students at the end of each of their 4 years of college and discovered several important ways in which the thinking of young adults differs from that of adolescents. As younger students, the subjects held rigid ideas about right and wrong, good and bad. This rigid, dualistic thinking gradually grew more flexible, however, when they began to realize that their opinions on many matters were as good as those of others. As they continued to accumulate knowledge and to better understand how their values affected their thinking, the young adults made their own commitments. That is, they reached their own decisions and committed to their own beliefs, while simultaneously accepting that other valid possibilities exist. (As you evaluate Perry's ideas and assess their universality, remember that his subjects were taken from a small, highly select and educated group.)

Among the theorists who concentrated on adult cognitive development was William Perry (1970, 1981), who interviewed 67 Harvard and Radcliffe students at the end of each of their 4 years of college and discovered several important ways in which the thinking of young adults differs from that of adolescents.

Another explanation of cognitive development in early adulthood was proposed by K. Warner Schaie (1977, 1994). Schaie believed that young adults differ from adolescents in the way that they *use* their cognitive abilities. The problems they encounter become more complex; the situations they face become more diverse; the decisions they make become more critical. Although young adults continue to acquire knowledge in specific, more restricted fields, their cognitive focus shifts more to the application of knowledge.

Another explanation of cognitive development in early adulthood was proposed by K. Warner Schaie (1977, 1994).

Schaie formulated several stages to trace and explain adult cognition. He termed the early adult stage the **achieving stage** to indicate how young adults apply their cognitive abilities to those circumstances that have profound long-term consequences, such as career, marriage, and family (**Table 66-1**).

Table 66-1 Theories of Cognitive Development in Early Adulthood

Piaget:	Formal operational thinking
Perry:	Rigidity–flexibility–commitment
Schaie:	Achieving stage (applying knowledge)

IMPLICATIONS FOR HEALTHCARE PROVIDERS

Young adults tend to be relatively healthy, which means that you need to be insightful and creative in suggesting care for this age group. Because they possess the cognitive abilities described in this chapter, they are more likely to comprehend treatment procedures you recommend. You will contact many individuals in this age group on college and university campuses. Consequently, you should try to advocate programs stressing positive health behaviors, perhaps in courses with a health education component or in peer counseling groups. Identify as many opportunities as possible for health promotion and protection in places where young adults gather.

SOURCES

Berk, L. (2008). *Development through the lifespan.* Needham Heights, MA: Allyn & Bacon.

Flavell, J., Miller, P., & Miller, S. (1993). *Cognitive development.* Englewood Cliffs, NJ: Prentice Hall.

Inhelder, B., & Piaget, J. (1958). *The growth of logical thinking from childhood to adolescence.* New York: Basic Books.

Perry, W. (1970). *Forms of intellectual and ethical development in the college years.* New York: Holt, Rinehart and Winston.

Perry, W. (1981). Cognitive and ethical growth. In A. Chickering (Ed.), *The modern American college.* San Francisco: Jossey-Bass.

Piaget, J. (1950). *The psychology of intelligence.* Oxon, Great Britain: Routledge and Kegan Paul.

Piaget, J. (1971). *Biology and Knowledge.* Chicago: University of Chicago Press.

Piaget, J., & Inhelder, B. (1969). *The psychology of the child.* New York: Basic Books.

Schaie, K. W. (1977). Toward a stage theory of adult cognitive development. *Aging and Human Development, 8,* 129–138.

Schaie, K. W. (1994). The course of adult intellectual development. *American Psychologist, 49,* 304–313.

Siegler, R., & Richards, D. (1982). The development of intelligence. In R. Sternberg (Ed.), *Handbook of human intelligence.* New York: Cambridge University Press.

- The early years of adulthood are often described as a "time of firsts."
- These years constitute Erikson's stage of "intimacy versus isolation."
- In his study of the lifespan, psychologist Daniel Levinson focused on the "seasons of a person's life."
- The Study of Adult Development has provided numerous insights into the aging process.

67

Early Adulthood: Psychosocial Development

TERMS
- ☐ Gender splitting
- ☐ Intimacy
- ☐ Isolation
- ☐ Seasons of life
- ☐ Study of Adult Development

The early adult years are often described as a "time of firsts": job, marriage, pregnancy, children, education of children, owning a home (**Table 67-1**). It is a testing period for any one or two individuals; they are now relatively independent, free to make their own mistakes. Psychiatrist George Valliant (1993), a well-known chronicler of the life span, referred to the "two anxieties" of the early adult years: commitment to another person and success in a chosen career. In a modern society that recognizes nonmarried couples coinhabiting, gay and lesbian lifestyles, high rates of divorce, a volatile economy, and shifting employment practices, change is a constant accompaniment to early adult development.

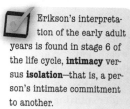

Psychiatrist George Valliant (1993), a well-known chronicler of the life span, referred to the "two anxieties" of the early adult years: commitment to another person and success in a chosen career.

INTIMACY AND ISOLATION

Erikson's (1959) interpretation of the early adult years is found in stage 6 of the life cycle, **intimacy** versus **isolation**—that is, a person's intimate commitment to another. Positive intimacy implies being with another person in an interdependent, committed, and intimate manner, while simultaneously retaining a needed core of independence. Reconciling these two opposites leads to the basic conflict of Erikson's stage 6. Resolving the crisis of this stage depends on both internal influences (a person's capacity for love) and external influences (one's partner).

Erikson's interpretation of the early adult years is found in stage 6 of the life cycle, **intimacy** versus **isolation**—that is, a person's intimate commitment to another.

During these years, an identity crisis may reemerge as a result of the struggle to resolve the independent–interdependent conflict. Without resolution, a person may define himself or herself through his or her partner, thus sacrificing self-esteem and initiative. A person who has achieved intimacy with another, however, transfers a sense of ease to other relationships, yet is perfectly fine when alone.

THE SEASONS OF A PERSON'S LIFE

Believing that there are four major **seasons of life**, Yale psychologist Daniel Levinson conducted two famous studies on life spans, one of men in 1978 and the other of women in 1996. A key concept in

Table 67-1 Tasks of Early Adulthood

Selecting a mate
Learning to live with a partner
Starting a family
Rearing children
Managing a home
Starting an occupation
Assuming civic responsibility
Finding a congenial social group

Levinson's work is the notion of life structure—that is, the basic pattern or design of a person's life at any given time. Life structure is whatever a person finds important—another person, an institution, an occupation. For most people, life structure is built around family and work. Levinson believed that men in the early adulthood years face several major tasks:

Believing that there are four major **seasons of life**, Yale psychologist Daniel Levinson conducted two famous studies on life spans, one of men in 1978 and the other of women in 1996.

- During these years, men develop a dream or vision that sparks vitality and provides motivation and energy for the tasks that lie ahead. For most men, the dream involves career choices and a blueprint detailing the road to success in their chosen occupations.
- Formulating a dream is tied tightly to a relationship with a mentor who is usually an older colleague, although occasionally a friend or relative may fill this role.
- During these years, men select a partner and determine the nature and quality of the relationship with that person.

At about age 30, men typically go through a transition period where they question the quality of their lives—their life structures—and speculate on ways to improve it. During the later years of the early adult period, men focus on consolidating their careers, establishing harmonious family relationships, and becoming more involved in community affairs.

Women's paths through these years, while similar, nevertheless follow a different timetable. **Gender splitting** (rigid divisions separating men and women) has declined owing to changed thinking about women's role in a modern society. As a result of the widespread adoption of birth control techniques and high divorce rates, the idea of a female homemaker and a male provider is no longer the standard for family life.

ADAPTING TO LIFE

In 1938, two physicians at Harvard University, Arlie Bock and Clark Heath (1945), received a grant from philanthropist William T. Grant to study healthy human lives. Two hundred sixty-eight sophomores were selected for the **Study of Adult Development**, most of whom were born about 1920. (On0 of the ly 2subjects dropped out over the course of the study.) These individuals were constantly followed (some of whom were still participating as recently as 2002) and queried about their work, families, and physical and psychological health.

In 1938, two physicians at Harvard University, Arlie Bock and Clark Heath, received a grant from philanthropist William T. Grant to study healthy human lives. Two hundred sixty-eight sophomores were selected for the **Study of Adult Development**, most of whom were born about 1920.

George Valliant (1977/1995) described a typical developmental path for most of the men: During their 20s and 30s, they established their independence from their parents and began their own families. Sometime in their 30s and 40s, after achieving a desired intimacy with a partner, they entered a stage of career consolidation; that is, they clearly defined their career choices and goals as being characterized by commitment, compensation, contentment, and competence. As Valliant noted, these four words distinguish a career from a job. Remarkably, 60% of this group have survived or will survive past their 80th birthdays.

IMPLICATIONS FOR HEALTHCARE PROVIDERS

The early adult years are typically a time of good health. However, more young adults are becoming increasingly aware of the preventive benefits of a good diet, exercise, and regular check-ups. Consequently, positive health behaviors, safety practices, diet, exercise, sexuality, addiction, and stress are widely discussed topics among today's young adults.

You should be alert to opportunities to encourage practices that are designed to prolong these years of good health. Colleges and universities are natural settings for lectures, seminars, and health fairs that both encourage and inform. In business settings, topics such as nutrition, stress management, blood pressure monitoring, smoking reduction, and employee relationships are among subjects suited for workers.

SOURCES

Erikson, E. (1950). *Childhood and society.* New York: W. W. Norton.

Erikson, E. (1959). *Identify and the life cycle.* New York: International Universities Press.

Havighurst, R. (1972). *Developmental tasks and education.* New York: McKay.

Heath, C. W. (1945). *What people are.* Cambridge, MA: Harvard University Press.

Levinson, D. (1978). *The seasons of a man's life.* New York: Knopf.

Levinson, D. (1996). *The seasons of a woman's life.* New York: Knopf.

Valliant, G. (1977/1995). *Adaptation to life.* Boston: Little, Brown & Company.

Valliant, G. (1993). *The wisdom of the ego.* Cambridge, MA: Harvard University Press.

- Stochastic theories propose that aging is random, cumulative, and microscopic.
- Nonstochastic theories interpret aging to be genetically programmed into the lives of cells.
- Weight gain is a common problem during the midlife years.
- Both vision and hearing decrease in middle adulthood.
- Cardiovascular disease is the leading cause of death among adults in the United States.
- Menopuse is the most significant physical change in women at midlife.

68

Middle Adulthood: Physical Health

TERMS

- ☐ **Cardiovascular disease (CVD)**
- ☐ **Free radical theory**
- ☐ **Melanin**
- ☐ **Menopause**
- ☐ **Nonstochastic**
- ☐ **Periodontal disease**
- ☐ **Stochastic**

THE AGING PROCESS

Nature brings life from conception to the peak of reproductive capacity. After that, there is no genetic plan for maintenance: Life runs on reserve power (see Chapter 65). Aging is not a disease, although the incidence of disease increases with age, and disease can make people age more quickly.

Stochastic theories propose that aging events are random, cumulative, and microscopic. For example, random exposure to radiation can induce mutations in DNA, causing cells to malfunction. The slow accumulation of damage to cell membranes by free radicals (the by-products of oxygen metabolism) is another stochastic theory. The **free radical theory** is related to the cross-link, or connective tissue, theory. It proposes that chemical reactions bind molecular structures that work best when separate, such as proteins, nucleic acid, and collagen. These structures change the composition of soft tissue, such as skin, muscles, and blood vessels, thereby compromising their effectiveness. **Nonstochastic** theories propose that aging is genetically programmed into the lives of cells. For example, a genetic timetable shuts down the ovaries, causing menopause.

> ✓ Aging is not a disease, although the incidence of disease increases with age, and disease can make people age more quickly.

> 🔍 **Stochastic** theories propose that aging events are random, cumulative, and microscopic. **Nonstochastic** theories propose that aging is genetically programmed into the lives of cells. For example, a genetic timetable shuts down the ovaries, causing menopause.

AGE-RELATED CHANGES

Weight

The ratio of lean body mass to fat decreases with time. Because the metabolic needs of lean tissue are greater than those of fat, metabolic needs decrease during midlife. Adults who do not compensate by eating fewer calories and less fat and by increasing exercise will gain weight.

> ✓ The ratio of lean body mass to fat decreases with time.

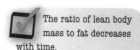

Skin, Hair, and Teeth

Exposure to sunlight—specifically ultraviolet rays—may hasten the normative overgrowth of elastin and loss of collagen in the dermis, the layer of skin beneath the epidermis. Wrinkles and sagging occur when the subcutaneous layer of connective tissue and fat shifts.

Hair is given its color by **melanin**, which is produced by cells called melanocytes in hair follicles. When these cells wear out during midlife, they are not replaced. As a consequence, hair loses its color and appears gray or white.

Periodontal disease first appears in midlife, initially as gingivitis. Plaque irritates the gums, making them tender, inflamed, and more likely to bleed. As plaque builds up, gums begin to recede from the teeth and open spaces appear between the teeth (periodontitis). Eventually, teeth become loose and the gums infected. Good oral hygiene is the best preventive measure.

Vision and Hearing

The need for reading glasses is a definitive marker of middle age. The lens within the eye thickens and the eyeball elongates. Refracted images fall short of the retina, and objects within 18 inches or so of the eye are out of focus, a condition called presbyopia. Presbycusis refers to a decreased ability to hear the higher frequencies (3000 to 4000 hertz). Adults in midlife occasionally miss consonant sounds found in this higher range. "Bed," "bet," and "vet" sound alike, especially against background noise.

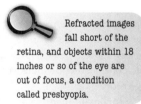

Refracted images fall short of the retina, and objects within 18 inches or so of the eye are out of focus, a condition called presbyopia.

Musculoskeletal Changes

By midlife, there is some loss of bone mass and muscle fibers as cells wear out and are not replaced. The water content of cartilage decreases, as does the manufacture of synovial fluid in joints. With less lubrication available, joints—especially the knees—stiffen. The rate of decline in strength and endurance varies greatly among individuals. Inactivity, nutrition, and disease rather than aging alone account for the rate of decline.

Cardiovascular Changes

Cells in the heart and diaphragm—two muscles that are in constant use—do not change much with age. However, the elastic properties of the heart and blood vessels are altered by other factors, related largely to diet, smoking, and inactivity. Fat and connective tissue infiltrate muscle and nerve cells in the heart and narrow arteries. Poorly oxygenated blood further starves the heart muscle. The decrease in the flow of oxygenated blood to the heart muscle, alterations in electrical conduction within the heart muscle, and the inefficiency of infiltrated muscle cells in the heart valves may all compromise the heart's functioning.

Cardiovascular disease (CVD) is the leading cause of death among adults in the United States. Since 1948, the Framingham Heart Study has monitored thousands of male and female volunteers, leading to the identification of the major risks factors for CVD, and elucidating the role of diet, exercise, and stress in the development and prevention of heart disease and stroke (**Table 68-1**). In 1991, the National Institutes of Health began the Women's Health Initiative to study CVD in postmenopausal women.

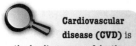

Cardiovascular disease (CVD) is the leading cause of death among adults in the United States.

The incidence of CVD is the same in women as in men, except that women develop the disease about 10 years later than men. Women seem to be protected against CVD by an "estrogen umbrella" prior to menopause. After menopause, their risk for CVD and osteoporosis increases, sparking the debate about the value of hormone replacement therapy for women in midlife.

Reproductive Changes

Menopause is the most significant physical change in women at midlife (review Chapter 55). The symptoms associated with menopause are related to the rate of decline in estrogen production.

Table 68-1 Cardiovascular Disease and Stroke: Risk Factors

Risk Factor	Explanation of Risk
Smoking[a]	Damaged lungs → poor oxygen exchange → less oxygen to major systems → increased workload on heart + hypertension
Hypertension[a] > 160/90 mm Hg	Decreased elasticity of blood vessels → increased workload on heart + impaired blood flow to brain (→ stroke) and impaired blood flow to heart muscle (→ myocardial infarction)
Diabetes (Type 1)[a]	High blood glucose → chronic damage to blood vessels → increased risk of peripheral vascular disease → impaired blood flow to and from extremities via the heart and lungs
High cholesterol: Total > 200 mg/dL LDL > 180 mg/dL	Increased plaque → narrowed diameter of arteries + clots in arteries + damage to blood vessel interior wall → hypertension + increased workload on heart + impaired blood flow to heart muscle (→ myocardial infarction) and to brain (→ stroke)
Obesity	Diet high in fats + less physical activity → increased workload of heart + increased risk for diabetes and hypertension
Stress	Increases heart rate and blood pressure; liver releases cholesterol and fatty acids into bloodstream
Alcohol overuse	Empty calories + poor dietary habits + lack of exercise → elevates arterial blood pressure → overload on heart

LDL = low-density lipoprotein.
a. Indicates major risk factors according to the Framingham Heart Study.

The faster the dropoff, the more severe the symptoms, such as heavy bleeding, hot flashes, night sweats, insomnia, and irritability. Women who have been heavy smokers reach menopause earlier, and they may have a sharper decline in estrogen than nonsmokers.

- During middle adulthood, individuals typically reach the peak of their influence and careers.
- Much of our knowledge concerning the stability of intellectual performance has come about through the use of cognitive tests.
- Basic tests of intelligence, coupled with the assessment of crystallized and fluid intelligence and longitudinal studies such as the Seattle Longitudinal Study, have yielded promising insights into the maintenance and decline of intelligence.

69

Middle Adulthood:
Cognitive
Development

TERMS
- ☐ **Crystallized intelligence**
- ☐ **Fluid intelligence**
- ☐ **Normality**
- ☐ **Stanford–Binet**
- ☐ **Wechsler Adult Intelligence Scale— Revised**

During the middle adulthood years, most men and women reach the peak of their influence in their careers, in their families, and in the community. At the same time, they may have established an intimate bond with a partner or taken steps to repair or resolve a troubled relationship. Physical changes during these years (increased risks of cardiac problems for men and breast cancer for women) lead to periods of self-evaluation, even self-doubt. Simultaneously, external pressures—career demands, family obligations, caring for aging parents—increase, causing many middle-aged adults to question their own ability.

THE INTELLIGENCE TESTING MOVEMENT

Intelligence—that fascinating, yet enigmatic "something" that promised to discriminate the able from the less able—defied definition for many years. Some researchers nevertheless believed that perhaps it could be quantified. With the advent of the 20th century and the influx of immigrants to the United States, there appeared to be a need to devise some means of classifying individuals for education, for work, and ultimately for military service.

> With the advent of the 20th century and the influx of immigrants to the United States, there appeared to be a need to devise some means of classifying individuals for education, for work, and ultimately for military service.

Binet and Mental Tests

The story of Alfred Binet (1857–1911) and his search for the meaning and measurement of intelligence has been hailed as a major event in the history of psychology. Devising an instrument to measure intelligence meant that Binet had to begin with a preconceived notion of intelligence, which he believed consisted of three elements:

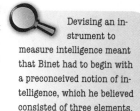

> Devising an instrument to measure intelligence meant that Binet had to begin with a preconceived notion of intelligence, which he believed consisted of three elements.

- *Mental processes possessing direction*—that is, directed toward the achievement of a particular goal
- *The ability to adapt by the use of tentative solutions*—that is, testing the relevance of ideas as one proceeds toward a goal
- *The ability to make judgments and to criticize solutions*—that is, objectively evaluating solutions

When a test item differentiated between normal and subnormal, Binet retained it; if no discrimination appeared, he rejected it. Binet defined **normality** as the ability to do the things that others of the same age usually do. A U.S. psychologist, Lewis Terman, ultimately adapted Binet's work for American usage. Called the **Stanford–Binet**, the test has been repeatedly revised and widely used.

Wechsler's Measures of Intelligence

David Wechsler, a clinical psychologist at New York's Bellevue Hospital, needed a reliable means for identifying the truly subnormal in his examination of criminals, neurotics, and psychotics. Consequently, Wechsler devised a series of tests designed to measure intelligence across the life span.

The adult version, which is known as the **Wechsler Adult Intelligence Scale—Revised**, consists of 11 subtests, 6 constituting the verbal scale and 5 forming the performance scale. Consequently, there are three possible intelligence scores: verbal, performance, and total IQ. Many clinicians have found the separation of intelligence components into verbal and performance assessments to be particularly valuable for diagnostic purposes.

Crystallized and Fluid Intelligence

Psychologists have long been intrigued by the notion of crystallized and fluid intelligence (**Figure 69-1**). **Crystallized intelligence** includes individual differences associated with family, school, and environmental opportunity. Thus crystallized intelligence is directed at the acquisition of factual knowledge, accumulated information, and basic skills. **Fluid intelligence**, by contrast, is active in problem solving and creative efforts. It is a more flexible and insightful tool than crystallized intelligence.

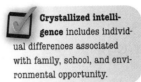

Crystallized intelligence includes individual differences associated with family, school, and environmental opportunity.

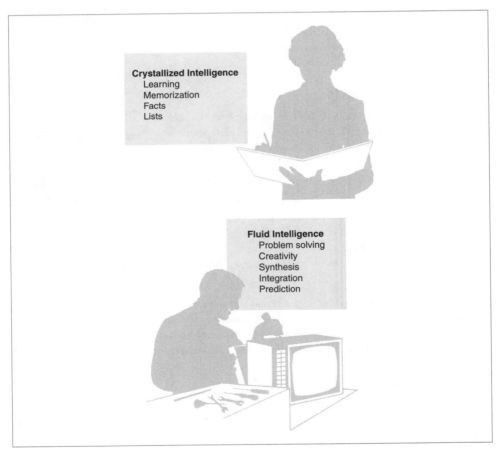

Figure 69-1 Cognitive Development in Middle Adulthood

Research indicates that crystallized intelligence continues to increase into late adulthood, whereas fluid intelligence begins to decline during the early adulthood years. In the Seattle Longitudinal Study, begun in 1956, Schaie studied 50 subjects, 25 men and 25 women, in each 5-year age bracket from ages 20 to 70. Approximately 5000 individuals in total participated in this research. One positive finding has been data showing that there is no cognitive collapse throughout the adult years. Most healthy adults begin to demonstrate some decline in fluid intelligence during their 60s and 70s, but crystallized intelligence either remains stable or actually increases until well into the 70s.

Even with this overall pattern, individual variation is typical. For example, some subjects showed a decline as early as their 30s, whereas others remained mentally alert through their 70s. Summarizing, then, cognitive ability holds up well during middle adulthood.

Fluid intelligence, by contrast, is active in problem solving and creative efforts. It is a more flexible and insightful tool than crystallized intelligence.

In the Seattle Longitudinal Study, begun in 1956, Schaie studied 50 subjects, 25 men and 25 women, in each 5-year age bracket from ages 20 to 70. Approximately 5000 individuals in total participated in this research.

IMPLICATIONS FOR HEALTHCARE PROVIDERS

As the middle years progress, the accumulated consequences of an individual's bodily constitution, the environmental forces that have been active over the years, and personality factors such as a positive or negative outlook on life are potent forces in shaping cognitive functioning. Absence of major diseases, a contented family life, and job satisfaction contribute to a stable, or enhanced, mental life. People in their middle years are also concerned about the younger generation and often assume a mentoring role with their own children and younger colleagues. In your work with middle-aged adults in clinic, hospital, or business settings, look for signs that suggest tension or stress in their lives.

SOURCES

Schaie, K. (1994). The course of adult intellectual development. *American Psychologist, 49,* 304–313.
Sternberg, R. (1995). *Successful intelligence.* New York: Simon and Schuster.
Weschler, D. (1939). *The measurement of adult intelligence.* Baltimore: Williams & Wilkins.
Weschler, D. (1997). *Weschler Adult Intelligence Scale®—Third Edition (WAIS®—III).* San Antonio, TX: Harcourt Assessment, Inc.

- Erikson has identified middle adulthood as the time of generativity.
- This period is typically characterized by maximum career achievement.
- Considerable doubt exists about the universality of the midlife crisis.
- The five-factor model of personality suggests that personality remains stable during these years.
- The Study of Adult Development identified seven factors that predict healthy aging.
- The ability to acquire self-efficacy is an insightful tool into a person's reactions to life's events.

70

Middle Adulthood: Psychosocial Development

TERMS

- ☐ Five-factor model of personality
- ☐ Generativity
- ☐ Midlife crisis
- ☐ Self-efficacy
- ☐ Study of Adult Development

Given today's concerns and safeguards about health—diet, exercise, sleep—it comes as no surprise that healthy 50-year-old women will live into their 90s and that healthy males who reach age 65 will survive into their 90s. Longitudinal studies of this age group consistently reveal that both men and women report that they feel at least 10 years younger than their actual age.

Psychologically speaking, Erikson (1950, 1959) identified the major task of middle adulthood as achieving **generativity** and avoiding stagnation. Generativity refers to a concern for guiding the next generation, the appearance of a sense of caring for the future of family, community, and country. It brings with it greater emphasis on the welfare of children and the assumption of more community and social responsibility.

During these years, the careers of most men will peak. Some men may be forced into early retirement by a trend toward downsizing; others may shift jobs for a variety of reasons; some may even change their career paths. For example, those who have chosen careers requiring great strength, speed, or unusual motor coordination (such as professional athletes, dancers, and pilots) must face the reality of a career change. Many women reenter the work force after an absence of many years as homemakers. Frequently, these women are not overly concerned with money or prestige, but by a desire to work effectively with other adults after spending years with children.

 Some men may be forced into early retirement by a trend toward downsizing; others may shift jobs for a variety of reasons; some may even change their career paths.

COHORT DIFFERENCES OR UNIVERSAL MODELS?

Given the possibility of these changes in middle adulthood, recent studies have focused on the stability of an individual's personality over the life span. For example, studies such as those by Costa and McCrae (1991, 1994) questioned widely accepted beliefs about middle adulthood, such as the inevitability of a **midlife crisis.** Research has shown that personality remains remarkably stable during these years. The work of Costa and McCrae, and others, indicates that five traits appear with sufficient regularity to create a **five-factor model of personality** (**Figure 70-1**). These five factors are consistently found in children, college students, and adults, and in both males and females.

Given today's concerns and safeguards about health—diet, exercise, sleep—it comes as no surprise that healthy 50-year-old women will live into their 90s and that healthy males who reach age 65 will survive into their 90s.

Generativity refers to a concern for guiding the next generation, the appearance of a sense of caring for the future of family, community, and country. It brings with it greater emphasis on the welfare of children and the assumption of more community and social responsibility.

The work of Costa and McCrae, and others, indicates that five traits appear with sufficient regularity to create a **five-factor model of personality** (**Figure 70-1**). These five factors are consistently found in children, college students, and adults, and in both males and females.

N Neuroticism (individuals who display considerable anxiety, hostility, depression)

E Extroversion (individuals who tend to be warm, positively assertive, active)

O Openness to experience (individuals who tend to be imaginative, creative, open to new ideas)

A Agreeableness (individuals who are trusting, modest, altruistic)

C Conscientiousness (individuals who are competent, self-disciplined, achieving)

Figure 70-1 Five-Factor Model of Personality

Trait theorists believe that these characteristics exhibit considerable continuity throughout the lifetime. Such experiences as menopause and retirement *do not* alter the basic personality of most people. Although an individual's personality as a whole remains stable over the years, changes—even dramatic changes—may nevertheless occur. Physical illness, psychiatric disorder, or catastrophic trauma, for example, can radically alter a person's personality.

For example, studies such as those by Costa and McCrae (1991, 1994) questioned widely accepted beliefs about middle adulthood, such as the inevitability of a **midlife crisis.**

THE MIDLIFE CRISIS

Most psychologists today question the inevitability of a midlife crisis. Age alone does not mean that some predetermined crisis looms ahead. There are stresses and strains common to these years, as is true of any age in human development.

In the **Study of Adult Development**, Valliant (2002) found that seven factors predict healthy aging:

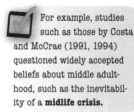

In the **Study of Adult Development**, Valliant found that seven factors predict healthy aging:

- Not being a smoker or stopping young
- Adaptive coping (mature defenses)
- Absence of alcohol abuse
- Regular exercise
- Healthy weight
- Stable marriage
- Years of education

When these factors are linked to a positive social network, the individual's prospects for avoiding a midlife crisis and looking forward to a long and happy life seem encouraging.

- Not being a smoker or stopping young
- Adaptive coping (mature defenses)
- Absence of alcohol abuse
- Regular exercise
- Healthy weight
- Stable marriage
- Years of education

SELF-EFFICACY AT MIDLIFE

Stanford psychologist Albert Bandura (1997) introduced the concept of **self-efficacy** as an insightful tool in understanding people's reactions to life's events. Unless individuals believe they can produce desired results by their actions, they have little incentive to act. Self-efficacy, then, is an excellent tool

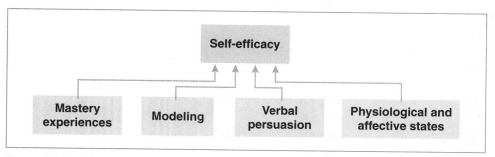

Figure 70-2 Sources of Self-Efficacy

with which to explore an individual's reactions to the events of middle adulthood. (**Figure 70-2** illustrates the sources of self-efficacy.)

By midlife, most adults have a realistic sense of their efficacy in the activities they feel are important. As Bandura (1997, p. 196) noted, a popular myth portrays midlife as a time when personal growth has peaked, youthful goals are abandoned, and efforts to adjust to a static life inevitably lead to an emotional crisis. Quite the reverse is true. The stability and control that maturity has brought to the lives of most people result in time and opportunity to explore new fields, leading to expanded feelings of self-efficacy. Life is never static.

 Unless individuals believe they can produce desired results by their actions, they have little incentive to act.

IMPLICATIONS FOR HEALTHCARE PROVIDERS

Working in a variety of settings—occupational clinics, outpatient clinics, health club settings—you are in an excellent position to help middle-aged adults maintain the quality of their lives by calling attention to risk factors (e.g., safety at work) and measures that promote health, in settings ranging from individual sessions to group counseling. Topics such as methods and diet to reduce heart attacks and strokes, and awareness of the signs of cancer and diabetes should be priorities.

SOURCES

Bandura, A. (1997). *Self-efficacy: The exercise of control.* New York: Freeman.

Costa, P. T., & McCrae, R. (1991). Trait psychology comes of age. In T. Sonderegger (Ed.), *Psychology and aging. Nebraska Symposium on Motivation* (pp. 169–204). Lincoln: University of Nebraska Press.

Costa, P. T., & McCrae, R. (1994). Set like plaster? Evidence for the stability of adult personality. In T. F. Heatherton & J. L. Weinberger (Eds.), *Can personality change*? Washington, DC: American Psychological Association.

Erikson, E. (1950). *Childhood and society.* New York: W. W. Norton.

Erikson, E. (1959). *Identity and the life cycle.* New York: International Universities Press.

Valliant, G. (2002). *Aging well.* Boston: Little, Brown.

- Height and weight decrease with age.
- Both vision and hearing decline in the later adult years.
- Osteoporosis is a decrease in the amount and quality of bone.
- Individuals who have osteoporosis are at greater risk for fractures.
- Cardiovascular changes become more apparent during later adulthood.
- Kidneys function at a reduced rate simultaneously with a decrease in bladder capacity.

71

Later Adulthood: Physical Health

TERMS
- ☐ Cataracts
- ☐ Collagen
- ☐ Elastin
- ☐ Epidermal
- ☐ Genitourinary
- ☐ Osteoporosis

PHYSICAL CHARACTERISTICS

Body Composition

After age 65, most adults experience a 46% to 60% decrease in lean body mass and loss of body water. The matrix of **collagen** and **elastin** that transports material between cells becomes cross-linked, resulting in a network of inefficient connective tissue. Collagen becomes insoluble and rigid; elastin becomes brittle and less resilient. The rate at which height is lost increases after age 65, owing to a combination of the loss of body water and bone mass, weakened muscle groups, and deterioration of spinal disks. On average, 1.2 cm (1.5 to 3.0 inches) in height is lost over a lifetime, with women typically losing more height than men.

Nutrition and Weight

Elders typically tend to lose weight, in part due to a loss of body water, fat, lean muscle mass, and bone mass. Weight loss may also be attributed to health problems, decline in capacity for self-care, loneliness, and poverty. A decrease in food intake, a decrease in water intake due to concerns about urinary frequency, slowing of peristalsis in the gastrointestinal tract, and lack of exercise may all increase the risk for malnutrition, dehydration, and constipation. Malnourishment increases vulnerability to even minor illness. An assessment of nutritional status is key to promoting good health later in life.

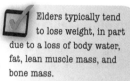

Elders typically tend to lose weight, in part due to a loss of body water, fat, lean muscle mass, and bone mass.

Malnourishment increases vulnerability to even minor illness. An assessment of nutritional status is key to promoting good health later in life.

Skin

Elders replace **epidermal** cells every 30 days or more, compared to 20 days or less in younger people. Loss of subcutaneous fat and collagen means that the dermis becomes thinner and loses elasticity. Older skin is more easily damaged, and wound healing is 50% slower than in midlife.

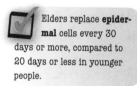

Elders replace **epidermal** cells every 30 days or more, compared to 20 days or less in younger people.

Vision and Hearing

A loss of cells along the optic nerve results in a decline in dynamic visual acuity (i.e., the ability to discriminate detail in moving objects). The reaction time of the pupil to changes in light slows, making it more difficult to negotiate the dark. **Cataracts** develop when the lens of the eye becomes more opaque owing to oxidative damage to the protein in the lens, a process hastened by exposure to sun.

Atrophy of the ear canal, degenerative changes in the bones of the middle ear, and thickening of the eardrum contribute to hearing loss in later life. The ability to detect higher frequencies (consonant sounds) first diminishes in midlife, followed later by loss in lower frequencies (vowel sounds), decreased ability to hear loud sounds, and difficulties locating the origin of a sound.

Musculoskeletal Changes

Osteoporosis is a decrease in the amount and quality of bone; the remaining bone is normal. Throughout life, bone is constantly being absorbed and rebuilt. With advanced age, however, more bone is reabsorbed than is replaced. As the bone thins, it becomes porous, increasing the risk for fractures. White women with small bone structure are at greatest risk; 15% will fracture a hip. The clinical causes of osteoporosis are related to decreased utilization of calcium in replacing bone, possibly related to estrogen deficiency. Bone density is maintained in women who undergo estrogen replacement therapy.

Cardiovascular Changes

During later adulthood, the heart muscles become less elastic, and the valves become thick and rigid because of infiltration by connective and fibrotic tissue. Contraction time is prolonged; the resting heart rate slows. Oxygen exchange is also less efficient, and aortic volume and systolic blood pressure may rise to compensate for this change. By age 60, the coronary arteries provide 35% less blood to the heart muscle. Half of all people older than age 60 have narrowing of the coronary arteries as the arterial walls thicken with connective tissue and fatty deposits; half do not. Of those individuals who do have this condition, half will develop coronary artery disease.

These changes are most noticeable with exertion or stress. It takes longer for an older person's heart to accelerate to meet the demand for increased blood flow and oxygenation. There is also a slower return to a resting heart rate when the demand ceases. The expected increase in heart rate in response to pain or anxiety may not be manifested as readily in elders due to the slower response time.

 Osteoporosis is a decrease in the amount and quality of bone; the remaining bone is normal. Throughout life, bone is constantly being absorbed and rebuilt. With advanced age, however, more bone is reabsorbed than is replaced. As the bone thins, it becomes porous, increasing the risk for fractures. White women with small bone structure are at greatest risk; 15% will fracture a hip. The clinical causes of osteoporosis are related to decreased utilization of calcium in replacing bone, possibly related to estrogen deficiency. Bone density is maintained in women who undergo estrogen replacement therapy.

By age 60, the coronary arteries provide 35% less blood to the heart muscle.

 These changes are most noticeable with exertion or stress. It takes longer for an older person's heart to accelerate to meet the demand for increased blood flow and oxygenation.

Genitourinary Changes

Genitourinary changes in late adulthood include a 50% reduction in the kidneys' rate of filtration, causing delays in the clearance of medications and glucose. At the same time, bladder capacity decreases, leading to greater urinary frequency. Older women may experience stress incontinence when they cough, but incontinence is not a normal part of aging and can be treated.

 Genitourinary changes in late adulthood include a 50% reduction in the kidneys' rate of filtration, causing delays in the clearance of medications and glucose.

Men continue to produce sperm well into old age, although the testes become smaller. A decrease in the production and concentration of testosterone results in a reduced sperm count and enlargement of the prostate gland. The enlarged prostate may block the flow of urine, causing older men to experience urinary frequency.

FUNCTIONAL ASSESSMENT

A functional assessment is a systematic evaluation of bodily activities of daily living (BADLs) and independent activities of daily living (IADLs) (**Figure 71-1**). A careful assessment can reveal manifestations of disease, open a dialog on one's living arrangements, and help set realistic goals for living life—not despite infirmity, but rather with it.

In Figure 71-1, the BADLs are listed vertically in order of acquisition (e.g., eating is mastered before self-bathing). Loss of ability occurs in reverse order, such that a person can perform activities above but not below his or her present level of ability. That is, attention to grooming typically fails before the ability to get dressed. Among IADLs, loss of ability often begins with managing finances. Individuals can usually perform activities below but not above their current level of competence.

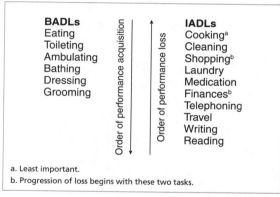

Figure 71-1   BADL and IADL Acquisition and Diminution

- A growing percentage of the U.S. population is living into their 80s and 90s.
- Cognitive performance encompasses many components that manifest both gain and loss.
- Various cognitive abilities show changes with increasing age.
- The distinction between cognitive mechanics and cognitive pragmatics helps to identify those functions that decline and those that remain stable.
- The memories of older adults vary in different situations.

72

Later Adulthood: Cognition

TERMS
- ☐ Cognitive mechanics
- ☐ Cognitive pragmatics
- ☐ Long-term memory
- ☐ Short-term memory
- ☐ Speed of response

Today, people who reach the age of 65 have a good chance of surviving into their 80s, with a 25% chance of making it to age 90. But it is the quality of these years that concerns most individuals as they approach later adulthood. Horror stories abound about the decline of cognitive abilities during the 60s, 70s, and 80s (even 90s), but fortunately recent studies (such as the Seattle Longitudinal Study) paint a more promising picture. They clearly show that individuals who maintain their levels of cognitive functioning continue to engage in mental activities, whether it is careful reading of newspapers, doing crossword puzzles, or facing new challenges (such as learning to use a computer).

Today, people who reach the age of 65 have a good chance of surviving into their 80s, with a 25% chance of making it to age 90.

COGNITIVE CHANGE: FACT OR FICTION?

Paul Baltes, long a thoughtful commentator on life span development, has proposed a division between those intellectual properties that decline and those that remain stable in later life. Specifically, he has suggested a division between **cognitive mechanics** and **cognitive pragmatics**. Cognitive mechanics refers to the structure of the brain and those areas that control such functions as speed of response, visual memory, and motor memory, which tend to decline in later adulthood. Cognitive pragmatics (e.g., language skills, acquired skills), by contrast, tend to retain good performance and may even improve in later adulthood.

Research suggests that as people enter these years, their physical stamina, memory, and cognitive processing do not decline as much as previously thought (for an example of this research, see the discussion of the Seattle Longitudinal Study). Although some aspects of cognitive functioning (e.g., speed of processing) lose a degree of efficiency, such losses in a healthy 60-, 70-, or 80-year-old are more than offset by gains in knowledge and skill due to greater experience.

Analysis of the causes of the apparent decline in intelligence (as measured by intelligence tests) leads to several conclusions:

- When physical health remains good, cognitive performance suffers only a slight decline.
- **Speed of response** is the time taken to perform any task that involves the central nervous system (CNS) such as perception, memory reasoning, and motor movement. It is the basis for efficient cognitive functioning—especially memory—and tends to decline with age.

Paul Baltes, long a thoughtful commentator on life span development, has proposed a division between those intellectual properties that decline and those that remain stable in later life. Specifically, he has suggested a division between **cognitive mechanics** and **cognitive pragmatics**. Cognitive mechanics refers to the structure of the brain and those areas that control such functions as speed of response, visual memory, and motor memory, which tend to decline in later adulthood. Cognitive pragmatics (e.g., language skills, acquired skills), by contrast, tend to retain good performance and may even improve in later adulthood.

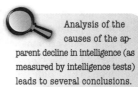

Analysis of the causes of the apparent decline in intelligence (as measured by intelligence tests) leads to several conclusions.

- Attitude, especially in a testing situation, affects cognitive performance. Test anxiety lowers test scores when older adults find themselves in strange settings, for example.

In assessing levels of intelligence, remember that cognitive functioning encompasses many components: sensory discrimination; attention; perceptual acuity; memory; extent of knowledge; speed of processing, integrating, and synthesizing facts; and the ability to recognize and attack problems. Cognitive performance is subject to both gain and loss with age. For example, reasoning, problem solving, and wisdom hold up well with age and may even improve. Speed of response and memory may show signs of slippage.

To summarize what seems to be happening cognitively during these years, let us again turn to the Seattle Longitudinal Study, remembering the distinctions between fluid and crystallized intelligence (see Chapter 69). Tests of crystallized intelligence (recognizing and understanding words, using numbers, retrieving words from long-term memory) indicate that older adults retain the meaning of words, can still apply numbers, and maintain stable levels of word fluency. Tests of fluid intelligence (identifying principles and rules, rotating objects mentally) show greater decline.

 Research suggests that as people enter these years, their physical stamina, memory, and cognitive processing do not decline as much as previously thought (for an example of this research, see the discussion of the Seattle Longitudinal Study).

Tests of crystallized intelligence (recognizing and understanding words, using numbers, retrieving words from long-term memory) indicate that older adults retain the meaning of words, can still apply numbers, and maintain stable levels of word fluency. Tests of fluid intelligence (identifying principles and rules, rotating objects mentally) show greater decline.

CHANGES IN MEMORY IN THE LATER YEARS

Psychologists today believe that memory, rather than being a single component of mind, consists of a variety of systems and processes. Each system relates to different neuronal networks that play a specialized role in remembering.

Two types of memories exist:

Two types of memories exist.

- **Short-term memory** enables brief retention of facts and information because of a system called working memory.
- **Long-term memory** enables storage of information indefinitely. The significance of long-term memory lies in its survival and adaptation value; humans require an enormous amount of information to survive in modern society.

Analyzing memory as a network of systems and as a key element in the intelligence of elders leads to an inescapable conclusion: The memories of older adults vary in different situations, ranging from improved performance in some fields, consistent performance in others, and a noticeable decline in still others. For example, after memorizing a list of familiar words, older adults (given no clues) tend to have difficulty remembering them (free recall). When shown a list of many words, however, they can identify which were on the original list (recognition) as well as college students can.

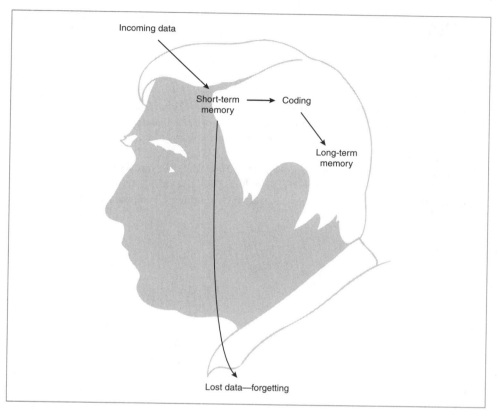

Figure 72-1 Cognitive Development in Later Adulthood

Summarizing these studies, we can say that as humans age, the richness of their memories for what happened last week or month declines. Older adults remember fewer details of their most recent experiences and rely more on general feelings of familiarity.

IMPLICATIONS FOR HEALTHCARE PROVIDERS

Recent findings suggest that mental decline is not as pronounced in the elderly as was once thought. In fact, many of today's elderly have maintained a high level of cognitive ability. Remember, however, that certain aspects of cognitive functioning, such as speed of processing information, show inevitable loss. If you are instructing elderly patients in the use of medication, for example, be sure to give them sufficient time to understand your meaning. In your contacts with older individuals, encourage them to read, keep in touch with others, and take seminars or classes if they are able. Your goal should be to urge them to keep their minds as active as possible.

SOURCES

Baltes, P., Smith, J., & Staudinger, U. (1992). Wisdom and successful aging. In J. Berman & T. Sonderegger (Eds.), *Psychology and aging. Nebraska Symposium on Motivation* 1991 (pp. 123–168). Lincoln: University of Nebraska Press.

Bandura, A. (1997). *Self-efficacy: The exercise of control.* New York: Freeman.

Birren, J., & Fisher, L. (1992). Aging and slowing of behavior. In J. Berman & T. Sonderegger (Eds.), *Psychology and aging. Nebraska Symposium on Motivation 1991* (pp. 1–38). Lincoln: University of Nebraska Press.

Papalia, D., & Olds, S. (2007). Human development. New York: McGraw-Hill.

Schacter, D. (1996). *Searching for memory.* New York: Basic Books.

Schaie, K. (1994). The course of adult intellectual development. *American Psychologist, 49*(4), 304–313.

- This phase of psychosocial development constitutes Erikson's final stage of integrity versus despair.
- Those individuals who believe they have achieved what they could and have adapted to the joys and disappointments of life possess a sense of integrity.
- Fisher's research led to a division of five separate periods of later development: continuity, early transition, revised lifestyle, later transition, and the final period.
- Baltes and his colleagues proposed the selective optimization with compensation theory.

73

Later Adulthood:
Psychosocial
Development I

TERMS
☐ Compensation
☐ Elective selection
☐ Integrity versus despair
☐ Loss-based selection
☐ Optimization
☐ Selection

The later years constitute Erikson's final stage of the life cycle: ego **integrity versus despair**. As Erikson stated (1950, p. 231), those who have taken care of people and things and have adapted to the joys and disappointments that accompany living can harvest the fruits of their lives. Lacking such adjustment leads to feelings of despair because little time remains to search for alternative life choices as well as to heightened fears of death. Individuals struggle to evaluate and give meaning to all that has occurred: Is there a meaningful pattern and satisfaction in a job well done, or a sense of despair that life should have been lived differently?

To understand how older people feel about their lives, Fisher (1993) interviewed 74 people aged 60 or older. In his analysis of the study results, he divided these years into five separate periods:

1. *Continuity with middle age.* Many of the elders interviewed did not feel any abrupt change with old age and retirement, but rather felt a sense of continuity with their behaviors and activities of middle adulthood. Fisher believed that the added time they could devote to leisure activities substituted for work activities.

2. *Early transition.* Awareness of change or transitions comes with the death of a spouse or a serious health problem. Such an abrupt shift made Fisher's subjects aware of the break with middle adulthood and the onset of old age, which occasionally led to feelings of loss and sadness.

3. *Revised lifestyle.* The transitions of the second period frequently required a change in lifestyle, such as a new residence if living alone or reduced activities if illness struck.

4. *Later transition.* In Fisher's study, many of the older adults had serious illnesses that dictated reduced mobility and loss of independence. Several of his subjects were forced to move in with their children or into retirement communities.

5. *Final period.* Individuals in this phase had to adjust to the circumstances in the fourth period and set new, realistic goals. Most of his subjects faced up to the challenges, but also recognized the inevitability of decline and death.

The later years constitute Erikson's final stage of the life cycle: ego **integrity versus despair**. As Erikson stated (1950, p. 231), those who have taken care of people and things and have adapted to the joys and disappointments that accompany living can harvest the fruits of their lives. Lacking such adjustment leads to feelings of despair because little time remains to search for alternative life choices as well as to heightened fears of death.

To understand how older people feel about their lives, Fisher (1993) interviewed 74 people aged 60 or older. In his analysis of the study results, he divided these years into five separate periods.

Awareness of change or transitions comes with the death of a spouse or a serious health problem. Such an abrupt shift made Fisher's subjects aware of the break with middle adulthood and the onset of old age, which occasionally led to feelings of loss and sadness.

SUCCESSFUL AGING

If we turn to the positive features of aging—expertise, wisdom, generativity, experience, and so on—we see characteristics that most older adults strive to attain. But are these positive markers the natural result of aging, or are they the benefits of a lifetime of conscious decision making and planned effort? Again, as we have seen so frequently, how individuals interpret the personal experiences of their lives leads to feelings of sadness or despair or a sense of satisfied culmination.

Paul Baltes (1991) identified three strategies that help older adults in their quest for successful aging: selection, optimization, and compensation (**Figure 73-1**).

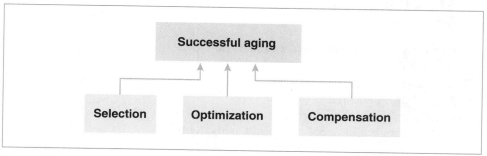

Figure 73-1 Psychosocial Development in Later Adulthood

The first component, **selection**, involves goals or outcomes. This category reflects the reduced capacity every older adult experiences and results in a more measured choice of goals—that is, selecting fewer, perhaps more meaningful, goals. Consequently, selection involves directionality, goals, and specification of outcomes. There are two kinds of selection:

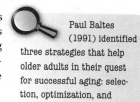

Paul Baltes (1991) identified three strategies that help older adults in their quest for successful aging: selection, optimization, and compensation.

- **Elective selection**, which is self-directed and considered desirable
- **Loss-based selection**, which implies a loss of function and making adjustments

The second component, **optimization**, refers to the attempt to achieve these goals or outcomes by making the maximum use of needed abilities and the adaptation of new technologies. As Baltes and his colleagues note, optimization can be active or passive, conscious or subconscious, and internal or external.

The third component, **compensation**, refers to a reduction in the means to achieve goals and desired outcomes and perhaps the selection of other meaningful goals. In this way, individuals can preserve a high level of performance by continued effort and added experience. Compensation reflects an adjustment in performance when tasks demand a level of response that taxes a person's capacity. Illness, which can be a frequent companion during the later adulthood years, frequently increases the need for compensation.

Using a television interview with pianist Arthur Rubinstein when he was in his 80s, Baltes and colleagues illustrated how selection, optimization, and compensation interact. Rubinstein described how he maintained a frantic schedule and superb performance as an older adult. First, he reduced the number of pieces he played—an example of selection. Next, he practiced more than he did as a younger man—an example of optimization. Finally, he devised new playing techniques such as slowing down before fast passages to emphasize the change in pace—an example of compensation.

SOURCES

Baltes, P. (1991). The many faces of human aging: Toward a psychological culture of old age. *Psychological Medicine, 21*, 837–854.

Erikson, E. (1950). *Childhood and Society.* New York: W. W. Norton.

Fisher, J. C. (1993). A framework for describing developmental change among older adults. *Adult Education Quarterly, 43*(2), 76–89.

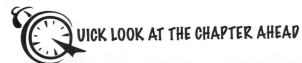

- The realization of death's approach affects people in different ways.
- Death can no longer be analyzed from a purely biological perspective.
- Kubler-Ross's initial statements about death brought the psychological needs of the dying to public attention.
- Individuals adjust to death in different ways at different times of their lives.
- Children need special consideration to help prevent lasting psychological damage as they learn about death.
- The advent of hospice has done much to make home care of the dying more acceptable.

74

Later Adulthood: Psychosocial Development II

TERMS
- ☐ **Causality**
- ☐ **Irreversibility**
- ☐ **Nonfunctionality**
- ☐ **Universality**

DEATH AND DYING

The later years are associated with thoughts of looming death. The realization of death affects different people in different ways. Some individuals face the reality of death calmly and with careful preparation. They draw up wills, dispose of assets, and solidify relationships. Others resist any thoughts about dying and grimly struggle to ignore what fate has foreordained. Still others succumb to thoughts of death by retreating into depression. As you can imagine, no matter how well prepared a person seems to be for the end, death anxieties inevitably creep in. How these worries are handled and evaluated goes far in determining whether one passes through these years in a state of integrity or despair.

The realization of death affects different people in different ways. Some individuals face the reality of death calmly and with careful preparation. They draw up wills, dispose of assets, and solidify relationships. Others resist any thoughts about dying and grimly struggle to ignore what fate has foreordained.

Death today is a complicated matter. No longer is it a matter of "not breathing." Modern technology has introduced ethical, legal, religious, and cultural matters into what was formerly a biological conclusion. For several decades, slow deaths disappeared from most people's immediate presence. Retirement homes, nursing homes, and hospitals were the most frequent locations for the death of an elderly person.

Death today is a complicated matter. No longer is it a matter of "not breathing."

More recently, the final scene of life has begun finding new terminal locations. As AIDS, drugs, and widespread violence have brought death to a steadily increasing number of younger people, the reality of death has once again returned to the community as families supported by hospice care, healthcare workers, police officers, and other parties become more involved in the dying process.

Whether one agrees with her views on death or not, Elizabeth Kubler-Ross (1969) is widely credited for her efforts to call attention to the psychological needs of the dying. After interviewing 200 terminally ill patients, she identified five stages that people pass through when they realize that death is inescapable (**Table 74-1**).

Kubler-Ross herself retreated from the rigidity of a stage theory of death. People simply do not follow a set formula in how they face death. In death, as in life, individual differences are the norm. Dying people exhibit many of these characteristics, but they do not unfailingly follow this prescribed pattern. People, as they did in their lives,

Kubler-Ross herself retreated from the rigidity of a stage theory of death.

Table 74-1 Kubler-Ross's Five-Stage Model of Death

Stage	Meaning
Denial	People refuse to believe they are terminally ill, especially when they still feel well.
Anger	People become angry at the "injustice of it all."
Bargaining	Accepting the truth of the diagnosis, people try to "make a deal." "If I do everything you tell me, can I get another year?"
Depression	When nothing works, feelings of futility set in.
Acceptance	Just before death, people usually accept the inevitable.

use individual techniques of coping with death. Also, different cultures make different interpretations of death. Some Native Americans, for example, are taught that death is part of nature's cycle, so it is not to be feared but rather faced with stoicism and composure. Still, to Kubler-Ross's credit, she created a sense of awareness and sensitivity to the feelings and emotions of those facing death.

ADAPTING TO DEATH

Death occurs constantly during the life span, which means that children, adolescents, and adults alike must learn to adapt to it. For adolescents, with their feelings of invincibility and immortality, the idea of death is almost irrelevant and something to be pushed to the back of their minds. Occasionally, the death of a friend or acquaintance brings it to a startling reality, but the pace of adolescent life helps youths to adjust fairly rapidly. Adults are increasingly aware of their own mortality, however, and death frequently becomes part of their long-range planning.

Children present a much different picture. For example, the limitations of preoperational thought are evident in the preschooler's notion of death. Studying 157 children aged 3 to 17 who had experienced a parent's illness and death, Christ (2000) discovered that children 3 to 5 years could not accept the finality of the parent's death. For months, they would ask when the parent was coming back. They needed repeated concrete explanations of what death meant.

Children present a much different picture. For example, the limitations of preoperational thought are evident in the preschooler's notion of death.

Many children aged 5 to 7 come in contact with death: the death of parents, the death of grandparents, the death of a pet, or the death of someone close to them. Books that discuss death in a developmentally appropriate manner may help children of these years to deal with their concerns. As with all aspects of their cognitive development, however, children only gradually grasp the concept of what death truly means, and as children develop, they face death in a different ways.

Reynolds et al. (1995) state that to fully grasp the meaning of death, children must grasp the essence of the following components of the death concept:

Reynolds et al. (1995) state that to fully grasp the meaning of death, children must grasp the essence of the following components of the death concept.

- **Irreversibility,** which conveys the conclusion that death is final and irrevocable
- **Universality,** which means that all living things die, whether humans, animals, or plants
- **Nonfunctionality,** which testifies to the realization that all living functions—our thinking, feeling, and sensing—cease
- **Causality,** which refers to comprehension of the actual causes of death: disease, accidents, and so forth

These interrelated elements develop in individual children depending on their cognitive development and level of maturity. In their early years, probably by the age of 3, children have some familiarity with the meaning of death, even if it entails the idea of "going away" or a "long sleep," which signifies an incorrect interpretation of irreversibility. Between the ages of 5 and 7, children typically acquire a true, albeit limited, meaning of these concepts.

Parents and nurses, while recognizing the cognitive limitations in their development of the death concept, should not be hesitant about preparing children to accept death by reading or suggesting books that are developmentally appropriate for them. Caution is needed, however. Although cognitive abilities are steadily improving, such limitations as egocentrism are still active and could cause children to think that they made the death happen.

HOSPICE CARE

Hospice has done much to make home care of the terminally ill person more acceptable. With its goal of providing appropriate care in a homelike atmosphere, its emphasis on meeting the range of a patient's needs, and its recognition of the importance of a dignified death, hospice care has become more appealing as people become familiar with its programs and goals.

Four characteristics have become the hallmark of a hospice program (Wentzel, 1981):

- Control of chronic pain, which consists of four essential parts: the right analgesic agent, in the least amount necessary, at the right time, and in the most effective manner
- Realism about death, which includes strong psychosocial support for the patient and family, coupled with realism and truthfulness
- The family as the primary unit of caring, which means a recognition that death is usually a social phenomenon—that is, the family context must be considered
- Staff support systems, implying that professionalism is compatible with compassion

IMPLICATIONS FOR HEALTH CARE PROVIDERS

One of the fastest-growing age groups in the United States is the older-than-85 category. With longer life spans, different perspectives about aging have appeared. Although many positive features of successful aging are now recognized, inevitable physical, cognitive, and psychosocial changes also occur. Increasing bouts with illness are common, and health maintenance becomes central to the quality of the older adult's lifestyle.

In working with older adults, be alert to any nutritional deficiencies, sleep problems, and lack of physical activity. Adjust your recommendations to the health and vigor of your clients. It is important to encourage their feelings of independence (and urge their family members to do likewise) so that they maintain a positive self-concept. Probably the most important consideration to remember is that these clients need as much psychological support as you can provide to help them adjust to declining functions and impending death.

SOURCES

Baltes, P., Smith, J., & Staudinger, U. (1992). Wisdom and successful aging. In T. Sonderegger (Ed.), *Psychology and aging. Nebraska Symposium on Motivation* (pp. 123–168). Lincoln: University of Nebraska Press.

Christ, G. (2000). *Healing children's grief.* New York: Oxford University Press.

Erikson, E. (1950). *Childhood and society.* New York: W. W. Norton.

Fisher, J. (1993). A framework for describing developmental change among older adults. *Adult Education Quarterly, 43*, 76–89.

Greer, S. (1991). Psychological response to cancer and survival. *Psychological Medicine, 21*, 43–49.

Kubler-Ross, E. (1969). *On death and dying*. New York: Macmillan.

Reynolds, L., et al. (1995). Anticipatory grief and bereavement. In M. Roberts (Ed.). *Handbook of pediatric psychology* (pp. 142–166). New York: Guilford Press.

Thompson, R. (1992). Maturing the study of aging. In T. Sonderegger (Ed.), *Psychology and aging. Nebraska symposium on motivation* (pp. 245–260). Lincoln: University of Nebraska Press.

Wentzel, K. (1981). *To those who need it most: Hospice means hope*. Boston: Charles River Books.

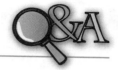

PART VII · QUESTIONS

For each of the following questions, choose the **one best** answer.

1. Which of the following is an example of health promotion in early adulthood?
   a. Breast self-examinations for women
   b. Stress management
   c. Using seat belts
   d. Being immunized against hepatitis B
2. What is the major reason for obesity during early adulthood?
   a. Maturing of muscles and bones
   b. Overindulgence in food and alcohol
   c. Lack of exercise
   d. Decline in the basal metabolic rate
3. A theorist who analyzed the cognitive workings of early adulthood was
   a. Freud.
   b. Skinner.
   c. Bandura.
   d. Piaget.
4. Schaie believed that young adults differ from adolescents in the way that they _____ their cognitive abilities.
   a. memorize
   b. neglect
   c. analyze
   d. use
5. The early adult years are often referred to as a
   a. time of firsts.
   b. time of crises.
   c. time of anxiety.
   d. time of regression.
6. Famous for his "seasons of life" concept is
   a. Freud.
   b. Maslow.
   c. Levinson.
   d. Valliant.
7. Which of the following is an example of a nonstochastic theory of aging?
   a. Exposure to radiation that causes mutation in DNA
   b. Damage to cell membranes by free radicals
   c. Genetically programmed changes (e.g., menopause)
   d. Increase in connective tissue

8. Which of the following is (are) the most significant risk factor(s) for cardiovascular disease?
   a. Smoking and hypertension
   b. Diabetes and high cholesterol
   c. Obesity and stress
   d. Being male
9. The person most responsible for the intelligence testing movement was
   a. Thorndike.
   b. Webster.
   c. Rorschach.
   d. Binet.
10. _____ intelligence tends to be more creative in nature.
    a. Fluid
    b. Crystallized
    c. Convergent
    d. Conceptual
11. An event long thought to be inescapable during middle adulthood is
    a. marriage.
    b. divorce.
    c. midlife crisis.
    d. health problems.
12. When people believe they possess the competence to do what needs to be done, they have a sense of
    a. confidence.
    b. self-fulfilling prophecy.
    c. self-expectation.
    d. self-efficacy.
13. What causes osteoporosis?
    a. Decrease in calcium in the diet
    b. Decreased utilization of calcium
    c. History of bone fractures
    d. Small bone structure
14. Which of the following is evidence of heart disease later in life?
    a. Prolonged contraction time of the heart muscle
    b. Increased rigidity of the heart valves
    c. Neither a nor b
    d. Both a and b
15. A cognitive ability that seems to decline with age is
    a. assimilation.
    b. speed of processing.
    c. notational accommodation.
    d. schema structuring.

16. Any loss in cognitive functioning in these years may be offset by acquired _____ and
    _____.
    a. assimilation, accommodation
    b. cognition, emotion
    c. introjection, regression
    d. knowledge, skill

17. These later years are Erikson's time of integrity or
    a. despair.
    b. transition.
    c. displacement.
    d. rationalization.

18. The person who is widely credited with making the needs of the dying more well known is
    a. Skinner.
    b. Piaget.
    c. Freud.
    d. Kubler-Ross.

PART VII • ANSWERS

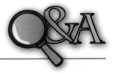

1. **The answer is b.** Primary prevention refers to efforts to prevent disease and injury in healthy people. Examples include immunizations, use of seat belts, and breast self-examinations. Health promotion is directed at increasing one's well-being, in part through healthy lifestyle choices, such as low-fat diet, regular exercise, and stress management.

2. **The answer is b.** A weight gain of 10 to 15 pounds between ages 18 and 30 is largely due to the maturing of muscles, bones, and internal organs and an increase in fatty tissue. Overindulgence in food and alcohol—and not a decline in the basal metabolic rate—is the major reason for obesity during this period.

3. **The answer is d.** Piaget's analysis of cognitive development has shed light on cognition at all ages. In early adulthood, for example, the characteristics of formal operational thinking help to explain the thought processes employed during these years.

4. **The answer is d.** Faced with more complex problems, young adults tend to apply their knowledge and cognitive abilities more than adolescents do.

5. **The answer is a.** So many "firsts" occur during these years (marriage, children, jobs) that this label is a natural.

6. **The answer is c.** Attempting to devise a technique that would encompass the varied happenings of the life span, Levinson turned to phases that he could identify because of the pattern or structure that characterized the various ages.

7. **The answer is c.** Stochastic theories propose that aging events are random, cumulative, and microscopic. For example, random exposure to radiation produces mutations in DNA, causing cells to malfunction. The slow accumulation of damage to cell membranes by free radicals (the by-products of oxygen metabolism) is another stochastic theory. The connective tissue theory proposes that chemical reactions bind molecular structures that work best when kept separate, such as proteins, nucleic acid, and collagen. Nonstochastic theories, by contrast, propose that aging is genetically programmed into the lives of cells. For example, a genetic timetable shuts down the ovaries, causing menopause.

8. **The answer is a.** Smoking, hypertension (blood pressure > 160/90 mm Hg), and Type 1 diabetes are the three major risk factors for cardiovascular disease (CVD). High cholesterol, obesity, stress, and overuse of alcohol are secondary risk factors. Men and women are at equal risk for CVD. However, men develop the disease almost 10 years earlier than women, and the manifestation of CVD in men and women is different.

9. **The answer is d.** Binet's ideas became the foundation for the acceptance and rapid growth of the intelligence testing movement. Unfortunately, Binet's ideas were misinterpreted and produced much of the mischief we have seen in the past several decades.

10. **The answer is a.** Fluid intelligence is what humans use when they are faced with problems. In a highly technological society, fluid intelligence is much needed.

11. **The answer is c.** Today, considerable skepticism greets the idea of an inevitable midlife crisis. Although crises do occur during these years, they result from typical causes—health problems, stress in the home, career concerns—that can appear at any age.

12. **The answer is d.** Self-efficacy—that feeling of justified confidence—is important at all ages, but especially during these years, when responsibilities have greatly increased.

13. **The answer is b.** Osteoporosis is a decrease in the amount of bone; the remaining bone is normal. Throughout life, bone is constantly being absorbed and rebuilt. With advanced age, more bone is reabsorbed than is replaced. As the bone thins, it also becomes more porous and its internal latticework is lost. Strength is compromised, increasing the risk for fractures. White women with small bone structure are at greatest risk; 15% will fracture a hip. The clinical causes of osteoporosis are thought to be related to decreased utilization of calcium in replacing bone, possibly as a consequence of estrogen deficiency.

14. **The answer is c.** Normative cardiovascular changes should not be confused with evidence of disease. With time and age, heart muscles become less elastic, and the valves become thick and rigid because of infiltration by connective and fibrotic tissue. Contraction time is prolonged; the resting heart rate slows. Oxygen exchange is also less efficient, and aortic volume and systolic blood pressure may rise to compensate for this phenomenon. By age 60, the coronary arteries provide 35% less blood to the heart muscle.

15. **The answer is b.** Research has shown that when the ability to process information slows, a person's memory is unable to extract as much information as in earlier years, when processing was speedier. More information simply drops out.

16. **The answer is d.** If a person remains healthy during these years, any cognitive deficits may be tempered by the greater amount of experience (i.e., knowledge and skill) acquired.

17. **The answer is a.** For those who have not adapted to the pain, joys, and reality of life (and death), despair looms large in these years. In a sense, it is a time of reconciliation with oneself.

18. **The answer is d.** Kubler-Ross's work, while challenged on a methodological basis, brought to the fore the need to recognize the needs of those facing death.

Index